CORE REVIEW FOR
Neonatal Intensive Care Nursing

CORE REVIEW FOR

Neonatal Intensive Care Nursing

Edited by

Robin L. Watson, RNC, MN, CCRN

Neonatal/Pediatric Clinical Nurse Specialist
Harbor-UCLA Medical Center
Torrance, California

AMERICAN
ASSOCIATION
of CRITICAL-CARE
NURSES

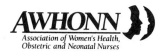
AWHONN
*Association of Women's Health,
Obstetric and Neonatal Nurses*

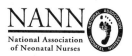
NANN
National Association
of Neonatal Nurses

W.B. SAUNDERS COMPANY
A Harcourt Health Sciences Company
Philadelphia   London   New York   St. Louis   Sydney   Toronto

W.B. SAUNDERS COMPANY
A Harcourt Health Sciences Company

The Curtis Center
Independence Square West
Philadelphia, Pennsylvania 19106

Library of Congress Cataloging-in-Publication Data

Core review for neonatal intensive care nursing/American Association of Critical-Care Nurses; edited by Robin L. Watson.

p.   cm.

ISBN 0–7216–9680–5

1. Neonatal intensive care—Examinations, questions, etc.   2. Infants (Newborn)—Diseases—Nursing—Examinations, questions, etc.   3. Intensive care nursing—Examinations, questions, etc.   I. Watson, Robin L. II. American Association of Critical-Care Nurses. [DNLM: 1. Intensive Care, Neonatal—methods—Examination Questions.   2. Nursing Care—methods— Examination Questions. WY 18.2 C7977 2001]

RJ253.5.C673 2001   618.92′01′076—dc21   2001020109

Vice President and Publishing Director, Nursing: Sally Schrefer
Executive Editor: Barbara Nelson Cullen
Senior Developmental Editor: Cindi Anderson
Production Manager: Frank Polizzano
Illustration Specialist: Lisa Lambert

CORE REVIEW FOR NEONATAL INTENSIVE CARE NURSING   ISBN 0–7216–9680–5

Printed in the United States of America.

Last digit is the print number: 9   8   7   6   5   4   3   2   1

For all of us

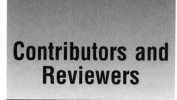
Wanda Todd Bradshaw, RNC, MSN, PNP, NNP, CCRN

Assistant Clinical Professor, Duke University School of Nursing; Neonatal and Pediatric Nurse Practitioner, Duke University Health System, Durham, North Carolina
Pharmacology

Lucinda B. Brzozowksi, RNC, BSN

Staff Nurse, Intensive Care Nursery, Thomas Jefferson University Hospital, Philadelphia, Pennsylvania
Neurologic Disorders

Sharon Conliffe-Torres, RN, MSN, CLC

Clinical Nurse Specialist and Education Coordinator, Regional Center for Newborn Intensive Care, Children's Hospital Medical Center, Cincinnati, Ohio
Pulmonary Disorders

Mila T. Flores, RNC, CNS, NNP

Neonatal Nurse Practitioner and Clinical Nurse Specialist, Presbyterian Intercommunity Hospital, Whittier, California
Immunologic Disorders and Infections

Janet Fogg, RNC, MSN

Instructor of Nursing, The Pennsylvania State University School of Nursing, Hershey, Pennsylvania
Orthopedic Disorders; Dermatologic Concerns; Ophthalmologic Disorders; Hydrops; Substance Abuse

Linda MacKenna Ikuta, RN, MN, CCNS, PHN

Neonatal Clinical Nurse Specialist, Neonatal Intensive Care Unit, Good Samaritan Hospital; Neonatal Clinical Adjunct, San Jose University; San Jose, California
Genetics

Robin M. Koeppel, MS, RNC, CNS, CPNP

Neonatal Clinical Nurse Specialist and Pediatric Nurse Practitioner, University of California, Irvine Medical Center, Orange, California
Nutrition and Feeding

Mary Mason-Wyckoff, RN, MSN, C-FNP, NNP

National Association of Neonatal Nurses, Board of Directors; American Association of Critical-Care Nurses, Neonatal Advisory Board, Advance Practice Advisory Board, North Miami Beach, Florida
Fluid and Electrolytes; Radiographic Interpretation

Sherri Garber Mendelson, RNC, MS, IBCLC

Clinical Nurse Specialist, Women's and Children's Services, Providence Holy Cross Medical Center, Mission Hills, California; Adjunct Instructor of Nursing, College of the Canyons, Santa Clarita, California
Assessment of Fetal Well-Being; Maternal-Fetal Complications

Rosemary Monaco, RN, MN

Clinical Nurse Specialist, Women's and Children's Services, Providence Saint Joseph Medical Center, Burbank, California
Assessment of Fetal Well-Being; Maternal-Fetal Complications

Tracy Pasek, RN, MSN, CCRN

Advanced Practice RN, Pediatric Intensive Care Unit, Children's Hospital of Pittsburgh, Pittsburgh, Pennsylvania
Physical Assessment; Gastrointestinal Disorders

Janet Pettit, MSN, RNC, NNP

Clinical Nurse Specialist and Neonatal Nurse Practitioner, Neonatal Intensive Care Unit, Doctors Medical Center, Modesto, California
Renal and Genitourinary Disorders

Valerie Bock Pinero, RN, BS
Manager, Education, Neonatal Intensive Care Unit, Childrens Hospital of Los Angeles, Los Angeles, California
Gestational Age Assessment

Diana J. Reiser, RN, MSN
Director, Inpatient Perinatal Services, Saint Luke's Hospital, Kansas City, Missouri
Adaptation to Extrauterine Life;
Thermoregulation

Karen Rohrs, RNC, MSN, CNS
Clinical Nurse Specialist, Neonatal Intensive Care Unit, Mercy Children's Hospital at St. Vincent Mercy Medical Center, Toledo, Ohio
Families in Crisis; Transition of the High-Risk Neonate to Home

Debbie Thompson, RNC, BA, BSN, CCRN
Perinatal Outreach Coordinator and Neonatal Nurse Educator, St. Vincent Mercy Medical Center, Toledo, Ohio
Metabolic/Endocrine Disorders

Marlene Walden, RNC, PhD, NNP, CCNS
Assistant Professor, The University of Texas Medical Branch at Galveston, School of Nursing, Galveston, Texas
Pain

Debbie Walter, RN, MSN, CRNP
Neonatal Nurse Practitioner, Children's Hospital of Pittsburgh, Pittsburgh, Pennsylvania
Gastrointestinal Disorders

Robin L. Watson, RNC, MN, CCRN
Neonatal/Pediatric Clinical Nurse Specialist, Harbor-UCLA Medical Center, Torrance, California
Physical Assessment; Gastrointestinal Disorders; Cardiovascular Disorders

Lucia D. Wocial, RN, PhD
Clinical Nurse Specialist, Neonatal Nursing, Mayo Medical Center, Rochester, Minnesota
Research; Ethical Issues in Neonatal Nursing

Della Daugherty Wrightson, RN, MSN
Clinical Nurse Specialist, Neonatal Intensive Care Unit and Special Care Nursery, Presbyterian Hospital of Dallas, Dallas, Texas
Developmental Care; Legal Issues in Neonatal Nursing

Lynda A. Wynsma, RNC, MSN, CNS
Neonatal Clinical Nurse Specialist, California Hospital Medical Center, Catholic Healthcare West, Los Angeles, California
Neonatal Resuscitation; Hematologic Disorders

Content Reviewers

Nancy Blake, RN, MN, CCRN, CNAA
Director of Clinical Care Services, Childrens Hospital Los Angeles, Los Angeles, California

Rita Allen Brennan, RNC, MS, CLE
Outcomes Manager, Women's and Children's Services, Central DuPage Hospital, Winfield, Illinois

Madge Buus-Frank, RNC, MS, ARNP
Neonatal Nurse Practitioner, The Children's Hospital at Dartmouth, Southern New Hampshire Medical Center; Consultant, Dynamic Neonatal Solutions, Hanover, New Hampshire

Jo Ann Casazza, RN, MSN, CS, LCCE, IBCLC
Clinical Specialist, Community Medical Center, Saint Barnabas Health Care System, Toms River, New Jersey

Ann Marie Dazé-Floyd, RN, MSN
Director, Department of Pediatrics, White Memorial Medical Center, Los Angeles, California

Cheryl DeGraw, RN, MSN, NNP
Nursing Instructor, Pediatrics and Pharmacology, Florence-Darlington Technical College, Florence, South Carolina

Laurie Gelardi, RNC, MSN, CPNP, CCNS
Nursing Care Specialist, Olive View-UCLA Medical Center, Sylmar, California

Margaret A. Jones, RN, MA
Director of Nursing for the Neonatal Service and Social Services, Texas Children's Hospital, Houston, Texas

Nadine A. Kassity, RN, BSN, MBA
Neonatal Outreach Coordinator, Children's Hospital and Health Center, San Diego, California

Ellen Mack, MN, RNC, CNS
Neonatal Clinical Nurse Specialist, Cedars-Sinai Medical Center, Los Angeles, California

Suzanne McLean, RNC, MSN
Neonatal Intensive Care Unit, California Hospital Medical Center, Catholic Healthcare West, Los Angeles, California

Susan Orlando, MSN, RNC, NNP
Neonatal Nursing Consultant, Destrehan, Louisiana

Cherrie M. Routon, RNC, MSN, CPHQ
Quality Systems Analyst, Childrens Hospital Los Angeles, Los Angeles, California

Patricia A. Waltman, RNC, EdD, NNP
Associate Professor of Nursing, School of Nursing, The University of Mississippi Medical Center, Jackson, Mississippi

Catherine L. Witt, MSN, NNP, RNC
Coordinator, Neonatal Nurse Practitioners, Columbia Presbyterian–St. Luke's Medical Center, Denver, Colorado

Reviewer, American Association of Critical-Care Nurses

Michelle Wolff, RN, MSN, CCRN
Professor of Nursing, Saddleback College, Mission Viejo, California

Reviewers, National Association of Neonatal Nurses

Wanda Todd Bradshaw, RNC, MSN, PNP, NNP, CCRN
Assistant Clinical Professor, Duke University School of Nursing; Neonatal and Pediatric Nurse Practitioner, Duke University Health System, Durham, North Carolina

Rita Allen Brennan, MS, RNC, CLE
Outcomes Manager, Women's and Children's Services, Central DuPage Hospital, Winfield, Illinois

Alison Brooks, MSN, RN, CS
Clinical Specialist, Alta Bates Medical Center, Berkeley, California

Margaret Conway Orgel, MSN, RNC, NNP
Nurse Practitioner, Medical University of South Carolina, Charleston, South Carolina

Lisa A. Dreyer, MSN, RNC, CNS
Consultant, Consultants with Confidence, Buffalo Grove, Illinois; Staff Nurse, Obstetrical Care, University Hospital, Cincinnati, Ohio

Linda MacKenna Ikuta, MN, RN, CCNS, PHN
Neonatal Clinical Nurse Specialist, Neonatal Intensive Care Unit, Good Samaritan Hospital; Neonatal Clinical Adjunct, San Jose University; San Jose, California

Linda J. Juretschke, PhD(c), RNC, NNP
Neonatal Nurse Practitioner, The Ronald McDonald Children's Hospital, Loyola University Medical Center, Maywood, Illinois

Jacqueline McGrath, PhD, RNC, NNP
Director of Neonatal Nurse Practitioner Program, College of Nursing, Arizona State University, Tempe, Arizona

Susan Orlando, MS, RNC, NNP
Neonatal Nursing Consultant, Destrehan, Louisiana

Ellen Tappero, MN, RNC, NNP
Neonatal Nurse Practitioner, Exempla Lutheran Medical Center, Wheat Ridge, Colorado; Executive Editor, Neonatal Network, Santa Rosa, California

Catherine L. Witt, MSN, NNP, RNC
Coordinator, Neonatal Nurse Practitioners, Columbia Presbyterian–St. Luke's Medical Center, Denver, Colorado

Foreword

Building on the unique partnership that was created to produce the second edition of the *Core Curriculum for Neonatal Intensive Care Nursing*, the American Association of Critical-Care Nurses, the Association of Women's Health, Obstetric and Neonatal Nurses, and the National Association of Neonatal Nurses have developed this companion text, the *Core Review for Neonatal Intensive Care Nursing*.

By tapping into the energy, talent, and expertise of practicing nurses from all three associations, editor Robin L. Watson has assembled an impressive team to write and review study questions for neonatal nursing core content.

We applaud the collaborative efforts of the editor, contributors, reviewers, and association staff whose commitment to cooperation, collegiality, and quality care for critically ill infants and their families has made this book possible.

Denise Thornby, RN, MS
President, American Association of Critical-Care Nurses

Janice E. Semler, RNC, MS
President, Association of Women's Health, Obstetric and Neonatal Nurses

Frances Strodtbeck, DNS, RNC, NNP
President, National Association of Neonatal Nurses

Preface

This text is the second collaborative project of three major nursing specialty organizations: the American Association of Critical-Care Nurses, the Association of Women's Health, Obstetric and Neonatal Nurses, and the National Association of Neonatal Nurses. Contributing authors from these three organizations from around the country have worked to create a comprehensive review of neonatal intensive care nursing. I applaud the leadership of these organizations for their pioneering and their partnership in creating learning resources for neonatal intensive care nurses.

The *Core Review for Neonatal Intensive Care Nursing* is a companion to the *Core Curriculum for Neonatal Intensive Care Nursing*. The *Core Review* validates the acquisition of knowledge of the core content for neonatal intensive care nursing practice and provides a mechanism for review and study of core content. This text is also designed to be a study guide and resource for nurses preparing to take national certification examinations in neonatal critical care nursing.

Three important resources were utilized in designing the structure and content of this text: *Core Curriculum for Neonatal Intensive Care Nursing, CCRN Certification Examination Blueprint–Neonatal Program,* and the *Guide to NCC Certification–Neonatal Intensive Care Nursing.* These resources guided the identification of content and distribution of items for each content area. The sections and chapters in this *Core Review* are similar to those in the *Core Curriculum.* The reader may notice that some content in the *Core Review* appears in a different chapter than it appears in the *Core Curriculum;* for example, hyperbilirubinemia is addressed in the Gastrointestinal Disorders chapter of the *Core Curriculum,* and in the Hematologic Disorders chapter of the *Core Review.* Differences in the location of specific content are primarily a result of where the content is categorized in either the *CCRN Certification Examination Blueprint* or the *Guide to NCC Certification.* Furthermore, nurses who are preparing for the CCRN examination will find the content in the Professional Issues and Family Care sections an appropriate review for the professional caring and ethical practice (Synergy Model) questions on the CCRN certification examination.

All study items are multiple choice with four options, giving the reader the practice to select a correct answer amidst three distractors. The answers to each item and explanations for the correct and incorrect answers can be found at the end of the text. References that support the correct answers and rationales are also provided.

Study items address various cognitive levels (e.g., knowledge/comprehension, application/analysis, and synthesis/evaluation), providing the readers the opportunity to recall, apply, and evaluate their knowledge of neonatal intensive care nursing. All phases of the nursing process are also represented by the study items. Every effort was made to ensure that each question represents universal knowledge and reflects core content of neonatal intensive and critical care nursing practice.

None of these questions has been or will be used on any certification examination. Because certification examinations are revised frequently, all nurses who are preparing for one are encouraged to contact the appropriate sponsoring agency to obtain the most up-to-date materials related to the areas of knowledge being tested on specific examinations. Information about CCRN certification can be found on the Web at www.certcorp.org; visit www.nccnet.org for NCC information.

I have many aspirations for this *Core Review for Neonatal Intensive Care Nursing.* I hope that novice nurses find this a useful tool as they begin the wonderful journey into neonatal intensive care nursing; that experienced nurses are able to use this text as a personal review of their professional development; that educators can use the *Core Review* as they design their own tools for assessing knowledge. And mostly, I hope that nurses who are studying for a national certification examination find this a helpful tool.

Robin L. Watson

Acknowledgments

I am forever grateful to the contributors for their persistence and patience. Without them, *Core Review for Neonatal Intensive Care Nursing* never would have materialized. I appreciate the suggestions from the many reviewers. Their constructive comments were a constant reminder of the importance of collaboration and teamwork. I thank my developmental editor at Harcourt Health Sciences, Cindi Anderson, for keeping me on track. And I thank all of the editorial staff for their wonderful assistance. I am indebted to Ellen French at the American Association of Critical-Care Nurses who provided unselfish support, encouragement, and guidance throughout this project. I respect and admire the caring neonatal intensive care nurses and neonatologists whom I have had the pleasure of working with for many years at Harbor-UCLA Medical Center. They have been a great inspiration. Finally, I thank Jo—for everlasting patience and endless trips to the post office.

Contents

SECTION III
PROFESSIONAL ISSUES • 83

SECTION IV
FAMILY CARE • 91

SECTION V
ANSWERS TO CORE REVIEW QUESTIONS • 99

SECTION
I

GENERAL ASSESSMENT AND MANAGEMENT

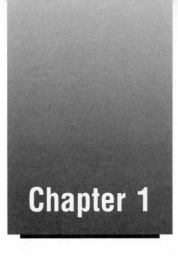

Chapter 1

Assessment of Fetal Well-Being

1. The test results on a pregnant woman indicate an elevated alpha-fetoprotein (AFP) level. This might indicate that the fetus has which of the following conditions?

   A. Abruptio placenta
   B. Down syndrome
   C. Amniotic bands
   D. Neural tube defect

2. The following biophysical profile results are from a 28-week gestation.

Fetal breathing movements	0
Gross body movement	0
Fetal tone	0
Quantitative amniotic fluid volume	2
NST	0

   Appropriate management of the woman with this score that promotes optimal fetal outcome would be:

   A. Repeat test in 4–6 hours or delivery if oligohydramnios is present.
   B. Delivery regardless of gestational age.
   C. Weekly biophysical profiles.
   D. Delivery if >36 weeks of gestational age with established lung maturity.

3. Which ultrasonographic measurement is used most frequently for establishing gestational age?

   A. Femur length
   B. Biparietal diameter
   C. Abdominal circumference
   D. Crown-rump length

4. Which of the following tests is the best choice for determining fetal lung maturity in a pregnant patient with diabetes?

   A. Lecithin/sphingomyelin (L/S) ratio
   B. Phosphatidylglycerol (PG)
   C. Fluorescence polarization NBD-PC
   D. Lamellar body count (LBC)

5. A nearly flat baseline is observed on a continuous fetal heart rate tracing. This type of pattern is associated with:

   A. A reassuring fetal heart rate.
   B. Fetal heart rate accelerations.
   C. Epidural anesthesia.
   D. Increased incidence of fetal compromise.

6. A symmetric fall in the fetal heart rate, beginning at or after the peak of the uterine contraction and returning to baseline only after the contraction has ended, is a (an):

   A. Late deceleration.
   B. Acceleration.
   C. Tetanic contraction.
   D. Baseline bradycardia.

7. A fetal monitoring strip indicates a baseline heart rate of 180. The most common cause of this heart rate is:

   A. Maternal analgesia.
   B. Fetal prematurity.
   C. Fetal sleep.
   D. Maternal fever.

8. A patient who currently has a 36-week gestation has been hospitalized for the past 2 weeks for tocolysis of preterm labor. Her amniotic membranes are intact. Vital signs are as follows: temperature, 36.4° C (97.6° F); pulse, 120 beats per minute; respirations, 18 per minute; blood pressure, 106/72. The fetal heart rate (FHR) tracing indicates a baseline of 180 beats per minute, minimal variability, and occasional accelerations to 200 beats per minute. Results of an L/S ratio are pending.

The increase in the FHR baseline is most likely due to:

   A. Maternal fever.
   B. Tocolysis with magnesium sulfate (MgSO₄).
   C. Tocolysis with terbutaline.
   D. Intact amniotic membranes.

9. A pregnant woman at term gestation is admitted in labor. She has just received epidural anesthesia. Her blood pressure prior to the procedure ranged from 110/60 to 126/80. Her blood pressure now is 80/58. What impact might you expect this drop in blood pressure to have on the fetus?

   A. Increased fetal activity.
   B. Decreased fetal oxygenation.
   C. Fetal hypothermia.
   D. Closure of the ductus arteriosus.

10. A newborn term infant is brought to the admission nursery following a forceps-assisted vaginal delivery. The physical assessment of the infant reveals semicircular bruising on both sides of the head, slight facial edema, and swelling on the scalp that feels "spongy" and does not cross suture lines. Based on these assessment findings, the infant must be monitored closely for signs of:

   A. Epilepsy.
   B. Polycythemia.
   C. Mental retardation.
   D. Hyperbilirubinemia.

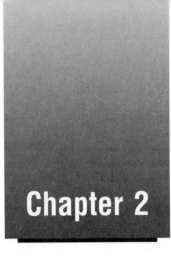

Chapter 2

Adaptation to Extrauterine Life

1. The Apgar score is:

   A. An initial assessment of an infant's transition to extrauterine life.
   B. A retrospective assessment tool to evaluate an infant at 1 and 5 minutes of age.
   C. An assessment to identify perinatal asphyxia in the newborn and predict eventual outcome.
   D. An assessment score to be determined prior to initiation of neonatal resuscitation.

2. Which of the following assessments is *not* indicative of perinatal asphyxia?

   A. Apgar scores of 0/1 minute, 1/5 minutes, and 3/10 minutes.
   B. Hypotonia.
   C. Initial pH of 7.18 on an umbilical artery sample.
   D. Oliguria with hematuria at 12 hours of life.

3. Timing of parental teaching about the newborn's specific behaviors, physical characteristics, feeding, and transitional process is most appropriately:

   A. Initiated as soon as possible after delivery, before the baby is put to breast.
   B. Not structured, but guided by questions from the mother and/or father.
   C. Included in the first hour to include feeding and bathing with the mother's participation with the caregiver.
   D. Guided by the mother's decision of her own readiness to interact with her baby and caregiver(s).

4. In fetal circulation, blood entering the right atrium from the inferior vena cava is shunted across the foramen ovale to the left atrium:

   A. To maintain pulmonary vascular resistance.
   B. To provide the highest oxygenated blood to the coronary, carotid, and subclavian arteries.
   C. To shunt deoxygenated blood to the placental circulation for reoxygenation by diffusion.
   D. To oxygenate the lower extremities, kidneys, and gut.

5. The three processes to facilitate the transition to extrauterine life are placental to pulmonary gas exchange and:

   A. Sustained high pulmonary vascular resistance, structural closures of fetal shunts.
   B. Closure of fetal shunts, equal pulmonary and systemic vascular resistance.
   C. Patency of the fetal shunts, equal pulmonary and systemic vascular resistance.
   D. Decreased pulmonary and increased systemic vascular resistance, functional closure of fetal shunts.

6. All of the following symptoms may indicate the earliest signs of illness in the transition period *except*:

   A. Poor feeding.
   B. Hypotonia.
   C. Diminished response to the environment.
   D. Sleep periods greater than 2 hours.

7. An infant is born vaginally at 36 3/7 weeks following rupture of membranes for 30 hours. Labor and delivery were unremarkable and the infant had Apgar scores of 7 and 8 at 1 and 5 minutes, respectively. On admission to the nursery at 45 minutes of age, the infant is pink with mild acrocyanosis and is noted to be tachypneic with a respiratory rate of 80/minute. There is no nasal flaring, grunting, or retractions. No maternal cultures were obtained. Since this infant is at risk for infection, the nurse's plan of care *at this time* includes:

   A. Initial and ongoing assessments to facilitate early identification of infection.
   B. Immediate gavage feeding.
   C. Initiating oxygen by hood to improve the infant's color.
   D. Routine care, as the infant does not appear to be ill.

8. Transient tachypnea of the newborn (TTN) is thought to be caused by:

   A. Surfactant deficiency.
   B. Aspiration.
   C. Delayed clearance of fetal lung fluid in term or near-term infants.
   D. Pneumothorax.

9. An infant exposed to maternal hepatitis B virus should be treated with administration of:

   A. Hepatitis B immune globulin (HBIG) if the mother is hepatitis B active.
   B. HBIG in the first 12 hours of life and hepatitis vaccine in the first week of life.
   C. Hepatitis vaccine if the mother is hepatitis B inactive.
   D. HBIG and hepatitis B vaccine only if the baby is surface antigen positive.

10. In the first hour of life, the infant is in an active alert state and in the initial period of reactivity. Nursing interventions during this period to facilitate bonding include:

   A. Giving eye prophylaxis and vitamin K injection while the infant is alert, then returning the infant to the parents.
   B. Giving eye prophylaxis and vitamin K injection in the delivery room and allowing parents to bond after the mother has been cleaned and repositioned.
   C. Giving eye prophylaxis, vitamin K injection, and other routine care in the nursery and returning the infant to the parents after the first hour of life.
   D. Providing time for parental bonding and breast-feeding in a quiet setting prior to eye prophylaxis and vitamin K injection.

11. At birth, an infant appears sleepy and is depressed with decreased respiratory effort, decreased tone, and a heart rate greater than 100 bpm. The mother received meperidine (Demerol) 3 hours prior to delivery. What would the appropriate nursing intervention be?

   A. Verify a negative history of substance abuse and prepare to administer naloxone (Narcan), and observe the infant for improved status.
   B. Administer naloxone (Narcan) and observe the infant for improved status, since administration of a narcotic in labor is confirmed.
   C. Provide supportive care for the infant until respiratory effort, tone, and responsiveness have improved.
   D. Provide stimulation for the infant until respiratory effort, tone, and responsiveness have improved.

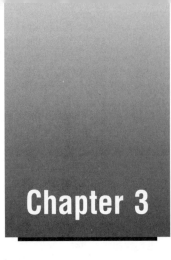

Chapter 3

Neonatal Resuscitation

1. Evaluation of the effect of resuscitation occurs:

   A. Immediately upon birth.
   B. After the initial steps have been completed.
   C. At the time of the 1- and 5-minute Apgar scores.
   D. Following each action.

2. When a neonate is found to be depressed, the most important component of preparation is:

   A. Institutional protocol that is annually reviewed by the staff.
   B. Personnel who are knowledgeable of their roles and able to function as a team.
   C. Equipment that is checked and within easy reach.
   D. Electrical equipment that is annually evaluated and maintained.

3. The obstetrician suctions thick, particulate meconium from the infant's mouth and nares after delivery of the head. Upon delivering the body, the physician hands the floppy pale infant to the resuscitation team. The infant is not breathing. The appropriate action at this point is to:

   A. Dry, stimulate, and position the baby and suction his hypopharynx.
   B. Dry the infant and then suction the hypopharynx and trachea.
   C. Position the infant and begin bag-and-mask ventilation.
   D. Position the infant, intubate, and perform tracheal suctioning.

4. In a 2-second period during interposed chest compressions and ventilations, which will occur?

   A. One compression and three ventilations.
   B. One ventilation and three compressions.
   C. One ventilation and five compressions.
   D. One compression and five ventilations.

5. Following 30 seconds of chest compressions with positive pressure ventilation (PPV) (100% F_{IO_2}), an 1800 g intubated infant has a heart rate of 58 beats per minute. The next appropriate intervention would be to:

   A. Administer 0.1 mL/kg 1:10,000 epinephrine through the endotracheal tube (ETT) followed by 1 mL of saline and PPV.
   B. Administer 0.1 mL/kg 1:1000 epinephrine through the ETT followed by 1 mL of saline and PPV.
   C. Insert a peripheral IV line and administer 0.1 mL/kg 1:1000 epinephrine quickly.
   D. Administer 1 mL/kg 1:10,000 epinephrine through the ETT followed by saline and PPV.

6. A 34-week pregnant woman has just been rolled into the operating room after being brought to the Emergency Room from a motor vehicle accident. A puddle of blood is on the gurney and the resuscita-

tion team is told that her abdomen was rigid upon admission. Which medication would be most specifically indicated for the resuscitation of this mother's newborn?

A. Epinephrine
B. Volume expanders
C. Sodium bicarbonate
D. Naloxone hydrochloride (Narcan)

7. A newborn infant is experiencing respiratory distress. He has 2+ retractions, a scaphoid abdomen, and persistent central cyanosis. Upon further examination, the nurse notes that bowel sounds are audible in the chest. After the initial steps of resuscitation, the most appropriate action would be to:

A. Administer continuous blow-by oxygen at 5 L per minute, 100% FiO$_2$.
B. Begin positive pressure ventilation via bag and mask.
C. Intubate the infant and begin positive pressure ventilation via the endotracheal tube.
D. Continue to stimulate the infant and suction the airway, providing whiffs of oxygen as needed.

8. The resuscitation team has been called for the delivery of an infant. The following report is given: The mother is Gravida 3, Para 1, and Spontaneous Abortion 1. She has not had any prenatal care. Her blood type is O negative. The fetal ultrasonogram shows cardiomegaly, ascites, and pleural effusion. In setting up for the resuscitation, the nurse should anticipate which of the following procedures?

A. A double volume exchange
B. Placement of a percutaneous central catheter
C. A partial volume exchange
D. A thoracentesis

9. Which of the following findings are suggestive of prolonged fetal hypoxia?

	Respiratory effort	Heart rate	Color
A.	Apnea	70	Pale
B.	Crying	128	Acrocyanosis
C.	Retractions	90	Cyanosis
D.	Apnea	120	Acrocyanosis

10. Upon birth, an infant experiences deep retractions and cyanosis when resting quietly. When he cries, his color changes to pink and he breathes more easily. The most likely condition that this infant may have is:

A. Respiratory distress syndrome.
B. Transient tachypnea of the newborn.
C. Bilateral choanal atresia.
D. Congenital heart disease.

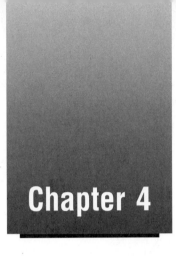

Chapter 4

Physical Assessment

1. Which of the following is a normal heart rate range for a newborn?

   A. 60–120 bpm
   B. 70–140 bpm
   C. 80–160 bpm
   D. 90–210 bpm

2. A newborn is suspected of having respiratory distress syndrome (RDS). The nurse should carefully assess for the onset of RDS for a minimum of how many hours?

   A. 1
   B. 2
   C. 4
   D. 6

3. To assess the degree of right-to-left ductal shunting, a nurse could compare oxygen values from which of the following?

   A. Umbilical artery line and left radial artery line
   B. Umbilical artery line and right dorsalis pedis artery line
   C. Left radial artery line and left dorsalis pedis artery line
   D. Umbilical artery line and right radial artery line

4. A 2-day-old newborn is noted to have breasts that are enlarged and with a milky secretion. This finding indicates the presence of:

   A. Infection.
   B. Maternal estrogen.
   C. Turner syndrome.
   D. Congenital adrenal hyperplasia.

5. Which of the following is the most common congenital heart malformation?

   A. Ventricular septal defect (VSD)
   B. Atrial septal defect (ASD)
   C. Atrioventricular (AV) canal
   D. Patent ductus arteriosus (PDA)

6. Infants born to mothers with insulin-dependent diabetes mellitus are at higher risk for developing which of the following cardiac disorders?

   A. Endocardial fibroelastosis
   B. Ebstein's malformation
   C. Hypertrophic cardiomyopathy
   D. Tetralogy of Fallot

7. A 37-week-old newborn was discovered to be cyanotic and tachypneic at 6 hours of age. A 100% oxygen administration test is performed. The results are as follows:

	Room Air	100% F_{IO_2}
Color	Blue	Blue
Pulse oximetry	65%	70%
Pa_{O_2}	33	36

   This infant would be suspected of having which of the following?

   A. Respiratory distress syndrome
   B. Cyanotic heart disease
   C. Pneumonia
   D. Acyanotic heart disease

8. Which chamber of the heart pumps against the highest pressure after successful transition from fetal to neonatal circulation?

   A. The left atrium
   B. The left ventricle

C. The right atrium

D. The right ventricle

9. An infant is born vaginally with forceps assist. He has a cone-shaped head. This will most likely evolve into a:

A. Cephalohematoma.

B. Caput succedaneum.

C. Skull fracture.

D. Subgaleal hemorrhage.

10. In a healthy term infant, by what age does functional closure of the ductus arteriosus usually occur?

A. 1 hour

B. 15 hours

C. 72 hours

D. 1 week

11. A newborn infant's visual acuity is estimated in the range of:

A. 20/80.

B. 20/100.

C. 20/200.

D. 20/400.

12. A red reflex test that is white indicates which of the following?

A. Retinoblastoma

B. Subconjunctival hemorrhages

C. Colobomas

D. Brushfield spots

13. A full-term infant has the following findings on physical examination: head circumference measuring less than the 5th percentile; closed sutures; anterior fontanel size and position are normal; head shape appears normal. What do these findings indicate?

A. Microencephaly

B. Cranioschisis

C. Hydroanencephaly

D. Aqueductal stenosis

14. All of the following are true of cephalohematomas *except*:

A. They occur only with vaginal deliveries.

B. They are contained within suture lines.

C. They can increase in size over the first 3 days following delivery.

D. They can be associated with linear skull fractures.

15. Premature closure of one or more cranial sutures is associated with which of the following conditions?

A. Cranioschisis

B. Craniosclerosis

C. Craniosynostosis

D. Overlapping suture

16. A full-term infant born by vaginal delivery with forceps is noted to have hoarseness and mild inspiratory stridor when crying. The infant is asymptomatic when at rest and quiet. This infant is most likely to have:

A. Choanal atresia.

B. A small glottic mass.

C. Bilateral vocal cord paralysis.

D. Unilateral vocal cord paralysis.

17. The triad of micrognathia, glossoptosis, and U-shaped cleft palate in the neonate is characteristic of:

A. VATER syndrome.

B. CHARGE syndrome.

C. Pierre-Robin syndrome.

D. Beckwith-Wiedemann syndrome.

18. A mother asks about several pearly white papules about 1 mm in size on her infant's chin and cheeks. The nurse should offer which of the following explanations?

A. They are normal and disappear during the first few weeks of life.

B. They are probably the result of bacteria and antibiotics should be started.

C. They are neonatal acne and a dermatologist should be consulted.

D. They will rupture within 48 hours, leaving small pigmented macules, which may take several months to disappear.

19. Which of the following is a result of mechanical trauma and paralysis to the spinal roots of the 5th cervical through the 1st thoracic nerves during delivery?

A. Torticollis

B. Brachial palsy

C. Phrenic nerve palsy

D. Calcified hematoma

20. Webbing of the neck is seen in which of the following syndromes?

    A. Trisomy 13
    B. Trisomy 18
    C. Turner syndrome
    D. Prader-Willi syndrome

21. An infant is born with moderate left shoulder dystocia. A radiograph is ordered to diagnose:

    A. Bell's palsy.
    B. Fractured clavicle.
    C. Brachial nerve palsy.
    D. Cervical spine fracture.

22. An infant has a skin rash composed of the following: 1–2 mm pustular lesions that are white to yellow-white in color; the lesions are firm and surrounded by an erythematous flare. This is most likely in which of the following conditions?

    A. Miliaria
    B. Nevus simplex
    C. Pustular melanosis
    D. Erythema toxicum

23. Dubowitz examination and scoring is performed to determine:

    A. Degree of asphyxia at birth.
    B. Estimate of gestational age at birth.
    C. Head sparing vs. non-head sparing growth retardation.
    D. Degree of placental function during pregnancy.

24. A 1-hour-old newborn has yellowish discoloration of the nailbeds, umbilical cord, and skin. This yellowish color indicates:

    A. Hepatitis.
    B. Jaundice.
    C. Intrauterine distress.
    D. Sclerema neonatorum.

25. The Barlow test is performed on the newborn infant to evaluate which of the following?

    A. Eyes
    B. Spine
    C. Hips
    D. Ears

26. A 2-hour-old, full-term infant suddenly becomes tachypneic with moderate cya-

nosis. Auscultation reveals absent breath sounds on the right. The nurse should suspect which of the following?

    A. Pneumonia
    B. Spontaneous pneumothorax
    C. Respiratory distress syndrome
    D. Persistent pulmonary hypertension of the newborn

27. All of the following are consequences of uncorrected cryptorchidism *except*:

    A. Infertility
    B. Epididymitis
    C. Inguinal hernia
    D. Tumor development

28. Which of the following signs would not be present in the affected arm of an infant with brachial palsy?

    A. Abduction
    B. Wrist flexion
    C. Forearm pronation
    D. Internal rotation

29. Which of the following techniques tests a neonate's masseter strength?

    A. Gentle touching of the eyelashes with a cotton ball
    B. Introducing a light into the peripheral visual field
    C. Opening the mouth and observing for jaw deviation
    D. Placing a gloved finger in the mouth and evaluating the biting portion of the suck

30. A newborn has micrognathia with an apparently normal size tongue. Airway obstruction is a problem. Once the airway is established, the nurse should proceed with assessing for all of the following conditions *except*:

    A. Pierre-Robin syndrome
    B. Treacher Collins syndrome
    C. Down syndrome
    D. Cornelia de Lange syndrome

31. The nurse notes a *lack* of fogging of a cold, flat metal object when held beneath an infant's nares. The infant's respirations are loud with periods of apnea. This infant most likely has which of the following conditions?

    A. A respiratory infection
    B. Choanal atresia

C. Cleft palate
D. Epstein pearls

32. The nurse examines a newborn and discovers the following: unequal level of knees, limited abduction, and buttocks asymmetry. With continued assessment, the nurse should expect which of the following?

A. A palpable clunk on abduction with the Barlow maneuver
B. An audible clunk with upward pressure with the Barlow maneuver
C. A palpable clunk with abduction with the Ortolani maneuver
D. An audible clunk with adduction with the Ortolani maneuver

33. Upon auscultating an infant's breath sounds, the nurse hears a noise at end inspiration that sounds like hair rubbing together. These sounds are best described as:

A. Stridor.
B. Rhonchi.
C. Vesicular.
D. Fine crackles.

34. Which of the following skin assessment findings warrant investigation?

A. Milia at 3 weeks of age
B. Epstein pearls at 2 weeks of age
C. Harlequin color change at 4 days of age
D. Circumoral cyanosis at 48 hours of age

35. When examining a full-term infant, an imaginary line from which of the following anatomic landmarks should be used to determine ear position?

A. The eyelids
B. The eyebrows
C. The bridge of the nose
D. The canthi of the eyes

36. A 1-hour-old infant delivered by elective cesarean section at 38 weeks' gestation becomes tachypneic to 76 breaths/minute. Mild-moderate intercostal retractions are noted. Chest radiograph reveals fluid in the interlobar fissures. This is most likely:

A. Pneumonia.
B. Respiratory distress syndrome (RDS).

C. Persistent pulmonary hypertension.
D. Transient tachypnea of the newborn (TTN).

37. A 7-day-old, 2.2 kg infant is admitted with vomiting and a rectal temperature of 39.0° C (102.2° F). Urine output over 24 hours is 264 mL. Urine specific gravity is 1.002. It is most important for the nurse to monitor all of the following except:

A. Serum electrolytes
B. Urine electrolytes
C. Gastric pH
D. Serum osmolarity

38. Which of the following should alert the nurse to consider the existence of neonatal hypoparathyroidism?

A. Warm extremities
B. Bradycardia
C. Hypertension
D. Prolonged bleeding

39. The best method to evaluate postural tone in the newborn is to:

A. Place the newborn supine and turn his head side to side.
B. Stimulate the palmar surface of the newborn's hand with a finger.
C. Hold the newborn upright and allow the soles of the feet to touch a flat surface.
D. Grasp the newborn's hands and pull him slowly from the supine to sitting position.

40. The nurse notices a small amount of blood-tinged vaginal discharge in a 1-day-old female infant. The most likely cause of this finding is:

A. Vaginal fissure.
B. Breech delivery.
C. Vitamin K deficiency.
D. Exposure to maternal hormones.

41. An infant's anterior fontanel measures 7 cm across and is flat and soft. This infant should be examined to rule out:

A. Hypothyroidism.
B. Down syndrome.
C. Intraventricular hemorrhage.
D. Intracranial arteriovenous malformation.

42. An infant has a port-wine stain over the forehead and left upper eyelid. Which syndrome must be ruled out?

A. Trisomy 13
B. Sturge-Weber
C. Kasabach-Merritt
D. Klippel-Trenaunay-Weber

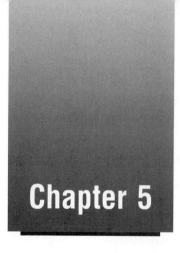

Chapter 5

Gestational Age Assessment

1. Full-term small for gestational age (SGA) infants are at risk for which of the following?

   A. Hypoglycemia, meconium aspiration, hypothermia
   B. Apnea, hyperbilirubinemia, respiratory distress syndrome
   C. Congenital heart malformation, hyperbilirubinemia, hyperglycemia
   D. Meconium aspiration, apnea, respiratory distress syndrome

2. A gestational age assessment is performed on a male infant estimated to be 28 weeks' gestation by dates. Which of the following physical characteristics should the nurse anticipate?

   A. Skin leathery, cracked, and wrinkled; full areola with 5–10 mm bud; testes pendulous
   B. Smooth pink skin with visible veins, abundant lanugo, scrotum empty with no rugae, and smooth plantar surface of the feet with faint red marks
   C. Cracking skin with rare veins, testes down with good rugae, raised areola with 3–4 mm bud
   D. Ear formed with instant recoil, very little lanugo, plantar creases cover entire sole

3. A major reason for determining gestational age is to:

   A. Prevent apnea.
   B. Provide statistical data.

   C. Prevent respiratory distress syndrome.
   D. Anticipate problems related to development.

4. An infant is determined to be large for gestational age (LGA). The nurse should assess this infant for which of the following conditions?

   A. Hypothermia
   B. Hypercalcemia
   C. Hypoglycemia
   D. Hypermagnesemia

5. Which of the following defines large for gestational age (LGA)?

   A. A post-term infant weighing more than the 75th percentile for gestational age
   B. A preterm infant weight more than the 10th percentile for gestational age
   C. A term infant weighing more than the 50th percentile for gestational age
   D. An infant weighing more than the 90th percentile for gestational age

6. A 40-week, 2000 g infant is admitted to the neonatal intensive care unit (NICU). The nurse should assess for which of the following conditions?

   A. Birth trauma
   B. Polycythemia
   C. Hyperglycemia
   D. Respiratory distress syndrome

7. An infant is lying in a frog-like position, the skin is cracking with few visible veins, the areola is raised with a 5–10 mm bud,

and the ears are formed and firm and have instant recoil. These findings are most consistent with which gestational age?

A. 28 weeks
B. 32 weeks
C. 36 weeks
D. 40 weeks

8. A 38-week-gestational infant is born weighing 1800 g. Which maturity classification best describes this infant?

A. Preterm large for gestational age
B. Preterm average for gestational age
C. Full-term average for gestational age
D. Full-term small for gestational age

9. The Ballard examination is based on assessment of:

A. Physical and neuromuscular characteristics.
B. Physical characteristics and cardiorespiratory criteria.
C. Electroencephalographic patterns and neurologic signs.
D. Anterior vascular capsule of the lens and neuromuscular characteristics.

10. Gestational age can be estimated using data from all of the following *except*:

A. Alpha-fetoprotein
B. Biparietal diameter
C. Dubowitz scoring system
D. Anterior vascular capsule of the lens

11. The square window sign demonstrates flexion of which joint(s)?

A. Knee
B. Hips
C. Wrist
D. Ankle

12. The arm recoil component of the Dubowitz scoring examination is performed to assess which of the following?

A. Posture
B. Muscle tone
C. Joint mobility
D. Symmetry of a primary reflex

13. After performing a Ballard examination, the nurse identifies a large discrepancy between the Ballard score and maternal dates. The nurse should:

A. Use maternal dates as the gestational age.
B. Use the data from the Ballard score as the gestational age.
C. Re-evaluate the infant after 24 hours using a more elaborate tool.
D. Calculate the average gestational age from the maternal dates and Ballard score.

14. When should a gestational age examination using the New Ballard Score be performed on an infant estimated to be less than 26 weeks' gestation by dates?

A. At less than 12 hours of age
B. Between 13 and 18 hours of age
C. Between 19 and 24 hours of age
D. At greater than 24 hours of age

15. Compared with infants with symmetric growth restriction, infants with asymmetric growth restriction have less associated morbidity because:

A. They have heavier birth weights.
B. Their head circumference is normal for gestational age.
C. They are usually born at full term.
D. Their lungs are more mature.

16. When performing the Ballard examination, which of the following describes the correct way to perform the arm recoil assessment?

A. Flex the arms then immediately release them.
B. Extend the arms for 10 seconds, then release them.
C. Extend the arms over the infant's head, then against the torso.
D. Flex the arms for 5 seconds, then fully extend and then release them.

17. Which of the following could the nurse expect to observe on an infant born at 32 weeks' gestation?

A. Creases over the entire sole of the foot
B. Gelatinous skin with very visible veins
C. An ear with a well curved and soft pinna that has a ready recoil
D. A scarf sign in which the elbow does not extend past the ipsilateral midclavicular line

18. A premature infant is admitted to the neonatal intensive care unit (NICU) following resuscitation in the delivery room. The infant is intubated and placed on a fentanyl drip. Which one of the following gestational age assessments would *not* be reliable in this situation?

    A. Nägele's rule
    B. Physical characteristics
    C. Neuromuscular characteristics
    D. Anterior vascular capsule of the eye

19. A newborn infant is determined to be below the 10th percentile for occipital frontal head circumference, weight, and length. Which of the following is the most likely cause of this infant's growth restriction?

    A. Gestational diabetes
    B. Maternal preeclampsia
    C. Congenital viral infection
    D. Decreased caloric intake in the third trimester

20. A healthy term infant displays which of the following?

    A. Hypotonicity
    B. Hypertonicity
    C. A relaxed posture
    D. A flexed posture

21. Which of the following is an obstetric method for determining gestational age?

    A. Amniotic fluid color
    B. Time of onset of labor
    C. Length of intrapartal period
    D. Last menstrual period (LMP) and menstrual history

22. Which of the following physical characteristics would you expect to see in a 30-week preterm neonate?

    A. Firm pinna
    B. Deep plantar creases
    C. Layers of subcutaneous fat
    D. Blood vessels visible over the chest and abdomen

23. The square window angle _____ with increasing gestational age.

    A. Flexes
    B. Decreases
    C. Increases
    D. Hyperextends

24. When assessing an infant who is projected to be 40 to 41 weeks' gestation, the nurse should expect to find vernix:

    A. In skin folds only.
    B. On legs and arms.
    C. Over chest and abdomen.
    D. In a thick layer all over the body.

25. A 42-week-gestation neonate is delivered. The nurse should expect which of the following findings during the gestational age assessment of this infant?

    A. Abundant lanugo
    B. Smooth plantar surfaces
    C. Thick vernix covering the body
    D. Desquamation at the ankles and wrists

26. A large for gestational age (LGA) infant is at a higher risk for all of the following complications *except*:

    A. Asphyxia
    B. Birth trauma
    C. Hypoglycemia
    D. Congenital infection

27. The following are all findings that the nurse should expect on a 23-week, extremely low birth weight neonate (ELBW) *except*:

    A. Fused eyelids
    B. Transparent skin
    C. Abundant lanugo
    D. Imperceptible breast buds

28. A 41-week, 4.2 kg neonate is born and taken to the nursery for observation after a difficult delivery. Upon physical examination, it is noted that the patient is not moving the left arm spontaneously. What is the most likely reason?

    A. Asphyxia
    B. Head trauma
    C. Hypoglycemia
    D. Peripheral nerve damage

29. A maternal history indicates chronic hypertension. What is a possible effect on the fetus/newborn from this condition?

    A. Birth trauma
    B. Hyperbilirubinemia
    C. Large for gestational age
    D. Intrauterine growth restriction

30. The New Ballard Score was developed to assess gestational age of infants:

    A. Who are extremely premature.
    B. Of drug abusing mothers.
    C. With congenital anomalies.
    D. With meconium-stained amniotic fluid.

31. Which of the following best describes the skin of an extremely premature infant?

    A. Sticky and transparent
    B. Flaky and like parchment
    C. Smooth with visible veins
    D. Thick with barely visible veins

32. The New Ballard Score includes assessment of:

    A. Grimace.
    B. Hand length.
    C. Hand creases.
    D. Eyelid separation.

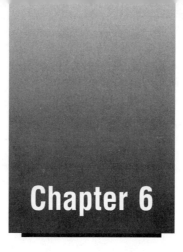

Chapter 6

Thermoregulation

Questions 1 and 2 refer to the following scenario: A full-term infant has an axillary temperature of 37.8° C (100.0° F). The infant's skin is cool to the touch and its temperature measures 35° C (95° F) by ISC probe. The infant is acrocyanotic with prolonged capillary refill. The infant is in a servocontrolled incubator.

1. The nurse's first action should be to:

   A. Assess the infant for signs of physiologic heat-losing mechanisms.
   B. Begin to cool the infant as quickly as possible by facilitating convective and evaporative heat loss.
   C. Check the function of the incubator and the placement of the skin probe.
   D. Turn the incubator off and open the port holes until thermal stability is attained.

2. This infant should be observed closely for signs of physiologic stress, which include:

   A. Hypoglycemia and dehydration.
   B. Decreasing blood pressure and bradycardia.
   C. Decreasing oxygen requirements.
   D. Respiratory and metabolic alkalosis.

3. An infant has an axillary temperature of 37.6° C (99.68° F). The infant's skin temperature is 38° C (100.4° F). The infant is flushed in appearance, irritable and sweating, and warm to touch. This baby is likely exhibiting:

   A. Physiologic incompetence secondary to endogenous heat production.

   B. Fever due to evolving sepsis.
   C. Thermal instability.
   D. Physiologic competence in response to overheating.

4. Head coverings made of insulated fabric are valuable in decreasing heat loss, especially in the delivery room, because:

   A. They prevent heat loss by radiation.
   B. The neonatal head accounts for one fifth of the total body surface area.
   C. They are effective under a radiant warmer.
   D. They will supplement heat production because they insulate a large surface area of the infant.

5. The greatest source of heat loss immediately after birth is by which process?

   A. Evaporation
   B. Convection
   C. Conduction
   D. Radiation

6. Warming an infant is effective when:

   A. The infant is placed in an environment where the air temperature is warmer than the infant's temperature.
   B. The infant's skin temperature is at least 2° C warmer than the rectal temperature.
   C. The infant is rewarmed by endogenous heat production.
   D. The infant is placed in a neutral thermal environment.

7. Servocontrol probes are appropriately placed:

    A. Over well-perfused, non-bony or non-excoriated areas free of clothing or bedding.
    B. On the upper thorax or intrascapular region.
    C. At any site appropriate for cardiac/apnea electrode placement.
    D. Over the infant's iliac crest if prone.

8. Hypothermia in an infant with sepsis is thought to be associated with:

    A. Immaturity of the infant's immune response.
    B. Shock and vasodilation and loss of homeothermic reactions.
    C. Peripheral vasoconstriction to increase perfusion to the vital organs.
    D. Immaturity of the hypothalamus for thermoregulatory function.

9. A full-term infant is at risk for heat loss three to four times greater than an adult because:

    A. The infant's thermoregulatory ability is not mature.
    B. The infant has a greater surface-to-body ratio.
    C. The infant has a limited ability to sweat.
    D. The infant cannot shiver.

10. A hypoxic infant may have thermal instability because:

    A. Organ damage to the gut or kidneys can alter the infant's metabolic processes.
    B. The normal neonatal intensive care unit (NICU) environment is too warm.
    C. Thermal receptors in the trigeminal area of the face fail to function.
    D. Hypoxia decreases the effect of norepinephrine or non-shivering thermogenesis (NST).

11. Brown fat is found in all of the following areas *except* which one?

    A. Intrascapular
    B. Paraspinal
    C. Perirenal
    D. Intraabdominal

12. Preterm infants are challenged in effective heat production by non-shivering thermogenesis (NST) because they have:

    A. Little protection from heat loss by the skin.
    B. Little subcutaneous fat.
    C. Immature function of the hypothalamus.
    D. Sparse brown fat stores.

13. Which of the following reflects the existence of a neutral-thermal state?

    A. Core temperature is 1° to 2° C greater than the skin temperature.
    B. There is normoglycemia with the core temperature within normal range.
    C. Core temperature is within normal range when the environment is maintained by servocontrol.
    D. Heat production, measured by oxygen consumption, is minimum and the core temperature is within normal range.

14. A cold-stressed hypoxic infant is at risk for developing:

    A. Respiratory acidosis.
    B. Hyperglycemia.
    C. Metabolic acidosis.
    D. Hypocarbia.

15. In addition to the neutral thermal environment (NTE), the addition of appropriate humidity to an infant's incubator may prevent heat loss by which mechanism?

    A. Radiation
    B. Convection
    C. Evaporation
    D. Conduction

16. The temperature of the environment and objects surrounding an infant in the microenvironment of an incubator is an important assessment because this can be a source of heat loss by which process?

    A. Convection
    B. Conduction
    C. Radiation
    D. Evaporation

17. An infant's incubator placed near a cooler exterior wall or window, or the use of a heat lamp, can cause thermal instability through which process?

A. Radiation
B. Evaporation
C. Conduction
D. Convection

18. The transfer of heat from the body core to the surface and to objects in contact with the infant's body is the process of which mechanism?

    A. Convection
    B. Radiation
    C. Evaporation
    D. Conduction

19. An infant receiving unwarmed oxygen by face mask is noted to be acrocyanotic. Which of the following might be the cause?

    A. Evaporative heat loss
    B. Inadequate oxygenation and anaerobic metabolism for heat production
    C. Stimulation of the thermal receptors in the trigeminal area of the face
    D. Radiant heat loss

20. An effective method of maintaining thermal stability in both average for gestational age (AGA) and small for gestational age (SGA) infants has been Kangaroo Care (skin-to-skin care). Which of the following explains the effect?

    A. Warm blankets surround and insulate the dyad, preventing evaporative heat loss.
    B. The mother will increase and decrease her skin temperature to keep her infant's temperature within normal limits.
    C. The mother radiates heat to the infant.
    D. Close monitoring during Kangaroo Care prevents the development of cold stress.

21. An infant is ready to wean from an incubator to an open crib when it is:

    A. 1600 g with occasional apnea and bradycardia requiring stimulation and oxygen.
    B. 34 weeks of gestational age, stable on a ventilator, gaining an average of 15 g 4 days a week.
    C. Thermally stable with stable weight loss no greater than 30 g on each of 3 consecutive days.
    D. At least 1500 g, medically stable with a consistent weight gain.

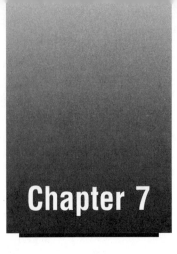

Chapter 7

Fluids and Electrolytes

1. During the diuretic phase, the preterm infant's urine output is:

   A. Increased and natriuresis occurs.
   B. Normal and insensible water loss is high.
   C. Minimal and insensible water loss is high.
   D. Normal and weight loss and body weight stabilizes.

2. A 26-week, 800 g infant is 2 days old and now weighs 660 g. Total fluids are 110 mL/kg/day. Urine output is 2.8 mL/kg/hour. Core temperature is 36.8° C (98.2° F). Incubator temperature is 37.0° C (98.6° F). Humidity is 45%. Which of the following is the most appropriate action?

   A. Change incubator and increase fluids.
   B. Increase humidity and fluids.
   C. Decrease fluids and increase humidity.
   D. No action is indicated, as this is a normal weight loss.

3. When assessing the appropriateness of medication doses in the premature infant, the nurse should consider which of the following postnatal developments?

   A. Renal blood flow decreases as renal vascular resistance rises.
   B. Antidiuretic hormone (ADH) is released by the hypothalamus and stimulates the kidneys.
   C. Preterm infants can not dilute urine, which may cause decreased excretion.
   D. Renal blood flow increases as renal vascular resistance falls.

4. A 900 g infant presents with necrotizing enterocolitis, generalized edema, and overwhelming septic shock. Which of the following is probably the cause of the edema?

   A. High colloid osmotic pressure
   B. Decreased capillary permeability to water and protein
   C. Increased hydrostatic pressure within the capillaries
   D. The abnormal accumulation of intracellular fluid (ICF) within the interstitial spaces

5. A 1200 g infant presents with oliguria and new-onset apnea. The infant has a history of diuretic use. Electrolytes are obtained. The results are Na^+ 121, K^+ 3.8, Cl^- 87, and CO_2 32. Which of the following is the most appropriate action?

   A. Provide KCl and NaCl supplementation to correct hyponatremia over 48 to 72 hours.
   B. Provide NaCl supplement to complete full correction in 24 hours.
   C. Discontinue diuretic and allow sodium to correct itself.
   D. Provide NaCl and KCl supplementation to correct hyponatremia over 24 to 48 hours.

6. A 1200 g infant presents with oliguria and new-onset apnea. The infant has a history of diuretic use. Electrolytes are obtained. The results are Na^+ 115, K^+ 3.8, Cl^- 87, and CO_2 32. This infant is at highest risk for which of the following?

A. Seizures
B. Syndrome of inappropriate diuretic hormone (SIADH)
C. Severe dehydration
D. Cardiopulmonary arrest

7. A 4-day-old, full-term infant is admitted to the neonatal intensive care unit (NICU) with a high-pitched cry, lethargy, irritability, and apnea. The infant has been at home for 2 days. The mother reports that the infant has been breast-feeding 10 to 12 times per day and has had two wet diapers per day. There is no history of fever or vomiting. The infant's symptoms are most likely secondary to which of the following?

A. Dehydration from breast-feeding malnutrition
B. Overhydration secondary to frequent feedings
C. Excessive insensible water losses
D. Sodium intake is less than sodium losses

8. A full-term infant with a history of atrial flutter has been on digoxin for the last 5 days. There have been no further episodes of flutter. The infant becomes apneic and the monitor shows a first-degree atrioventricular block. Electrolytes are sent stat. The nurse should evaluate the electrolytes for which of the following?

A. Hyperchloremia
B. Hypernatremia
C. Hyponatremia
D. Hypokalemia

9. A premature infant of 25 weeks' gestation suffered a traumatic delivery. The infant has generalized bruising. Which of the following is the anticipated pathophysiologic response regarding potassium?

A. Normal postnatal shift of potassium from the extracellular compartment to the intracellular compartment is intensified.
B. Metabolic alkalosis shifts potassium out of the cells.
C. Endogenous release of potassium from tissue destruction, hypoperfusion, hemorrhage, and bruising will take place.
D. Owing to increased glomerular filtration rate (GFR), potassium clearance will be higher.

10. Insensible water loss (IWL) in the preterm infant can be decreased by which of the following?

A. Phototherapy
B. Administering fluids at 1 1/2 times maintenance
C. Increasing environmental temperature above the neutral thermal zone
D. Transferring infant from a radiant warmer to an incubator as soon as possible after birth

11. A stable, 665 g, 26-week infant has a heart rate of 180 bpm. The following laboratory values were obtained from an umbilical catheter, which has dextrose 10% fluids infusing without additives:

Na^+ 149
K^+ 8.1
Cl^- 119
CO_2 17
Calcium 7.5
BUN 30
Creatinine 1.3

The most appropriate intervention would be to notify the physician and anticipate all of the following interventions *except*:

A. Infusion of glucose/insulin solution.
B. Administration of Kayexalate.
C. Infusion of calcium gluconate.
D. Administration of sodium chloride.

12. A full-term, 4.875 kg, large for gestational age infant presents to the neonatal intensive care unit (NICU) with jitteriness, seizure activity, and a high-pitched cry. This presentation would correlate with which of the following diagnoses?

A. Hyperkalemia
B. Hypercalcemia
C. Hypokalemia
D. Hypocalcemia

13. A 4.9 kg infant has a serum calcium level of 6.5 mg/dL. The physician writes an order to administer calcium gluconate. The nurse administering the calcium correction should know that:

A. Calcium chloride is the drug of choice to correct hypocalcemia.
B. Calcium gluconate should be given rapidly over 5 minutes.
C. Calcium gluconate does not require

cardiac monitoring during administration.

D. Calcium gluconate can cause intestinal necrosis and liver necrosis when administered via umbilical catheters.

14. A 36-week, 3.6 kg infant presents with hypoplastic left heart syndrome. The infant's calcium levels are consistently low with a continuous calcium drip of 500 mg/kg/day. Which of the following is the syndrome associated most frequently with hypocalcemia?

   A. Trisomy 13
   B. DiGeorge syndrome
   C. Trisomy 18
   D. Down syndrome

15. An 865 g, 28-week infant is receiving dextrose 7.5% at 70 mL/kg/day. This is:

   A. A sufficient quantity of glucose at 3.5 mL/hr, 5 mg/kg/min of glucose.
   B. Not a sufficient quantity of glucose at 2.5 mL/hr, 3.6 mg/kg/min of glucose.
   C. Not a sufficient quantity of glucose at 3.5 mL/hr, 5 mg/kg/min of glucose.
   D. A sufficient quantity of glucose at 2.5 mL/hr, 3.6 mg/kg/min of glucose.

16. Which of the following describes composition of body water in preterm infants compared with full-term infants. The preterm infant has:

   A. Greater total body water and less extracellular fluid.
   B. Greater total body water and greater extracellular fluid.
   C. Less total body water and less extracellular fluid.
   D. Less total body water and greater extracellular fluid.

17. Which of the following statements is accurate about a preterm infant weighing 965 g with a urine output of 160 mL/24 hours?

   A. It is normal in the diuretic phase to have an output of 5 mL/kg/hour.
   B. It is normal in the post-diuretic phase to have an output of 6.9 mL/kg/hour.
   C. It is abnormal in the post-diuretic phase to have an output of 5 mL/kg/hour.
   D. It is common in the diuretic phase to have an output of 6.9 mL/kg/hour.

18. A 1.265 kg preterm infant is receiving total parenteral nutrition (TPN), dextrose 15% at 3.9 mL/hour and 12 mL of 24-calorie formula every 3 hours. How many mL/kg/day is this?

   A. 150
   B. 125
   C. 135
   D. 105

19. A full-term infant of a diabetic mother weighing 4.9 kg presents with tremors, irritability, and hyperreflexia. The calcium level is 4.5 mg/dL. Multiple calcium gluconate boluses of standard doses have been administered, but the repeat calcium level is 5.5 mg/dL. What is the next consideration?

   A. Obtain a sodium level and prepare to administer a normal saline solution.
   B. Obtain a potassium level and prepare to administer a potassium correction.
   C. Prepare to administer a calcium chloride bolus.
   D. Obtain a magnesium level and prepare to administer magnesium.

20. A 30-day-old premature infant, born at 24 weeks' gestation, has a chest radiograph, which indicates undermineralized bones. Measurement of calcium, phosphorus, and alkaline phosphatase levels is obtained. What are the expected results?

   A. Low calcium, high phosphorus, and high alkaline phosphatase
   B. High calcium, high phosphorus, and high alkaline phosphatase
   C. Normal calcium, low phosphorus, and high alkaline phosphatase
   D. Low calcium, low phosphorus, and high alkaline phosphatase

21. At 36 hours of age, a full-term infant's electrolyte results are Na^+ 142 mEq/L, K^+ 3.5 mEq/L, calcium 6.5 mg/dL, and Cl^- 102 mEq/L. The skin is pale, cool, and mottled and the infant is jittery. These results are most consistent with which of the following?

   A. Hypocalcemia
   B. Hypokalemia
   C. Hyponatremia
   D. Hyperchloremia

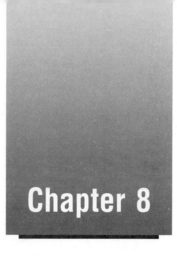

Chapter 8

Nutrition and Feeding

1. Iron supplementation in the first 2 months of life is required when a preterm infant is receiving which of the following?

   A. Intravenous lipids
   B. Erythropoietin
   C. Parenteral nutrition
   D. Enteral feedings

2. Portagen is a formula frequently used for infants with which of the following conditions?

   A. Feeding intolerance
   B. Allergy to cow's milk
   C. Fatty acid metabolism
   D. Renal insufficiency

3. A mother of a preterm infant is undecided about breast-feeding. In discussing the issue with her, which of the following should the nurse emphasize?

   A. Breast-milk has a high protein content.
   B. Infants fed breast-milk have fewer infections.
   C. There is no difference for preterm infants if they are breast-fed or bottle-fed.
   D. Breast-milk provides the preterm infant all the nutrients for adequate growth.

Questions 4, 5, and 6 refer to the following scenario: An infant at 23 weeks' gestation is admitted to the neonatal intensive care unit (NICU) and placed on a radiant warmer. The infant's skin is gelatinous. The physician orders phototherapy on admission as prophylaxis for hyperbilirubinemia. At 4 hours of age, a chemistry panel is drawn and the results are as follows:

   Sodium 156
   Potassium 5.8
   Chloride 120
   Calcium 8.0
   BUN 45
   Creatinine 0.6
   Bilirubin 4.8

4. The chemistry panel results are indicative of which of the following?

   A. Hypocalcemia
   B. Renal failure
   C. Dehydration
   D. Fluid volume overload

5. Calcium gluconate is added to the IV fluid due to which of the following?

   A. Dehydration
   B. Renal failure
   C. Hypocalcemia
   D. Low body stores of calcium at this gestational age

6. In planning care for this patient, the nurse considers that:

   A. Urine output will decrease in dehydration.
   B. Frequent chemistry panels will be avoided to minimize blood loss.
   C. The phototherapy light and radiant warmer will increase the infant's fluid requirements.
   D. Decreasing the relative humidity inside the incubator to less than 30% will decrease insensible water loss.

7. A 1-month-old infant born at 30 weeks' gestation has been stable in room air and tolerating small amounts of enteral feedings. A centrally placed PICC in her right arm supplies additional calories from total parenteral nutrition (TPN). During an assessment, the nurse notes acute respiratory distress and cyanosis. An arterial blood gas on 50% oxygen via nasal cannula is pH 7.19, $PaCO_2$ 80, PaO_2 50, and HCO_3^- 24. A chest radiograph is obtained and demonstrates right lung opacity. Which of the following is the most probable cause for the infant's deterioration?

   A. Sepsis
   B. Pneumonia
   C. Pneumothorax
   D. Pleural effusion

8. A true statement about vitamin E is that it is:

   A. Fat soluble.
   B. Plentiful in the low birth weight infant.
   C. Effective as an oxidant.
   D. Absorbed readily when given in formula.

9. Pregestimil is indicated for infants with which of the following conditions?

   A. Neurologic disease
   B. Renal disease
   C. Malabsorption
   D. Indirect hyperbilirubinemia

10. To have adequate growth and development, a healthy full-term infant requires how many kcal/kg/day?

    A. 50–60
    B. 70–80
    C. 100–120
    D. 150–180

11. Positive reducing substance in the stool is indicative of which of the following conditions?

    A. Slow gastrointestinal motility
    B. Hepatobiliary disease
    C. Necrotizing enterocolitis
    D. Possible carbohydrate malabsorption

12. Similac PM 60/40 is frequently used for infants with which of the following conditions?

    A. Lactose intolerance
    B. Renal insufficiency
    C. Cardiac disease
    D. Fatty acid metabolism defect

13. A 31-week preterm infant is receiving intermittent gavage feedings. Prior to feeding, the nurse checks for a residual and finds one third of the feeding remaining. The residual is green in color. The nurse's next action is to:

    A. Hold feeding and notify MD.
    B. Remove and replace gavage tube.
    C. Discard residual and feed as usual.
    D. Re-feed residual, subtract residual amount from feeding, and feed as usual.

14. The most limiting factor in providing enteral feedings to the premature newborn is:

    A. Small gastric capacity.
    B. Gastoesophageal reflux.
    C. Gastrointestinal motility.
    D. Limited absorption of nutrients from gastrointestinal tract.

15. An elevated alkaline phosphatase level may be indicative of which of the following conditions?

    A. Sepsis
    B. Malabsorption
    C. Bone demineralization
    D. Low calcium and phosphorus levels

16. Complications from total parenteral nutrition (TPN) administration include all of the following *except*:

    A. Cholestasis
    B. Hypoglycemia
    C. Hyperglycemia
    D. Necrotizing enterocolitis

17. Early minimal feeding of the premature newborn is associated with which of the following conditions?

    A. Intestinal perforation
    B. Apnea and bradycardia
    C. Improved calcium and phosphorus retention
    D. Increased incidence of necrotizing enterocolitis

18. Carnitine supplementation is required in the preterm infant who is NPO for all of the following reasons *except*:

    A. Preterm infants have low carnitine stores.
    B. Carnitine is essential to fat metabolism and energy production.
    C. Carnitine supplementation is associated with decreased incidence of necrotizing enterocolitis.
    D. Preterm infants may be missing the necessary enzymes involved in carnitine synthesis.

19. A side effect of intravenous lipid administration is:

    A. Increased binding of bilirubin to albumin.
    B. Increased pulmonary diffusion of gases.
    C. Hypophospholipidemia.
    D. Alteration in leukocyte function.

20. Preterm infant formulas differ from full-term infant formulas in that preterm formulas have:

    A. A soy base and increased fat and protein content.
    B. Increased calcium and phosphorus and decreased carnitine content.
    C. Increased calories and decreased minerals to lower osmolarity.
    D. Increased medium chain triglycerides, reduced amount of lactose, and increased protein content.

21. Soy-based formulas are indicated for infants with which of the following conditions?

    A. Bloody stools
    B. Frequent emesis
    C. Lactase deficiency
    D. Birth weight less than 1800 g

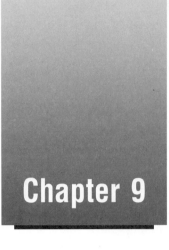

Chapter 9

Developmental Care

1. Obtaining a balance among the subsystems of the synactive theory of development, described by Heidelise Als and colleagues, is known as:

    A. Behavioral organization.
    B. State organization.
    C. Developmental organization.
    D. Self-regulatory organization.

2. An appropriate nursing intervention to assist an infant with poor suck/swallow/breathing coordination would be to:

    A. Allow longer feeding periods.
    B. Pace feedings with short sucking bursts.
    C. Limit the number of gavage feedings.
    D. Increase the liquid flow rate.

3. The fundamental premise of providing developmental care relies on:

    A. Observing, interpreting, and responding to infant behaviors.
    B. Establishing a structured care routine.
    C. Performing tasks that lead to growth and development.
    D. Providing a minimal stimulation environment.

4. If an infant displaying "time-out" signals is exposed to continuing sensory stimulation, what might occur next if someone does not intervene?

    A. Habituation
    B. Self-regulation
    C. Approach behavior
    D. Physiologic instability

5. In which state is it most appropriate to interact with an infant?

    A. Active alert
    B. Quiet alert
    C. Drowsy transitional
    D. Light sleep

6. Poor flexor tone, stimuli overload, shoulder retraction and neck extension, and decreased oral tone make it difficult for premature infants to:

    A. Sleep well.
    B. Mouth-breathe.
    C. Feed efficiently.
    D. Comfort themselves.

7. Some of the variables that should be assessed to determine oral feeding readiness include all of the following *except*:

    A. Medical condition
    B. Oral-motor control
    C. Head control
    D. Weight gain pattern

8. A sucking pattern that occurs at a rate of two sucks per second, satisfies sucking desire, and has a high ratio of sucking to swallowing describes what?

    A. Non-nutritive suck
    B. Nutritive suck
    C. Preterm suck
    D. Dysfunctional suck

9. Coordination of sucking, swallowing, and breathing may be seen as early as:

    A. 29–31 weeks' gestation.
    B. 32–34 weeks' gestation.

C. 35–37 weeks' gestation.
D. 38–40 weeks' gestation.

10. A nurse has just finished starting a peripheral IV line on a 35-week-gestation, 2-day-old infant. She observes that the infant is dusky, flailing his arms, and arching. An appropriate *developmental* intervention would be to:

   A. Provide external containment.
   B. Stroke the infant's chest while whispering soothing words.
   C. Turn on the infant's favorite musical stuffed animal.
   D. Take the infant out of his bed to rock him.

Questions 11 and 12 refer to the following scenario: A nurse notices that 30 minutes after repositioning an infant, the infant has moved to the corner of the bed and is pressed up against the plastic walls.

11. This example demonstrates what type of behavior?

   A. Escape
   B. Cuddling
   C. Avoidance
   D. Self-regulating

12. What can be done to prevent the infant from repeating this behavior?

   A. Use restraints
   B. Keep the bed flat
   C. Provide boundaries
   D. Provide Kangaroo care

13. Decreasing the feeding volume while increasing the number of feedings is one strategy that might be used for what feeding problem?

   A. Poor weight gain pattern
   B. Poor oral motor tone
   C. Uncoordinated suck/swallow/breathing
   D. Tiring before finishing

14. Interventions that support developmentally appropriate nursing care include all of the following *except*:

   A. Altering care schedules to match the infant's state.
   B. Teaching parents to interpret and understand their infant's behavior.

C. Allowing parents to continuously stroke the infant during a 60-minute visit.
   D. Positioning to achieve proper alignment and flexion.

15. Proper prone positioning can be beneficial because it promotes all of the following *except*:

   A. Improved lung mechanics
   B. External rotation of the hips
   C. Lower energy expenditure
   D. Physiologic flexion

16. Constantly monitoring an infant's response to stimulation and providing care activities according to behavioral capability can prevent which of the following?

   A. Self-regulation
   B. Organization
   C. Overstimulation
   D. Stabilization

17. Smooth body movements, hand-to-face actions, relaxed facial expression, and alertness indicate what type of self-regulation behaviors?

   A. Attentive
   B. Coping
   C. Time out
   D. Approach

Questions 18 and 19 refer to the following scenario: A parent begins tapping on the incubator to wake up a sleeping infant for a visit.

18. The most appropriate intervention at this time is to:

   A. Encourage the parent's interactions with her infant.
   B. Assist the parents with a state-appropriate activity.
   C. Gently discourage the parent by stating, "The baby doesn't like that."
   D. Suggest the parent wait until the infant is awake.

19. What might be an appropriate activity for the parent in this situation?

   A. Gently jiggling the baby to wake her up
   B. Talking loudly to the baby

C. Quietly encircling the infant with the parent's hands

D. Coming back to visit at another time

20. Primary goals of auditory interventions in the neonatal intensive care unit (NICU) are to:

A. Provide constant stimulation using a variety of sources.

B. Provide auditory stimulation, but only when the infants are awake.

C. Assess all infants' hearing levels and provide ear muffs.

D. Assess current noise levels and decrease sound decibels wherever possible.

21. Disrupted circadian rhythms, altered sleep cycles, decreased socialization, and decreased oxygenation are side effects primarily associated with what environmental stimulus?

A. Vibration

B. Smell

C. Light

D. Temperature

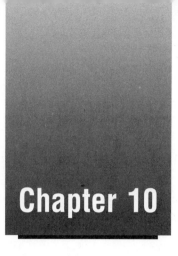

Chapter 10

Radiographic Interpretation

1. A chest radiograph described as bilateral diffuse alveolar infiltrates with a reticulogranular pattern and air bronchograms would be diagnostic of which of the following conditions?

   A. Meconium aspiration syndrome
   B. Transient tachypnea of the newborn
   C. Respiratory distress syndrome
   D. Pulmonary interstitial emphysema

2. A chest radiograph that shows alveolar overdistention with multiple small cyst-like radiolucencies that are unilateral would be diagnostic of which of the following conditions?

   A. Bronchopulmonary dysplasia
   B. Meconium aspiration syndrome
   C. Pneumonia
   D. Pulmonary interstitial emphysema

3. A chest radiograph described as bilateral asymmetric, with areas of atelectasis and a patchy appearance, hyperaeration with flattened hemidiaphragms, and atelectasis would be diagnostic of which of the following conditions?

   A. Bronchopulmonary dysplasia
   B. Pulmonary interstitial emphysema
   C. Pneumomediastinum
   D. Meconium aspiration syndrome

4. A chest radiograph that describes an irregular gas collection with air outlining the undersurface of the thymus gland and creating a "sail sign" is diagnostic of which of the following conditions?

   A. Pneumothorax
   B. Pneumopericardium
   C. Pneumoperitoneum
   D. Pneumomediastinum

5. A full-term infant presents to the neonatal intensive care unit (NICU) after being transferred from the newborn nursery. The infant presents with mild tachypnea and oxygen saturation of 91%. A chest radiograph shows a unilateral flattened diaphragm and a band of hyperlucency between the chest wall and the lung. The primary intervention is to:

   A. Prepare for immediate chest tube insertion.
   B. Provide oxygen to the infant.
   C. Position the infant with the affected side down.
   D. Obtain another chest radiograph with a lateral view.

6. The delivery team responds to the delivery room for a full-term infant with acute distress and apnea on delivery. Of note is a scaphoid abdomen, a potential for CDH. The initial intervention is to:

   A. Auscultate for bilateral breath sounds and supply oxygen via bag valve mask.
   B. Stimulate vigorously and supply blow-by oxygen.
   C. Call for a stat radiograph to evaluate the infant's problem.
   D. Intubate and provide ventilation via endotracheal tube (ETT) and bag.

7. On a chest and abdominal radiograph, the umbilical arterial catheter is noted tracking down toward the pelvis and making an acute turn into the internal iliac artery and common iliac artery, moving up into the aorta and slightly to the left of the vertebral column. The tip termination is at the eleventh thoracic vertebrae. This catheter is:

   A. Too high and needs to be pulled back to the third lumbar vertebra.
   B. In the appropriate position and does not need to be moved.
   C. In poor position and needs to be advanced to high placement at the fifth thoracic vertebra.
   D. Too high and needs to be pulled back to the fifth lumbar vertebra.

8. A 36-week infant on initial feed presents with vomiting episodes in the first few hours of life. The infant has some abnormal appearing features, which are suspicious of a congenital anomaly. The abdominal radiograph shows dilation of the stomach and proximal duodenum producing the characteristic "double bubble" pattern. The anticipated diagnosis includes which of the following?

   A. Duodenal atresia
   B. Meconium ileus

C. Pyloric stenosis
D. Malrotation

9. A preterm twin infant of 32 weeks' gestation on full breast-milk feeds with human milk fortifier presents with acute distress, abdominal distention, and bilious vomiting. Peripheral pulses are weak and thready; tachycardia began approximately 1 hour ago. The stat abdominal radiograph shows generalized distention, asymmetric distribution of bowel gas, and localized distention of bowel loops. The management of this infant includes which of the following?

   A. Continue enteral feeding and supplement with intravenous fluids.
   B. Insert a nasogastric tube to gravity drainage and hold feeds temporarily for 6 hours.
   C. Institute NPO, nasogastric tube to intermittent suction, and serial radiographs.
   D. Eliminate human milk fortifier from feeds and start antibiotics.

10. For a radiograph to evaluate endotracheal tube placement, the infant should be positioned supine with the head:

   A. Midline and neutral.
   B. Rotated toward one side.
   C. Midline and fully flexed.
   D. Midline and fully extended.

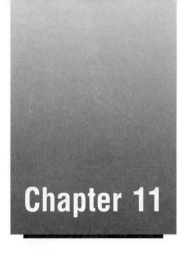

Chapter 11

Pharmacology

1. All of the following medications exhibit sympathomimetic effects *except*:

   A. Dopamine (Intropin)
   B. Isoproterenol (Isuprel)
   C. Methylprednisolone (Solu-medrol)
   D. Albuterol (Proventil, Ventolin)

2. Which of the following is the most serious side effect of Alprostadil (Prostin VR Pediatric Injection) administration in neonates?

   A. Apnea
   B. Bleeding tendencies
   C. Hypotension
   D. Pyrexia

3. Medications bound to protein have which of the following effects?

   A. Enhancement of drug availability
   B. Rapid distribution of the drug to receptor sites
   C. Less available drug for desired effect
   D. Increased metabolism of the drug by the liver

4. Which mechanism appears to be the principal method for transfer of most clinically relevant drugs across the placenta?

   A. Active transport
   B. Simple diffusion
   C. Pinocytosis
   D. Facilitated transport

5. A 23-year-old woman with a prolonged history of seizures treated with phenobarbital (Luminal) and phenytoin (Dilantin) delivers a 38-week-gestation infant. On examination 4 hours after birth, the infant may be expected to exhibit which of the following conditions?

   A. Seizures
   B. Digit and nail hypoplasia
   C. Omphalocele
   D. Drug withdrawal

6. An infant with a ventricular septal defect has been maintained on digoxin (Lanoxin). Furosemide (Lasix) was recently added to the pharmacologic regimen to treat symptoms of increasing congestive heart failure. The clinician must be alert for which of the following conditions?

   A. Hypothyroidism
   B. Hyperaldosteronism
   C. Hypokalemia
   D. Hyperinsulinemia

7. A 30-year-old woman presents to the obstetric floor with delivery imminent. She reports no prenatal care and a prior history of several sexually transmitted diseases. Before further information can be obtained, a 2155 g infant is delivered without respiratory effort. The infant is suctioned, dried, and stimulated and begins to exhibit gasping respiratory effort. Naloxone (Narcan) is:

   A. Indicated to facilitate respiratory effort.
   B. Not indicated because emergent intubation is needed.
   C. Not indicated due to the possibility of maternal infection.
   D. Not indicated due to unknown maternal illicit drug status.

8. A 35-week-gestation infant is delivered by cesarean section secondary to nonimmune hydrops fetalis due to supraventricular tachycardia. He has bilateral pleural effusions. Bilateral thoracenteses collectively removed 40 mL of effusate. He is digitalized and placed on furosemide (Lasix) 2 mg/kg every 8 hours. Ampicillin (Omnipen, Polycillin) and gentamicin (Garamycin) are initiated. Appropriate management consists of which of the following?

   A. An initial daily fluid intake of 130 to 140 mL/kg to replace fluid removed via thoracentesis
   B. Monitoring serum drug levels of gentamicin at 1 week of age
   C. Obtaining an auditory evoked response test on day 1 of life to detect hearing loss secondary to ototoxic drug administration
   D. Expecting an altered volume of water-soluble drug distribution

9. An infant returns to the neonatal unit intubated, with a left tube thoracotomy following surgical ligation of a patent ductus arteriosus. The infant is placed on a warmer bed, attached to a ventilator, pulse oximeter, and cardiorespiratory monitors, and given fentanyl for pain control. The infant suddenly exhibits desaturation followed by decreasing heart rate. The infant remains intubated without a pneumothorax. Which of the following is a possible cause of this infant's deterioration?

   A. Chest wall rigidity
   B. Rapid elimination of anesthetic gases
   C. Vagal response
   D. Hypotension

10. An acutely ill neonate with beta-streptococcal sepsis and persistent pulmonary hypertension is receiving maintenance IV fluid containing calcium through port one of an umbilical venous catheter (UVC). Dopamine and dobutamine are infusing through port two of the umbilical venous catheter. Normal saline is infusing through a peripheral arterial line in the right radial artery. A vecuronium (Norcuron) drip is infusing through a femoral venous line. No other IV sites could be accessed despite multiple attempts. The infant requires multiple medication administration including a sodium bicarbonate bolus followed by the regularly due dose of penicillin. What administration option should be considered?

   A. Infuse sodium bicarbonate through the maintenance fluid line and the penicillin through the peripheral arterial line.
   B. Infuse vecuronium and the inotropes through port two of the UVC, thus freeing the femoral venous line for medication administration.
   C. Give both sodium bicarbonate and penicillin through the peripheral arterial line.
   D. Give penicillin concurrently with the inotropes.

SECTION II

Pathophysiology

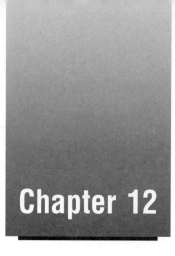

Chapter 12

Cardiovascular Disorders

1. Which of the following statements regarding fluid-filled pressure monitoring systems is *true*?

   A. Zeroing referencing ensures accuracy of the transducer and monitor.
   B. Soft, flexible tubing should be used between the patient and the transducer.
   C. The longer the tubing is between the patient and the transducer, the better the waveform is.
   D. Zero referencing negates the effect of atmospheric pressure on physiologic measurements.

2. A patient with a ventricular septal defect is *least* likely to develop which of the following?

   A. Polycythemia
   B. Hepatomegaly
   C. Congestive heart failure
   D. Frequent respiratory infections

3. Which two vessels does the Blalock-Taussig shunt connect?

   A. Aorta and pulmonary vein
   B. Aorta and pulmonary artery
   C. Subclavian artery and pulmonary artery
   D. Superior vena cava and pulmonary artery

4. In the case of which of the following congenital heart defects should the nurse expect the child to have cyanosis?

   A. Tricuspid atresia
   B. Atrial septal defect

   C. Patent ductus arteriosus
   D. Ventricular septal defect

5. Right heart preload is assessed in the clinical setting by evaluating which pressure?

   A. Central venous pressure
   B. Arterial systolic pressure
   C. Arterial diastolic pressure
   D. Pulmonary artery systolic pressure

6. A neonate with a congenital heart defect is at risk for which of the following?

   A. Endocarditis
   B. Rheumatic fever
   C. Kawasaki disease
   D. Primary cardiomyopathy

7. An infant with a suspected congenital heart defect is being evaluated in the neonatal intensive care unit (NICU). As part of the education provided to the parents, the nurse explains that echocardiography is a useful diagnostic tool because it:

   A. Measures electrical activity of the heart.
   B. Evaluates adequacy of myocardial perfusion.
   C. Measures intracardiac pressures and oxygen saturation.
   D. Visualizes heart structures and measures heart function.

Questions 8 and 9 refer to the following scenario: A previously stable 2-day-old 1000 g, 30-week-gestation infant develops an active precordium, widened pulse pressure, bounding pulses, and a murmur heard best at the left upper sternal border.

8. The nurse suspects this infant has which of the following conditions?

   A. Sepsis
   B. Pneumonia
   C. Patent ductus arteriosus
   D. Intraventricular hemorrhage

9. Which of the following is the most appropriate medical management of this infant?

   A. Antibiotics
   B. Indomethacin
   C. Prostaglandin E_1
   D. High-frequency oscillatory ventilation

10. Which of the following is true about the relationship between systemic and pulmonary pressures during fetal life?

    A. Systemic and pulmonary pressures are equal.
    B. Systemic pressure is less than pulmonary pressure.
    C. Systemic pressure is greater than pulmonary pressure.
    D. Systemic and pulmonary pressures are the same as after birth.

11. Which of the following correctly describes transposition of the great vessels?

    A. Pulmonary artery and aorta arise from the same ventricle.
    B. Pulmonary artery arises from the left ventricle, aorta arises from the right ventricle.
    C. Pulmonary artery arises from the right atrium, aorta arises from the left atrium.
    D. Pulmonary artery arises from the right ventricle, aorta arises from the left ventricle.

Questions 12 and 13 refer to the following scenario: A 2-week-old, 5 kg neonate demonstrates the rhythm illustrated below. The patient is alert, color is slightly pale, and capillary refill is 2 seconds.

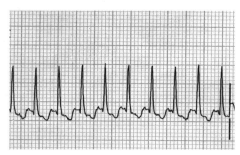

12. Which of the following best describes this rhythm?

    A. Sinus tachycardia
    B. Normal sinus rhythm
    C. Ventricular tachycardia
    D. Supraventricular tachycardia

13. Which of the following interventions would be appropriate for the patient demonstrating this rhythm?

    A. Verapamil
    B. Adenosine
    C. Defibrillation
    D. Eyeball massage

14. Which of the following statements accurately reflects the Frank Starling Law of the Heart?

    A. Increasing preload will increase cardiac output.
    B. Increasing preload will decrease cardiac output.
    C. Decreasing preload will increase cardiac output.
    D. Increasing afterload will increase cardiac output.

15. Which of the following is the most common cause of myocarditis in infants?

    A. Coxsackievirus
    B. *Escherichia coli*
    C. Cytomegalovirus
    D. Beta-hemolytic *Streptococcus*

16. In the absence of tricuspid valve disease, central venous pressure reflects:

    A. Arterial diastolic pressure.
    B. Right ventricular systolic pressure.
    C. Left ventricular end-diastolic pressure.
    D. Right ventricular end-diastolic pressure.

17. An umbilical artery catheter was placed 1 hour ago. The nurse notes the toes on the right foot to be bluish. The nurse's first intervention should be to:

    A. Administer oxygen.
    B. Massage the right foot vigorously.
    C. Remove the umbilical artery catheter.
    D. Apply a warm compress to the left foot.

18. A critically ill infant has the following invasive lines: radial artery line, umbilical

venous line with the tip in the inferior vena cava, right hand peripheral intravenous line, left foot peripheral intravenous line. Which of the following is the most optimal site to begin a dopamine infusion?

A. Umbilical venous line
B. Radial artery line
C. Left foot peripheral intravenous line
D. Right hand peripheral intravenous line

19. The nurse should expect prostaglandin E_1 to be initiated in an infant with which of the following congenital heart lesions?

A. Tricuspid atresia
B. Atrial septal defect
C. Ventricular septal defect
D. Isolated patent ductus arteriosus

20. A 2-week-old neonate with tetralogy of Fallot (TOF) suddenly develops hyperpnea and becomes agitated and cyanotic. The nurse tries to calm the infant but the infant becomes progressively cyanotic. Which of the following interventions is *most* appropriate at this time?

A. Intubate
B. Administer morphine
C. Administer indomethacin
D. Perform percussion and postural drainage

21. Nursing interventions for the neonate with congestive heart failure (CHF) might include all of the following *except*:

A. Position in semi-Fowler.
B. Keep in a quiet environment.
C. Maintain neutral thermal environment.
D. Administer fluids at one and half times maintenance.

22. What is the mechanical event that produces S_2?

A. Opening of the aortic and pulmonic valves
B. Opening of the mitral and tricuspid valves
C. Closing of the mitral and tricuspid valves
D. Closing of the aortic and pulmonic valves

23. In which of the following conditions would the nurse expect to assess pulsus paradoxus?

A. Cardiac tamponade
B. Hypovolemic shock
C. Congestive heart failure
D. Ventricular septal defect

24. A 3-week-old infant is admitted with congestive heart failure. The admission weight was 4235 g. Twenty-four hours later, the weight is 4400 g. Which of the following statements is true about the weight change?

A. The weight gain is normal for an infant of this age.
B. The weight gain is too little for an infant with a cardiac defect.
C. The weight gain is excessive for an infant of this age.
D. The weight gain is normal for an infant with a cardiac defect.

25. An infant with transposition of the great vessels (TOGV) underwent a cardiac catheterization. During the catheterization, a balloon septostomy was performed. The purpose of the balloon septostomy was to:

A. Increase mixing of blood at the atrial level.
B. Make the opening of the pulmonic valve larger.
C. Increase mixing of blood at the ventricular level.
D. Redirect blood flow from the subclavian artery to the pulmonary artery.

26. The most effective mechanism for increasing cardiac output in the neonate is by increasing:

A. Preload.
B. Afterload.
C. Heart rate.
D. Contractility.

27. A 6-hour-old infant demonstrates the following rhythm.

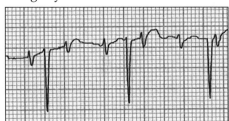

What maternal medical problem should the nurse suspect?

A. Substance abuse
B. Diabetes mellitus
C. Systemic lupus erythematosus
D. Pregnancy-induced hypertension (PIH)

28. A rhythm strip from a 1-day-old infant shows evidence of tall, peaked T waves. The nurse should evaluate this infant for which of the following conditions?

    A. Hypocalcemia
    B. Hypercalcemia
    C. Hypokalemia
    D. Hyperkalemia

29. A 3-day-old full-term infant has the following laboratory results: sodium, 140 mEq/L; K, 3.8 mEq/L; Ca, 6.5 mg/dL; Cl, 95 mEq/L. The nurse should evaluate this infant's ECG for:

    A. Peaked T waves.
    B. Flattened T waves.
    C. Prolonged QT interval.
    D. Presence of prominent U waves.

30. The care plan for an infant with a cyanotic heart defect with decreased pulmonary blood flow should reflect that the infant is at high risk for which of the following?

    A. Pneumonia
    B. Polycythemia
    C. Pneumothorax
    D. Pulmonary edema

31. Congestive heart failure can lead to which type of renal failure?

    A. Prerenal failure
    B. Intrarenal failure
    C. Postrenal failure
    D. Obstructive renal failure

32. The nurse would expect to assess which of the following findings in a neonate in early septic shock?

    A. Hypotension, bradycardia, pallor
    B. Tachycardia, normotension, warm extremities
    C. Bradycardia, decreased urine output, pallor
    D. Tachycardia, cool extremities, hypotension

33. A 2-hour-old full-term infant is admitted with complete heart block. Vital signs include a ventricular rate of 90; RR, 30; BP, 60/45; O_2 saturation, 100%. Extremities are warm and peripheral capillary refill is 2 seconds. What intervention is appropriate?

    A. Observe infant
    B. Defibrillation
    C. Administer adenosine
    D. Synchronized cardioversion

34. An intubated neonate has an intravenous line in the right antecubital fossa that is infusing 10% dextrose in water, an umbilical artery catheter (UAC) infusing half-normal saline, and a heplock in the left foot. When administering adenosine to this patient, the nurse should administer it:

    A. In the UAC over 1 to 2 seconds and followed by a normal saline flush.
    B. Diluted with normal saline and given via the left foot over 20 to 30 seconds.
    C. Diluted with normal saline and given via the endotracheal tube over 2 to 3 seconds.
    D. In the right antecubital vein over 1 to 2 seconds and followed by a normal saline flush.

35. Which of the following cyanotic congenital heart defects is associated with increased pulmonary blood flow?

    A. Tricuspid atresia
    B. Tetralogy of Fallot
    C. Transposition of the great vessels
    D. Pulmonary atresia with intact ventricular septum

36. A preceptor-orientee team is caring for a neonate with tetralogy of Fallot. The infant is in oxygen 25% FIO_2 via hood and is pink. The orientee asks why the baby is not cyanotic. During the explanation, the nurse preceptor should include which of the following statements?

    A. The supplemental oxygen is preventing hypoxemia.
    B. Tetralogy of Fallot is not usually associated with cyanosis.
    C. Infants with tetralogy of Fallot do not typically become cyanotic until about 6 weeks of life.
    D. The degree of cyanosis is dependent on the degree of right ventricular out-

flow tract obstruction and the amount of shunting across the ventricular-septal defect (VSD).

37. Intravenous indomethacin should be administered over 30 minutes to:

    A. Minimize risk of infiltration.
    B. Improve distribution of the drug.
    C. Improve efficacy of closing the ductus arteriosus.
    D. Minimize adverse effects on cerebral, gastrointestinal, and renal blood flow velocities.

38. What is the most significant recognizable side effect of indomethacin?

    A. Apnea
    B. Hypotension
    C. Hyponatremia
    D. Transient renal dysfunction

39. A 4-day-old, 1200 g infant has had one dose of indomethacin for treatment of a patent ductus arteriosus. Twelve hours after the first dose, the nurse's assessment includes the following: active precordium, bounding pulses, murmur, distended and erythematous abdomen. A radiograph of the abdomen shows evidence of pneumotosis intestinalis. The second dose of indomethacin is due. The nurse should:

    A. Hold indomethacin and notify the doctor.
    B. Administer indomethacin and observe the infant.
    C. Assess platelet level, then administer indomethacin if the platelet count is over 50,000.
    D. Assess renal function, then administer indomethacin if urine output is greater than 0.6 mL/kg/hr.

40. The nurse is preparing to initiate a prostaglandin E_1 (PGE_1) infusion. The nurse should be sure to have which of the following items readily available?

    A. Lidocaine
    B. Defibrillator
    C. Indomethacin
    D. Bag-valve-mask

41. The primary clinical effect of dopamine administered at 2.5 μg/kg/min is increased:

    A. Heart rate.
    B. Urine output.
    C. Blood pressure.
    D. Capillary refill.

42. Dobutamine improves cardiac output primarily by:

    A. Increasing heart rate.
    B. Decreasing preload.
    C. Improving cardiac contractility.
    D. Decreasing systemic vascular resistance.

43. Digoxin, dobutamine, and epinephrine are all drugs that:

    A. Increase heart rate.
    B. Are antiarrhythmics.
    C. Improve cardiac output.
    D. Decrease blood pressure.

44. The tip of an umbilical catheter is determined to be in the inferior vena cava just above the diaphragm. Which physiologic pressure is monitored when this line is connected to a transducer?

    A. Arterial pressure
    B. Left atrial pressure
    C. Central venous pressure
    D. Pulmonary artery pressure

45. The nurse notices that the umbilical artery waveform is dampened. Troubleshooting strategies will include all of the following *except*:

    A. Check for kinks in the line.
    B. Check tightness of all connections.
    C. Attempt to aspirate blood, then flush.
    D. Add an additional extension tubing to the line.

46. What are two important goals in the management of an infant with congestive heart failure (CHF)?

    A. Minimize heart rate; maximize blood pressure
    B. Optimize cardiac contractility; minimize cardiac demands
    C. Decrease systemic vascular resistance; increase preload
    D. Decrease cardiac output; increase oxygen consumption

Questions 47 and 48 refer to the following scenario: A 2-week-old infant with a ventricular septal defect (VSD) is admitted with a diagnosis of congestive heart failure (CHF). The parents have been giving digoxin and furosemide (Lasix) to the infant at home. The nurse obtains a rhythm strip and notices the following characteristics: ventricular rate 125, regular R-R interval, PR interval 0.18 seconds, no dropped beats.

47. These characteristics are associated with which of the following?

    A. Wenckebach phenomenom
    B. Sinus bradycardia
    C. Normal sinus rhythm
    D. First-degree atrioventricular (AV) block

48. What is the most likely cause of the rhythm in this patient?

    A. Dehydration
    B. Hypokalemia
    C. Digoxin toxicity
    D. Ventricular septal defect

Questions 49 and 50 refer to the following scenario: A 4-week-old infant with an atrioventricular (AV) canal defect is admitted to the neonatal intensive care unit (NICU). Vital signs are HR 180, RR 50, BP 60/45, O_2 saturation 95%. Assessment findings include the following: color is pale, capillary refill is 3 seconds, extremities are cool to the touch, grade III/VI murmur, rales bilaterally, liver 4 cm below the right costal margin.

49. Which of the following conditions does the nurse suspect?

    A. Sepsis
    B. Dehydration
    C. Congestive heart failure
    D. The ductus arteriosus has opened

50. Pharmacologic management of this infant may include all of the following *except*:

    A. Digoxin.
    B. Furosemide.
    C. Dobutamine.
    D. Hydralazine.

51. A characteristic finding in neonates with coarctation of the aorta is:

    A. Cyanosis at birth.
    B. Boot-shaped heart on radiograph.

C. Cyanosis of only the upper half of the body.
D. Upper extremity pulses stronger than lower extremity pulses.

52. During fetal life, oxygenated blood is shunted from the liver to the inferior vena cava via the:

    A. Hepatic vein.
    B. Foramen ovale.
    C. Ductus venosus.
    D. Ductus arteriosus.

53. What is the purpose of the ductus arteriosus in the fetus?

    A. It shunts blood from the umbilical vein to the inferior vena cava.
    B. It shunts blood from the pulmonary artery to the aorta.
    C. It shunts blood from the right to left atrium.
    D. It shunts blood from the left to the right ventricle.

54. A full-term, small for gestational age (SGA) infant is admitted to the unit. Admission laboratory results are glucose 45 mg/dL, venous hemoglobin 23 g/dL. The infant is on room air and has no signs of respiratory distress. At 4 hours of life, the mother visits and asks the nurse why the infant looks blue. The nurse's explanation is based on which of the following?

    A. Cyanosis is the best predictor of hypoxemia.
    B. SGA infants frequently have cyanotic heart lesions.
    C. Central cyanosis is common during the first 24 hours of life.
    D. An infant who is polycythemic may be cyanotic without being hypoxemic.

55. Which of the following is the most common cause of hypertension in neonates?

    A. Low cardiac output
    B. Left-to-right shunting
    C. Renal vein thrombosis
    D. Congestive heart failure

56. All of the following are indicated for the ongoing medical management of hypoplastic left heart syndrome (HLHS) *except*:

    A. Diuretics.
    B. Dopamine.
    C. 100% oxygen.
    D. Prostaglandin E_1.

57. The nurse notices a pool of blood underneath an infant. It is ascertained that the infant kicked out his umbilical artery catheter. The infant is pale, peripheral pulses are weak, extremities are cool, capillary refill is 3 seconds, and the heart rate is 180 bpm. Which of the following is a clinical sign of improvement following the administration of a normal saline fluid bolus?

    A. Warm extremities
    B. A heart rate of 190
    C. Thready peripheral pulses
    D. Capillary refill of 4 seconds

58. How will the arterial pressure reading be affected if the air-fluid interface of the zeroing stopcock on an umbilical artery line is placed below the phlebostatic axis during zeroing?

    A. The pressure reading will accurately reflect the patient's actual pressure.
    B. The pressure reading will be lower than the patient's actual pressure.
    C. The pressure reading will be higher than the patient's actual pressure.
    D. The pressure reading will reflect central venous pressure.

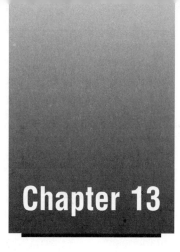

Chapter 13

Pulmonary Disorders

1. The formation of respiratory bronchioles (i.e., acini) during the canalicular stage of fetal lung development is significant because it heralds:

   A. Primitive development of the gas exchange section of the lung.
   B. Creation of alveolar ducts and alveoli.
   C. Initiation of surfactant synthesis.
   D. Rapid proliferation of pulmonary vasculature.

2. Which of the following statements is the most accurate description of fetal lung development during the terminal sac stage of fetal lung development?

   A. Decrease in pulmonary vascularization occurs.
   B. Surface-active phospholipid (lecithin) is first detected.
   C. Progressive increase in respiratory surface area is necessary for gaseous exchange.
   D. Adult component of alveoli is obtained.

3. Although surfactant production may be insufficient to prevent respiratory distress syndrome, at what gestational age is the fetal lung first capable of supporting extrauterine life?

   A. 19–23 weeks
   B. 24–25 weeks
   C. 26–28 weeks
   D. 29–33 weeks

4. Lung development is completed by what age?

   A. 38–40 weeks of gestation
   B. 12–15 months of age
   C. 5 years of age
   D. 8–10 years of age

5. Surfactant improves lung function by:

   A. Reducing surface tension forces at the air-liquid interface in the alveolus.
   B. Promoting structural maturation of the lung.
   C. Inhibiting alveolar fluid clearance.
   D. Increasing opening pressure.

6. By 36 weeks of gestation, the risk for the development of respiratory distress syndrome due to surfactant deficiency is low except for which of the following infants?

   A. Infants of heroin-addicted mothers
   B. Infants of mothers with hypertension
   C. Infants with intrauterine growth retardation (IUGR)
   D. Infants of class A/B/C diabetic mothers

7. Surfactant is produced in the lungs by:

   A. Type I pneumocyte.
   B. Type II pneumocyte.
   C. Surfactant protein-A.
   D. Acinus.

8. Early signs of respiratory distress in a neonate include:

   A. Acrocyanosis.
   B. Respiratory rate of 30 to 40 breaths per minute.
   C. Hypotension.
   D. Grunting, flaring, retractions.

9. The incidence of respiratory distress syndrome:

   A. Is inversely related to gestational age.
   B. Affects 40% of infants born at less than 28 weeks.
   C. Is 2:1 female to male ratio.
   D. Is increased in first-born twin.

10. A 1200 g infant at 30 weeks' gestation was born via precipitous vaginal delivery after a 24-hour period of spontaneously ruptured membranes. The mother was afebrile at the time of delivery but was treated with one dose of intravenous antibiotics 1 hour prior to delivery for unknown group B *Streptococcus* (GBS) status. The infant was cyanotic, floppy, and apneic with a heart rate less than 100 beats per minute. Positive pressure ventilation by bag and mask was administered for 2 minutes, at which time the infant began to cry and color improved. By 5 minutes of life, the infant was tachypneic with respirations 88, expiratory grunting, and nasal flaring. Intercostal and substernal retractions were moderate to severe. Breath sounds were diminished bilaterally despite respiratory effort. A 100% oxygen blow-by failed to improve respiratory status, with oxygen saturation less than 88% via pulse oximetry. Intermittent periods of apnea were observed with heart rate drops below 85 beats per minute. The infant was intubated and prepared for transport to the neonatal intensive care unit (NICU) for ongoing management.

    Based on the history and clinical presentation, the nurse suspects this patient has:

    A. Transient tachypnea of the newborn (TTN).
    B. Meconium aspiration syndrome (MAS).
    C. Respiratory distress syndrome (RDS).
    D. Pulmonary air leak syndrome.

11. Expiratory grunting represents the infant's attempt to:

    A. Prevent alveolar collapse at the end of expiration.
    B. Decrease upper airway resistance.
    C. Decrease functional residual capacity.
    D. Overcome large airway obstruction.

12. To rule out the possibility of group B streptococcal infection as an underlying cause of respiratory distress, which of the following studies would be most appropriate?

    A. Eye cultures
    B. Blood cultures
    C. Nasal pharyngeal cultures
    D. Axillary and rectal cultures

13. The clinical picture of grainy lungs and prominent air bronchograms characteristic of respiratory distress syndrome represents which of the following conditions?

    A. Pulmonary air leaks
    B. "Wet lungs"
    C. Aerated bronchioles superimposed over nonaerated alveoli
    D. Hyperinflated lungs

14. Results of an infant's arterial blood gases (ABG) assessment are as follows:

pH	7.25	O_2 saturation	88%
PaO_2	50	HCO_3	21
$PaCO_2$	70	Base excess	-4

    These blood gases are indicative of which condition?

    A. Metabolic acidosis
    B. Metabolic alkalosis
    C. Respiratory acidosis
    D. Respiratory alkalosis

15. An infant is being mechanically ventilated for respiratory failure associated with respiratory distress syndrome. Arterial blood gas (ABG) results indicate a rising $PaCO_2$ level on current ventilator settings of:

Intermittent mandatory ventilation (IMV)	40
Positive inspiratory pressure (PIP)	16
Positive end-expiratory pressure (PEEP)	+5
Fractionated concentration of oxygen (FIO_2)	70%

    Breath sounds are coarse bilaterally, with bubbling of secretions observed in the endotracheal (ET) tube. The infant is extremely restless, with "see-saw" respirations. The ventilator is consistently alarming for high inspiratory pressure. The nurse's first action should be to:

A. Silence ventilator alarms.
B. Assess breath sounds, suction, reassess breath sounds.
C. Administer sedation.
D. Reposition the infant.

16. By 72 hours of life, a small preterm infant with severe respiratory distress syndrome develops a loud continuous "machinery-like" murmur. Bilateral rales are heard on auscultation of breath sounds. Bounding peripheral pulses with widened pulse-pressure are present. Urine output is less than 2.0 mL/kg/hr. Blood gases reveal increasing hypoxemia, hypercarbia, and metabolic acidosis with subsequent need for increased ventilatory support. These findings are most consistent with which condition?

A. Pulmonary interstitial emphysema (PIE)
B. Pneumonia
C. Patent ductus arteriosus
D. Sepsis

17. Medical management of the infant with respiratory distress syndrome complicated by patent ductus arteriosus would include all of the following *except*:

A. Prostaglandin E_1
B. Indomethacin
C. Fluid restriction
D. Diuretics

18. The clinical presentation of tachypnea, hypercarbia, tissue mottling, diminished capillary refill, and oliguria associated with patent ductus arteriosus (PDA) is the result of which of the following conditions?

A. Right-to-left shunting of blood
B. Left-to-right shunting of blood
C. Pulmonary hypoperfusion
D. Systemic hypertension

19. Pulmonary complications associated with patent ductus arteriosus (PDA) include all of the following *except*:

A. Pulmonary interstitial emphysema
B. Long-term ventilatory dependency
C. Pulmonary hemorrhage
D. Pulmonary hypoplasia

20. Nursing management of a preterm infant with acute respiratory distress syndrome should be directed toward:

A. Maintaining the infant in a neutral thermal environment.
B. Liberalization of fluids.
C. Frequent handling to provide developmental stimulation.
D. Weaning FIO_2 for oxygen saturation values less than 90%.

21. When assessing an infant with respiratory distress syndrome, the nurse calculates the infant's urine output to be greater than 5 mL/kg/hr for an 8-hour period of time. The nurse suspects that the increase in urine output is indicative of which of the following conditions?

A. Worsening pulmonary status
B. Recovery phase of respiratory distress syndrome
C. The development of chronic lung disease
D. Renal failure

22. A maternal history of chorioamnionitis, fever, premature rupture of membranes greater than 24 hours, prolonged labor with intact membranes, and excessive obstetric manipulations are predisposing factors of which of the following conditions?

A. Transient tachypnea of the newborn (TTN)
B. Respiratory distress syndrome (RDS)
C. Meconium aspiration syndrome (MAS)
D. Congenital pneumonia

Questions 23 and 24 refer to the following scenario: A 39-week large for gestational age (LGA) neonate was delivered by repeat cesarean section. Apgar scores were 8 and 9 at 1 and 5 minutes, respectively. Initial vital signs were: temperature 37° C (98.6° F), heart rate 130 beats per minute, respiratory rate 50 breaths per minute. During breast-feeding 2 hours later, the mother reported that the infant was "breathing hard and turning blue." Physical examination revealed respiratory rates above 90 accompanied by nasal flaring, slight duskiness of mucous membranes, and minimal intercostal retractions. Expiratory grunting was noted on auscultation of breath sounds. Pulse oximetry reading was 88% in room air. Blow-by oxygen was provided with oxygen saturation rising to 95 to 96%. A chest radiograph, arterial blood gas assessment, complete blood cell count with differential, serum electrolytes, and blood cultures were obtained. Initial blood gases revealed: PaO_2 of 65, $PaCO_2$ of 36, pH of 7.36, and a bicarbonate level of 24.

23. Appropriate management for this infant would include which of the following interventions?

    A. Provision of supplemental oxygen to maintain PaO_2 above 70 to 80 mm Hg
    B. Intubate and mechanically ventilate
    C. Surfactant
    D. Nitric oxide

24. The initial chest radiograph for the infant reveals diffuse haziness with prominent perihilar streaking bilaterally. This radiographic picture is consistent with which diagnosis?

    A. Respiratory distress syndrome (RDS)
    B. Meconium aspiration syndrome (MAS)
    C. Transient tachypnea of the newborn (TTN)
    D. Persistent pulmonary hypertension of the newborn (PPHN)

25. The underlying clinical pathology of transient tachypnea of the newborn (TTN) is respiratory distress resulting from which of the following conditions?

    A. Retained lung fluids
    B. Progressive atelectasis
    C. Aspiration
    D. Pulmonary hypoplasia

26. The differential diagnosis of transient tachypnea of the newborn (TTN) includes all of the following *except*:

    A. Pneumonia
    B. Pulmonary edema
    C. Respiratory distress syndrome
    D. Pneumothorax

27. Asphyxia is characterized by:

    A. Progressive hypoxemia, hypocarbia, and acidosis.
    B. Progressive hypoxia, hypocarbia, and alkalosis.

    C. Progressive hypoxia, hypercarbia, and acidosis.
    D. Progressive hypoxemia, hypercarbia, and alkalosis.

28. A 38-week infant presented at delivery with apnea, hypotonia, cyanosis, and a heart rate of less than 100 beats per minute. When tactile stimulation and blow-by oxygen fails to induce spontaneous respiration, the nurse initiates positive-pressure bag and mask ventilation, suspecting that the infant has experienced which of the following conditions?

    A. Primary apnea associated with asphyxia
    B. Secondary apnea associated with asphyxia
    C. Persistent pulmonary hypertension of the newborn (PPHN)
    D. Aspiration pneumonia

29. Severe asphyxia of the full-term infant in the early neonatal period may result in which of the following conditions?

    A. Transient tachypnea of the newborn
    B. Left-to-right shunting through the ventricular-septal defect (VSD)
    C. Pneumonia
    D. Persistent pulmonary hypertension of the newborn (PPHN)

30. Central apnea is defined as:

    A. Absence of airflow with continued respiratory effort.
    B. Absence of airflow and respiratory effort.
    C. Cyclic respirations of breathing for 10 to 15 seconds, followed by apnea for 5 to 10 seconds, occurring at least three times in succession.
    D. "Mixed" apnea.

31. The neonate's "unique" response to hypoxemia and carbon dioxide retention is characterized by:

    A. A brief period of increased respiration followed by respiratory depression.
    B. A 10- to 20-fold increase in minute ventilation above baseline.
    C. An initial decrease in respiratory effort.
    D. Prolonged sustained increase in alveolar ventilation.

32. Causes of apnea include all of the following *except*:

    A. Impaired oxygenation
    B. Inhibitory reflexes
    C. Metabolic disorders
    D. Hypertension

33. Which of the following factors is thought to be responsible for the increased prevalence of apnea during active or REM sleep?

    A. Increased minute ventilation
    B. Hering-Breuer inflation reflex
    C. Paradoxical chest wall movements
    D. Increased muscle tone of tongue and pharynx

34. Nursing interventions to prevent or decrease the incidence of "iatrogenic" apnea in preterm infants includes all of the following *except*:

    A. Positioning with small rolls under neck and shoulder
    B. Environmental temperature control
    C. Limiting loud noises
    D. Weighing on cold scale

35. Apnea or respiratory depression is a possible side effect for which of the following medications?

    A. Prostaglandin E_1
    B. Furosemide
    C. Aminophylline
    D. Epinephrine

36. Which of the following medications is used to treat apnea that is refractory to methylxanthine therapy?

    A. Aminophylline
    B. Doxapram
    C. Theophylline
    D. Caffeine

37. As the nurse prepares to administer a dose of theophylline to a preterm infant, the nurse determines that the infant is tachycardic, with a heart rate of 190 beats per minute. The infant is resting quietly in the incubator. The nurse should:

    A. Administer the dose of theophylline.
    B. Withhold the dose and notify the physician.
    C. Retake the heart rate and administer the dose if heart rate is less than 180 beats per minute.
    D. Wait 5 minutes before administering the dose.

38. The recommended dose for theophylline is:

    A. 5 mg/kg loading dose followed by 1–2 mg/kg every 8–12 hours.
    B. 5 mg/kg loading dose followed by 1–2 mg/kg every 6 hours.
    C. 10 mg/kg loading dose followed by 2.5 mg/kg every 12 hours.
    D. 10 mg/kg loading dose followed by 5 mg/kg every 24 hours.

39. What are the advantages to the use of caffeine citrate over theophylline in the management of apnea of prematurity?

    A. Caffeine can only be given by mouth.
    B. Caffeine has a longer half-life, resulting in smaller changes in its plasma concentration.
    C. Caffeine requires twice-a-day dosing.
    D. Caffeine is excreted more rapidly by the kidneys.

40. When an apnea monitor alarms after 20 seconds following the cessation of breathing, the most appropriate immediate response is to:

    A. Assess breath sounds.
    B. Provide gentle tactile stimulation of chest and/or extremities.
    C. Bang loudly on the top of the incubator.
    D. Administer positive pressure ventilation with bag and mask.

41. Parents of a preterm infant are preparing to take their infant home on an apnea monitor. The nurse's discharge teaching regarding monitor care is effective if the parents:

    A. Respond appropriately to monitor alarms.
    B. Disconnect or silence the monitor because of annoyance with monitor alarms.
    C. State intention to use apnea monitor only when infant is asleep at night.
    D. Are observed bathing the infant in a tub with apnea monitor leads intact.

42. Side effects of methylxanthine therapy include all of the following *except*:

    A. Increased wakefulness
    B. Hypotension
    C. Gastroesophageal reflux
    D. Urinary retention

43. Important nursing interventions for the care of the infant receiving nasal continuous positive airway pressure (CPAP) include all of the following *except*:

    A. Monitor vital signs and pulse oximetry
    B. Assess nares for signs of skin breakdown
    C. Maintain nasogastric tube to gravity drainage
    D. Monitor and document CPAP pressure

44. Exclusion criteria for the use of extracorporeal membrane oxygenation (ECMO) for the treatment of respiratory failure include which of the following?

    A. Birth weight greater than 2500 g
    B. Sepsis
    C. Gestational age less than 34 weeks
    D. Absence of major intraventricular hemorrhage

45. Which of the following conditions are indications for the use of extracorporeal membrane oxygenation (ECMO)?

    A. Transient tachypnea of the newborn (TTN)
    B. Bilateral pulmonary hypoplasia
    C. Bronchopulmonary dysplasia (BPD)
    D. Persistent pulmonary hypertension of the newborn

46. Which of the following statements regarding extracorporeal membrane oxygenation (ECMO) is false?

    A. ECMO is rapidly replacing nitric oxide therapy (NO) for the therapeutic management of PPHN (persistent pulmonary hypertension of the newborn).
    B. Positive pressure ventilation can be reduced to minimal settings during VA ECMO (venoarterial perfusion).
    C. ECMO can be safely used for full-term infants with coagulopathy associated with sepsis.

D. ECMO may be indicated for congenital diaphragmatic hernia.

47. What complication is the most frequent cause of death during extracorporeal membrane oxygenation (ECMO) therapy?

    A. Fluid and electrolyte balance
    B. Renal failure
    C. Cardiovascular collapse
    D. Thrombocytopenia and low platelet function

48. After exclusion criteria have been ruled out, the final determining factor for extracorporeal membrane oxygenation (ECMO) eligibility is based on objective criteria that predict which of the following?

    A. 80% mortality risk
    B. Survival rates
    C. Complications associated with ECMO
    D. Positive outcomes

49. Long-term complications associated with extracorporeal membrane oxygenation (ECMO) include all of the following *except*:

    A. Developmental delay
    B. Chronic lung disease
    C. Necrotizing enterocolitis
    D. Failure to thrive

50. Surfactant is recommended for the treatment of which of the following conditions?

    A. Transient tachypnea of the newborn
    B. Meconium aspiration
    C. Respiratory distress syndrome
    D. Pneumonia

51. Which of the following statements about surfactant replacement is false?

    A. Surfactant replacement increases pulmonary compliance.
    B. Surfactant replacement increases pulmonary vascular resistance.
    C. Surfactant replacement reduces the distending pressures needed to inflate the lung.
    D. Surfactant replacement decreases right-to-left shunting.

52. The administration of surfactant at the time of delivery is termed:

A. Rescue therapy.
B. Prophylactic therapy.
C. Chemical resuscitation.
D. Assisted ventilation.

53. A 1000 g infant of 30 weeks' gestation is receiving surfactant. During the first dosing, the infant suddenly becomes dusky and bradycardic, with an oxygen desaturation below 85%. What is the most appropriate step to take?

A. Interrupt dosing and allow infant to recover.
B. Obtain arterial blood gases.
C. Continue administration of surfactant.
D. Suction endotracheal tube.

54. Important nursing interventions for the care of the infant receiving surfactant include all of the following *except*:

A. Assist with positioning during dosing
B. Monitor vital signs and pulse oximetry before, during, and after dosing
C. Suction immediately following dosing
D. Monitor for signs of complications

Questions 55 and 56 refer to the following scenario: A 2.5 kg, post-date infant was born via cesarean section for prolonged fetal bradycardia and thick meconium-stained fluid. The infant was suctioned on the perineum. The infant was limp, apneic, cyanotic, and bradycardic. The infant was intubated and a thick, green substance was aspirated from the trachea. The procedure was repeated twice; the infant also required repeated oral and nasal suctioning for residual meconium.

55. Upon admission, the admitting nurse recognizes that this infant is at high-risk for which of the following conditions?

A. Transient tachypnea of the newborn (TTN)
B. Meconium aspiration syndrome (MAS)
C. Nonspecific respiratory distress syndrome
D. Pulmonary edema

56. Upon arrival to the neonatal intensive care unit (NICU), the infant is placed in a 100% oxygen hood. Initial arterial blood gases revealed pH of 7.28; PCO_2, 56; PO_2, 150; HCO_3^-, 11; base excess, − 14. These

blood gases are indicative of which condition?

A. Respiratory acidosis
B. Metabolic acidosis
C. Hypoxemia
D. Mixed or respiratory and metabolic acidosis

57. At 1 hour of age, an infant with thick meconium at delivery developed grunting, flaring, and retractions with poor aeration and hypoxemia. The chest radiograph revealed white fluffy infiltrates consistent with meconium aspiration syndrome. The infant was intubated and placed on conventional ventilation. At 3 hours of age, the cardiorespiratory monitor alarms for bradycardia and hypotension. The infant is extremely restless and cyanotic, with diminished breath sounds on the left side, poor peripheral pulses, asymmetrical chest rise, and a mediastinal shift toward the right. The nurse should suspect the development of which of the following conditions?

A. Pleural effusion
B. Pulmonary hemorrhage
C. Tension pneumothorax
D. Pulmonary interstitial emphysema (PIE)

58. A 38-week-gestation infant is being treated in the neonatal intensive care unit for group B streptococcal pneumonia. The infant was initially stable in an oxygen hood at 60% FIO_2 with pulse oximeter readings above 95%. At 6 hours of age, the infant becomes increasingly tachypneic and cyanotic, with desaturation below 80% on pulse oximeter during handling or crying. The oxygen concentration is increased to 100% by head hood. Arterial blood gases reveal a PO_2 of 50 mm Hg despite the infant's receiving 100% oxygen. Pulse oximeter readings from the right wrist probe site are higher than readings obtained from the right ankle probe site. On the basis of this clinical presentation, the nurse suspects the development of persistent pulmonary hypertension of the newborn (PPHN) as characterized by:

A. Left-to-right shunting across the ductus arteriosus.

B. Right-to-left shunting across the foramen ovale and ductus arteriosus.
C. Shunting through the ductus venosus.
D. Shunting through a ventral septal defect.

59. The conventional management of infants with persistent pulmonary hypertension of the newborn includes all of the following *except*:

A. Hypoventilation
B. Hyperoxygenation
C. Pharmacologic vasodilators
D. Muscle relaxants, vasopressors, and sedatives

60. Why is inhaled nitric oxide (iNO) useful in the treatment of persistent pulmonary hypertension (PPHN)?

A. Inhaled nitric oxide promotes bronchodilation.
B. Inhaled nitric oxide is a potent selective pulmonary vasodilator.
C. Inhaled nitric oxide decreases systemic arterial pressure.
D. Inhaled nitric oxide supports cardiac function.

61. Potent complications of nitric oxide therapy include all of the following *except*:

A. Methemoglobinemia
B. Pulmonary edema
C. Platelet dysfunction
D. Apnea

62. Which of the following is a complication associated with persistent pulmonary hypertension of the newborn (PPHN)?

A. Renal failure
B. Hyperglycemia
C. Intraventricular hemorrhage
D. Systemic hypertension

63. Which of the following statements about the care of an infant with a chest tube is accurate?

A. Tube patency, fluctuation, and bubbling in the drainage system should be monitored and documented hourly.
B. Milking and stripping of the chest tube are routine interventions to ensure tube patency.
C. Repositioning of the patient should be minimized.

D. Continuous bubbling in the water seal chamber is an indication that the chest tube is functioning effectively.

64. A preterm infant being treated with mechanical ventilation for severe respiratory distress syndrome suddenly presents with hypotension, muffled heart sounds, and severe bradycardia. Chest radiograph reveals a halo appearance surrounding the heart. The nurse should suspect which of the following conditions?

A. Pneumothorax
B. Pneumomediastinum
C. Pneumopericardium
D. Pulmonary interstitial emphysema

Questions 65, 66, and 67 refer to the following scenario: A 37-week-gestation infant is delivered vaginally following an uncomplicated labor and delivery. Immediately after birth, the infant becomes cyanotic with severe grunting, retracting, and nasal flaring. The infant is intubated and given positive pressure ventilation. On physical examination, it is noticed that breath sounds are diminished on the left side with displacement of cardiac sounds toward the right. The abdomen is scaphoid in appearance. Chest radiograph reveals dilated loops of bowel in the thoracic space with right mediastinal shift.

65. The nurse should suspect that the infant has which of the following conditions?

A. Congenital diaphragmatic hernia
B. Pneumothorax
C. Pneumomediastinum
D. Cystic adenomatoid malformation

66. Which of the following factors places this infant at risk for the development of persistent pulmonary hypertension of the newborn (PPHN)?

A. Left-to-right shunting
B. Increased size of pulmonary vessels
C. Pneumothorax
D. Pulmonary hypoplasia

67. Important nursing interventions for this infant include all of the following *except*:

A. Monitor for signs of pneumothorax
B. Position infant on affected side with head of bed raised 45 degrees
C. Monitor pre- and post-ductal oxygen

saturations by pulse oximetry and/or arterial blood gases

D. Maintain orogastric tube for gravity drainage

68. The nurse anticipates that an infant will be scheduled for surgical reduction of a congenital diaphragmatic hernia:

A. Immediately after delivery.
B. Following surfactant therapy.
C. Once pulmonary stabilization has been achieved.
D. After a trial period on nitric oxide.

69. Pulmonary disorders with clinical presentations similar to congenital diaphragmatic hernia (CDH) include all of the following *except*:

A. Congenital lobar emphysema
B. Eventration of the diaphragm
C. Cystic adenomatoid malformation
D. Pulmonary interstitial emphysema

70. Which of the following is a long-term complication associated with congenital diaphragmatic repair?

A. Gastroesophageal reflux
B. Necrotizing enterocolitis
C. Potter's syndrome
D. Chylothorax

71. Clinical presentation of pulmonary hemorrhage includes which of the following conditions?

A. Congestive heart failure
B. Pink or red frothy pulmonary secretions
C. Pulmonary interstitial emphysema
D. Pneumothorax

72. Emergency management of pulmonary hemorrhage includes which of the following interventions?

A. Aggressive airway suctioning
B. Positive pressure ventilation with positive end-expiratory pressure
C. Surfactant administration
D. Diuretic therapy

Questions 73 and 74 refer to the following scenario: A full-term infant is noted to be cyanotic with intermittent periods of apnea during rest. When stimulated, the infant be-

gins to cry with immediate improvement in cyanosis. The nurse is unable to pass a 6 French catheter into the nasal passages.

73. The nurse suspects that the infant has which of the following conditions?

A. Small nasal passage
B. Bilateral choanal atresia
C. Cleft palate
D. Mucus plugging

74. The nurse should expect the diagnostic work-up for this infant to include which of the following tests?

A. Echocardiogram
B. Pulmonary function
C. Head ultrasonogram
D. Abdominal radiograph

75. Micrognathia, glossoptosis, and cleft palate are characteristics of which of the following conditions?

A. Pierre Robin sequence
B. Beckwith-Wiedeman syndrome
C. Down syndrome
D. CHARGE association

76. Infants with micrognathia and glossoptosis are at risk for all of the following complications *except*:

A. Obstructive apnea
B. Cor pulmonale
C. Failure to thrive
D. Subglottic stenosis

77. The parents of a 600 g infant ask what the chance is of their infant developing bronchopulmonary dysplasia (BPD). In response, the nurse explains that the incidence of BPD in infants weighing less than 700 g is approximately:

A. 65%.
B. 75%.
C. 85%.
D. 95%.

78. Factors that predispose an infant to bronchopulmonary dysplasia include which of the following?

A. Oxygen and mechanical ventilation
B. Full-term birth
C. Transient tachypnea of the newborn
D. Hypovolemia

79. Signs and symptoms of bronchopulmonary dysplasia (BPD) include all of the following *except*:

    A. Rales, rhonchi, wheezing
    B. Bronchospasm
    C. Respiratory alkalosis
    D. Retractions

80. Radiographic findings characteristic of severe bronchopulmonary dysplasia (BPD) include which of the following?

    A. Cystic lung fields with hyperinflation and atelectasis
    B. Alveolar infiltrates
    C. Pleural effusion
    D. Dark areas without parenchymal markings

Questions 81 and 82 refer to the following scenario: A preterm infant being mechanically ventilated for bronchopulmonary dysplasia suddenly becomes cyanotic and agitated. The infant is tachycardic with apical pulse above 180 beats per minute. Breath sounds are "tight" with audible inspiratory and expiratory wheezing. The infant continues to demonstrate increased work of breathing and desaturation despite increasing oxygen concentration delivered by ventilator.

81. The nurse suspects that the infant:

    A. Has extubated.
    B. Is experiencing a bronchospasm.
    C. Needs to be suctioned.
    D. Has a pneumothorax.

82. What medication might be appropriate for this infant?

    A. Furosemide
    B. Albuterol
    C. Dexamethasone
    D. Digoxin

83. Signs and symptoms of right-sided congestive heart failure include all of the following *except*:

    A. Weak femoral pulses
    B. Hepatomegaly
    C. Diminished capillary refill
    D. Respiratory distress

84. Nephrocalcinosis is a complication associated with which medication?

    A. Lasix
    B. Aldactone
    C. Dexamethasone
    D. Indomethacin

85. A 33-day-old, former 27-week-gestation infant with bronchopulmonary dysplasia (BPD) presents with the following arterial blood gas results: pH, 7.31; $Paco_2$, 69; Pao_2, 49; BE, +6; HCO_3^-, 35.

    What is your interpretation?

    A. Respiratory acidosis
    B. Partially compensated metabolic acidosis
    C. Hypoxemia and respiratory alkalosis
    D. Partially compensated respiratory acidosis and hypoxemia

86. Nursing care for the infant receiving corticosteroids should include monitoring for which of the following side effects?

    A. Hypertension
    B. Hypoglycemia
    C. Hypercalcemia
    D. Pulmonary edema

87. What are the caloric requirements for infants with severe bronchopulmonary dysplasia (BPD)?

    A. 100 kcal/kg/day
    B. 110–120 kcal/kg/day
    C. 120–140 kcal/kg/day
    D. 150–200 kcal/kg/day

88. After extubation, infants with bronchopulmonary dysplasia (BPD) often require long-term oxygen supplementation to:

    A. Prevent cor pulmonale.
    B. Prevent respiratory infection.
    C. Minimize use of diuretics.
    D. Promote surfactant secretion.

89. Which of the following statements about pulmonary physiology is accurate?

    A. Functional residual capacity (FRC) is defined as the volume of gas that remains in the lungs after a normal expiration.
    B. Tidal volume (TV) is defined as the volume of air maximally inspired and maximally expired.
    C. Vital capacity (VC) is defined as the amount of air that moves into or out of the lungs with each single breath at rest.
    D. Physiologic dead space is defined as the volume of gas within the area of the pulmonary conducting airways that cannot engage in gas exchange.

90. Radiographic findings associated with pulmonary interstitial emphysema (PIE) include all of the following *except*:

    A. Microcystic areas
    B. Grainy lungs
    C. Hyperinflation
    D. Flattened diaphragm

91. Which of the following statements about the hemoglobin-oxygen dissociation curve is inaccurate?

    A. The hemoglobin-oxygen dissociation curve reflects the affinity of hemoglobin to oxygen.
    B. The pH, temperature, and hemoglobin structure influence hemoglobin's affinity for oxygen.
    C. The absence of cyanosis indicates a well-oxygenated infant.
    D. A right-shifted curve indicates decreased affinity of hemoglobin for oxygen.

92. Which of the following factors can lead to inaccurate oxygen saturation values displayed by pulse oximetry?

    A. Decreased peripheral perfusion
    B. Vasodilating drugs
    C. Prematurity
    D. Cyanotic heart disease

93. When assessing the oxygen delivery system for a neonate receiving supplemental oxygen by oxygen hood, the nurse notes that the oxygen flow rate is set at 4 L/min. An appropriate nursing intervention would be to:

    A. Decrease flow to 3 L/min.
    B. Do nothing, because no intervention is required.
    C. Increase flow to 5–7 L/min.
    D. Increase flow to >10 L/min.

94. Which of the following signs is indicative of endotracheal tube (ETT) extubation?

    A. Breath sounds audible in stomach
    B. Breath sounds louder on the right
    C. Fogging in endotracheal tube
    D. Hypotension

95. Which of the following statements is an inaccurate description of high frequency oscillatory ventilation (HFOV)?

    A. Breathing rates or frequency are expressed in Hertz.
    B. Breaths are delivered by a vibrating diaphragm, where inspiration and exhalation are active processes.
    C. CO_2 elimination is controlled only by oscillatory amplitude.
    D. Oxygenation is controlled by adjusting mean airway pressure (MAP).

96. A sudden decrease in chest wall vibration for infants receiving high frequency ventilation may indicate:

    A. Plugged endotracheal tube.
    B. Decreased cardiac output.
    C. Need to increase mean airway pressure (MAP).
    D. Need to increase amplitude.

97. A preterm infant with severe respiratory distress syndrome is diagnosed with pulmonary interstitial emphysema (PIE) at 36 hours of age. Chest radiographic findings indicate localized PIE throughout the left lower lobe. Treatment may include all of the following options *except*:

    A. Selective intubation of right mainstem bronchus
    B. Left side-lying position
    C. Extracorporeal membrane oxygenation (ECMO)
    D. High frequency ventilation (HFV)

98. An infant with respiratory distress syndrome has the following arterial blood gases:

    pH 7.50
    Pao_2 75
    $Paco_2$ 30
    HCO_3 22

    These blood gases are indicative of which of the following conditions?

    A. Metabolic acidosis
    B. Metabolic alkalosis
    C. Respiratory acidosis
    D. Respiratory alkalosis

99. Which of the following would be the appropriate management for ventilator-induced respiratory alkalosis?

    A. Increase ventilator rate
    B. Decrease ventilator rate
    C. Increase peak inspiratory pressure
    D. Decrease positive end-expiratory pressure

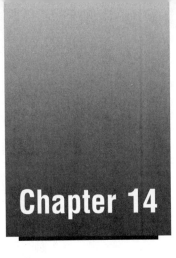

Chapter 14

Metabolic/Endocrine Disorders

1. An infant is to be born to an insulin-dependent diabetic mother. The nurse should be prepared to do which of the following after the infant is born?

   A. Keep on NPO status until serum blood glucose level is obtained.
   B. Provide early feeding if medically stable.
   C. Immediately start an intravenous infusion of D$_5$W.
   D. Wait to perform glucose screen until infant is 6 hours of age.

2. Short-term treatment of an infant with an acute hypercalcemic episode includes giving which of the following calciuretic agents?

   A. Furosemide
   B. Calcitonin
   C. Chloramphenicol
   D. Hydralazine

3. Rapid intravenous infusion of calcium to correct hypocalcemia can result in which of the following conditions?

   A. Tremors
   B. Tachycardia
   C. Bradycardia
   D. Tachypnea

4. Currently all states and the District of Columbia require screening of PKU and what other disease prior to discharge of a newborn infant?

   A. Hypothyroidism
   B. Galactosemia

   C. Maple syrup urine disease
   D. Cystic fibrosis

5. An infant presents with irritability, tremors, intrauterine growth retardation, and hyperthermia. The mother has a history of Graves disease. The most likely diagnosis of the infant's condition is:

   A. Hypothyroidism.
   B. Hyperthyroidism.
   C. G6PD deficiency.
   D. Adrenal hyperplasia.

6. The nurse caring for an infant diagnosed with SIADH (syndrome of inappropriate antidiuretic hormone) would expect to see which combination of findings?

   A. High urine output, high urine specific gravity, high urine sodium
   B. Low urine output, low urine specific gravity, low urine sodium
   C. Low urine output, high urine specific gravity, high urine sodium
   D. High urine output, low urine specific gravity, low urine sodium

7. The primary cause of metabolic bone disease in the premature infant is:

   A. Vitamin D deficiency.
   B. Inadequate calcium and phosphorus intake.
   C. Inadequate magnesium and calcium intake.
   D. Vitamin C deficiency.

8. The nurse caring for the infant of a diabetic mother should assess the infant for

signs and symptoms of which of the following conditions?

A. Hypercalcemia
B. Hyponatremia
C. Hypocalcemia
D. Hypermagnesemia

9. At birth an infant should have a serum glucose level that is about what percentage of the mother's?

A. 20%
B. 40%
C. 60%
D. 80%

10. A newborn infant presents with vomiting and diarrhea after feedings with lactose-based formula are initiated. Which of the following should the nurse consider the cause to be?

A. Maple syrup urine disease
B. Galactosemia
C. Cystic fibrosis
D. Glycogen storage disease

11. A preterm infant with hypophosphatemia has a radiograph that shows skeletal deformities. What would the most likely diagnosis be?

A. Osteogenesis imperfecta
B. Osteomyelitis
C. Rickets
D. Osteochondrodysplasia

12. An appropriate plan of care for a premature infant with osteopenia of prematurity would include all of the following except:

A. Gentle handling.
B. Avoiding chest physiotherapy.
C. Monitoring calcium and phosphorus levels.
D. Giving vitamin D supplements.

13. The neonate with an inborn error of metabolism can appear normal at birth because of effective removal of toxins by what structure?

A. Placenta
B. Liver
C. Pancreas
D. Gall bladder

14. Which type of inheritance pattern is characteristic of inborn errors of metabolism?

A. Autosomal recessive
B. Autosomal dominant
C. X-linked dominant
D. Y-linked recessive

15. Which of the following is the most common cause of ambiguous genitalia in the newborn?

A. Turner syndrome
B. Congenital adrenal hyperplasia
C. G6PD deficiency
D. Klinefelter syndrome

16. The nurse caring for the newborn infant less than 24 hours old should recognize that treatment for hypoglycemia should be started for which of the following serum glucose results?

A. 65 mg/dL
B. 55 mg/dL
C. 50 mg/dL
D. 35 mg/dL

17. Which of the following is the most serious complication of untreated congenital hypothyroidism?

A. Sepsis
B. Thyrotoxicosis
C. Mental retardation
D. Cortisol insufficiency

Chapter 15

Gastrointestinal Disorders

1. The classic "double bubble" on an abdominal radiograph is a diagnostic sign for which of the following?

   A. Jejunal atresia
   B. Gastric perforation
   C. Duodenal atresia
   D. Imperforate anus

2. Duodenal atresia is commonly associated with which genetic condition?

   A. Trisomy 13
   B. Noonan syndrome
   C. Trisomy 21
   D. Turner syndrome

3. Intestinal obstruction from meconium ileus is the result of which of the following?

   A. Formed meconium with abnormally low concentrations of albumin and macro proteins
   B. Formed meconium with high water content
   C. Hypersecretion of water and electrolytes by the intestines and pancreas
   D. Meconium with high protein content and an abnormal mucous glycoprotein

4. All of the following physiologic factors interfere with normal gastrointestinal function in the preterm infant (<36 weeks) *except*:

   A. Poor suck and swallow coordination
   B. Shorter gastric emptying time
   C. Decreased gastric acidity
   D. Incompetent lower esophageal sphincter

5. Risk factors that are strongly associated with the pathogenesis of necrotizing enterocolitis (NEC) are:

   A. Minimal enteral feedings and prematurity.
   B. Immature gut motility and increased gastric acidity.
   C. Immature gastrointestinal tract and rapid advancement of enteral feeding.
   D. Bacterial colonization of the gastrointestinal tract and breast-milk feedings.

6. An infant is admitted to the neonatal intensive care unit (NICU) with an esophageal malformation. The nurse suspects that it will most likely be which of the following?

   A. Upper pouch fistula
   B. Isolated tracheoesophageal fistula
   C. Isolated esophageal atresia; no tracheal communication
   D. Esophageal atresia with lower segment tracheoesophageal fistula

7. An infant born at 39 weeks' gestation had an omphalocele repaired 3 weeks ago. The infant had progressed to full feedings and was tolerating feedings. Forty-eight hours before discharge, the infant presents with bilious vomiting and abdominal distention. The nurse should report these findings immediately because he/she suspects which condition?

   A. Malrotation
   B. Incarcerated inguinal hernia
   C. Lactobezoar
   D. Mild protein allergy

8. Which syndrome is commonly associated with tracheoesophageal fistula (TEF)?

   A. Pierre Robin
   B. CHARGE
   C. VATER
   D. DiGeorge

9. Which abdominal wall defect is most frequently associated with other congenital anomalies?

   A. Umbilical hernia
   B. Inguinal hernia
   C. Omphalocele
   D. Gastroschisis

10. The nurse is caring for an infant who has had a staged reduction of a gastroschisis. This was the final reduction and the abdominal wall is closed. Four hours after the final reduction and closure of the abdominal wall, the infant's lower extremities become dusky and urine output is decreased. What action should the nurse take?

    A. Immediately call the surgical team
    B. Elevate the infant's legs and insert a Foley catheter
    C. Administer a 5% albumin bolus
    D. Reposition the infant and administer a narcotic

11. A previously stable premature infant demonstrates signs and symptoms consistent with necrotizing enterocolitis (NEC). What should be the first priority of the nurse?

    A. Place infant on NPO status
    B. Obtain blood cultures
    C. Administer antibiotics
    D. Insert a urinary drainage catheter

12. Malrotation with midgut volvulus is a surgical emergency because of the high risk of which of the following?

    A. Mesenteric artery rupture
    B. Intestinal ischemia
    C. Intestinal perforation
    D. Disseminated intravascular coagulation

13. During the daily reduction after staged closure of gastroschisis with a silo, the nurse should be alert for the development of which of the following signs?

    A. Hyperthermia
    B. Hypocarbia
    C. Hypoxemia
    D. Hypoglycemia

14. During the immediate postoperative period after a staged closure of gastroschisis with a silo, the nurse should expect to perform all of the following interventions except:

    A. Administer antibiotics
    B. Replace nasogastric drainage
    C. Maintain NPO status
    D. Initiate kangaroo care (skin-to-skin)

15. Which section of intestine, if removed, results in overgrowth of colonic bacteria in the small intestine?

    A. Ileum
    B. Jejunum
    C. Ileocecal valve
    D. Transverse colon

16. Upon inspecting the umbilicus of a neonate, the nurse notes an abnormal thickening of the umbilical cord. This infant should be further evaluated for which of the following conditions?

    A. Granuloma
    B. Omphalocele
    C. Patent urachus
    D. Prune belly syndrome

17. Which of the following is the single most important risk factor for the development of necrotizing enterocolitis (NEC)?

    A. Male gender
    B. Polycythemia
    C. Prematurity
    D. Formula feeding

18. A 38-week-gestation infant is admitted to the neonatal intensive care unit (NICU). The nurse notes extrusion of abdominal contents to the right of the umbilical cord. There is no sac covering the extruded contents. The nurse suspects this infant has which of the following conditions?

    A. Omphalocele
    B. Gastroschisis
    C. Prune belly syndrome
    D. Congenital diaphragmatic hernia

19. A nurse is caring for a 48-hour-old full-term neonate. Upon noting that the neo-

nate has abdominal distention, the nurse inserts a sump tube, which drains bilious materials. Maternal history is notable for polyhydramnios. The infant has not stooled yet. These findings are most consistent with what diagnosis?

A. Esophageal atresia
B. Intestinal obstruction
C. Prune belly syndrome
D. Necrotizing enterocolitis

20. A full-term infant with a maternal history of polyhydramnios is noted to have excessive drooling. The nurse inserts an orogastric tube. A radiograph shows the orogastric tube ending in a pouch high above the stomach. What is the primary problem the nurse should be concerned about in this infant?

A. Aspiration
B. Dehydration
C. Midgut volvulus
D. Poor feeding habits

21. A 4-day-old 30-week-gestation infant is noted to have abdominal distention, bilious vomiting, and increasing episodes of apnea and bradycardia. A cross-table radiograph shows a pneumoperitoneum. Which of the following interventions should the nurse expect?

A. Surgery
B. Insertion of a chest tube
C. Loading dose of aminophylline
D. Placement of an orogastric tube for gravity drainage

22. A 28-week-gestation infant is now 35 days old. The infant is receiving premature formula and parenteral nutrition. The infant is noted to have abdominal distension and bile-stained emesis. Vital signs have been stable and there are no episodes of apnea and bradycardia. Past history reveals that the infant had necro-

tizing enterocolitis on day 8 of life and was kept NPO for 10 days. Which of the following is the most likely cause of this infant's gastrointestinal dysfunction?

A. Intestinal stricture
B. Milk protein allergy
C. Gastroesophageal reflux
D. Recurrent necrotizing enterocolitis

23. A previously well full-term neonate presents with bilious vomiting. What is the first disorder that should be ruled in or out?

A. Pyloric stenosis
B. Imperforate anus
C. Necrotizing enterocolitis
D. Malrotation with midgut volvulus

24. Metochlopramide may be useful in the treatment of gastroesophageal reflux (GER) because it:

A. Suppresses nausea.
B. Increases gastric pH.
C. Enhances gastric emptying.
D. Increases lower esophageal peristalsis.

25. Infants who are preterm, have congenital diaphragmatic hernia, or have neurologic damage are all at risk for which of the following conditions?

A. Malrotation
B. Short bowel syndrome
C. Gastroesophageal reflux
D. Necrotizing enterocolitis

26. The outcome for infants with anorectal anomalies is primarily determined by which of the following?

A. Gender
B. Presence of a rectourethral fistula
C. The age at which the defect is corrected
D. Level of the upper rectal pouch in relation to the puborectal muscle

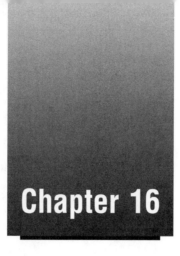

Chapter 16

Hematologic Disorders

1. The fetus of a mother with pregnancy-induced hypertension may experience chronic deprivation of oxygen and nutrition. As a result, which of the following colony-stimulating factors may be increased in utero?

   A. G-CSF
   B. M-CSF
   C. Erythropoietin
   D. Interleukin 4–9

2. The hemoglobin-oxygen dissociation curve is shifted to the right in which of the following situations?

   A. Increased carbon dioxide
   B. Decreased temperature
   C. Increased pH
   D. Decreased 2,3-diphosphoglycerate

3. A 28-week-old infant is admitted to the neonatal intensive care unit (NICU). Physiologic jaundice of the preterm infant is anticipated for all of the following reasons except:

   A. The red blood cells of preterm infants have a shorter life span than those of term infants.
   B. The enterohepatic circulatory system is less mature in preterm infants than term infants.
   C. Preterm infants have decreased glucuronyl transferase activity in their livers.
   D. Preterm infants have an increased level of albumin for bilirubin transport in their blood.

4. All of the following factors would increase the blood volume in the neonate except:

   A. Placement of the newborn baby below the level of the placenta prior to the cord being clamped
   B. Chronic placental insufficiency
   C. Cord compression in the 30 minutes prior to delivery
   D. Product of a maternal-fetal transfusion

5. Sepsis increases the risk of kernicterus in hyperbilirubinemia primarily because sepsis:

   A. Decreases the number of acceptor proteins at the wall of the liver.
   B. Alters the integrity of the blood-brain barrier.
   C. Decreases bilirubin conjugation in the liver.
   D. Increases enterohepatic circulation.

6. A nurse is caring for a 34-week-old septic infant with an indirect bilirubin of 23.8 mg/dL. The infant is intubated and on synchronized intermittent mechanical ventilation. Over the last 6 hours, his pH has varied between 7.20 and 7.29 with a base deficit of −6. He is receiving 4 μg/kg/min of dopamine. Which action is most important prior to starting a double volume exchange transfusion?

   A. Ensure that the infant is restrained.
   B. Give a bolus of albumin so that the dopamine can be discontinued.
   C. Correct the metabolic acidosis.
   D. Ensure that emergency equipment is available at the bedside.

7. Infants with an increased direct bilirubin need to be evaluated for:

   A. ABO incompatibility.
   B. Liver function.
   C. Extravasation of blood.
   D. Constipation.

8. The administration of vitamin K most directly affects which coagulation test?

   A. Platelet count
   B. Prothrombin time (PT)
   C. Partial thromboplastin time (PTT)
   D. Fibrinogen level

9. A Gravida 1 Para 1 female has O+ blood. Her 38-week-gestation infant is A+. Which set of findings will this infant most likely exhibit at four days of life?

   A. A bilirubin of 7 mg/dL, hematocrit of 45%, and white blood cell count of 10 mm³.
   B. Petechiae, a prothrombin time of greater than 25 seconds, and oozing from intravenous insertion sites.
   C. Mild hemolysis, anemia, and reticulocytosis.
   D. Ascites, pleural effusion, and hepatosplenomegaly.

Questions 10 and 11 refer to the following scenario: A 32-week 1700 g infant has an umbilical arterial line in place. Fifteen minutes following radiograph of the infant, the nurse notices a large pool of blood on the bed next to the infant. The estimated blood loss is 45 mLs.

10. Which set of signs and symptoms is most likely to reflect the infant's condition in the first 30–60 minutes following this acute loss of blood?

	Blood		
Hematocrit	Pressure	Heart Rate	Multisystem
A. Decreased	Hypotension	Tachycardia	Tachypnea, pallor
B. Same as before incident	Hypotension	Tachycardia	Pallor, capillary refill 3 sec, respiratory distress
C. Same as before incident	Hypotension	Bradycardia	Apnea, cyanosis
D. Decreased	Same as before incident	Same as before incident	Hepatosplenomegaly

11. What is the most critical immediate intervention for this baby?

   A. Increasing the percentage of inspired oxygen to 100%.
   B. Placing the infant in a Trendelenburg position.
   C. Sending down a blood specimen for type and cross-match.
   D. Administering a rapid infusion of isotonic saline or 5% albumin.

12. A 26-week-old, 650 g neonate was admitted 10 hours ago in critical condition to the neonatal intensive care unit (NICU). Maternal history is significant for ruptured membranes for 18 hours. Antibiotics have been started. He has petechiae on his trunk and prolonged oozing from heel stick sites. Blood is being suctioned from the endotracheal tube. The most recent hematocrit is 44%. Coagulation panel results have just returned and are as follows:

Platelets	66,000 mm/L
PT	22 seconds
PTT	65 seconds
Fibrinogen	80 mg/L

The next priority in drug/transfusion therapy is to:

   A. Administer 10 mL/kg fresh frozen plasma.
   B. Administer 10 mL/kg packed red blood cells.
   C. Administer 10 mL/kg of platelets.
   D. Administer 10 mL/kg cryoprecipitate.

13. The role of phototherapy in the treatment of hyperbilirubinemia is to:

   A. Increase the amount of ligand at the liver wall, thus facilitating uptake.
   B. Cause oxidation and isomerization of bilirubin into a water-soluble, excretable form.
   C. Increase the amount of glucuronyl transferase so that bilirubin can be more easily conjugated.
   D. Cause movement of extravascular bilirubin into the vascular space, thus facilitating albumin binding.

14. To rule out idiopathic thrombocytopenic purpura in the neonate with thrombocytopenia, the physician needs to consider which of the following?

A. The presence of fetal platelets in the maternal circulation
B. The presence of fetal hemorrhage prior to delivery
C. The mother's platelet count
D. The mother's blood type

15. Which set of maternal characteristics is associated with the greatest risk of polycythemia in the neonate?

Gestational age	Maternal condition
A. 28 weeks	pregnancy-induced hypertension
B. 36 weeks	prolonged rupture of membranes
C. 39 weeks	status post motor vehicle accident
D. 41 weeks	gestational diabetes

16. A 38-week-old small for gestational age newborn has a venous hematocrit of 62%. The infant has had some jitteriness and is not nipple-feeding well. She is not experiencing any respiratory difficulties and her blood glucose level is 54 mg/dL. Her urinary output is 2.1 mL/kg/hr. Anticipatory management at this time would include which of the following interventions?

A. Performing a partial exchange transfusion with normal saline or 5% albumin
B. Closely monitoring her respiratory status, glucose levels, and hydration while encouraging feeds
C. Putting her on NPO status and beginning maintenance IV fluids at 80 mL/kg/day
D. Continuing current care

17. A 95-day-old infant (current weight, 2.2 kg; postconceptual age, 36 weeks) is being cared for in the neonatal intensive care unit (NICU). He has bronchopulmonary dysplasia and is receiving oxygen at 0.2 LPM, 100% F_{IO_2} via nasal cannula. He is pale and lethargic and has had six apneic episodes in the past 24 hours. His heart rate is 176 beats per minute. Complete blood cell count (CBC) results include:

WBC count: 15,000/mm³
Hemoglobin: 8.5 g/dL
Hematocrit: 27%
Reticulocyte count: 1.8%
Platelet count: 265,000/mm³

Based on the clinical picture and laboratory results, what would the appropriate action be?

A. Begin a course of Epogen (recombinant human erythropoietin)
B. Begin a course of supplemental iron with feeds
C. Transfuse the infant with 10 mL/kg packed red blood cells
D. Continue current care

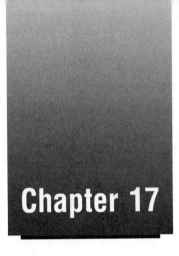

Chapter 17

Neurologic Disorders

1. What is the normal range of head circumference growth per week for a preterm newborn?

   A. 0.25 cm
   B. 0.5–1 cm
   C. 1–2 cm
   D. 10% increase

2. Large or numerous cafe-au-lait spots on the skin may be associated with which condition?

   A. Hemangiomas
   B. Neurofibromatosis
   C. Neural tube defects
   D. Chromosome abnormalities

3. Limited autoregulation in premature infants predisposes them to which condition?

   A. Apnea
   B. Hypothermia
   C. Bradycardia
   D. Intraventricular hemorrhage

Questions 4, 5, and 6 refer to the following scenario: A full-term infant is admitted following prolonged fetal bradycardia necessitating a stat cesarean section and delivery room resuscitation. Apgar scores were 0, 4, 4, and 8 at 1, 5, 10, and 20 minutes of life. Results of an arterial blood gas (ABG) assessment at 30 minutes of life are:

   pH 7.02.
   P_{CO_2} 38.
   P_{O_2} 78.
   BE −16.
   94% O_2 saturation.

The infant required continuous positive airway pressure (CPAP) initially then weaned to room air. The infant has stable vital signs and is hypotonic.

4. What is the infant at risk for?

   A. Sepsis
   B. Kernicterus
   C. Respiratory failure
   D. Hypoxic ischemic encephalopathy

5. The infant is now staring and lip-smacking and has elevated blood pressure. This most likely represents which condition?

   A. Seizure activity
   B. Hypercalcemia
   C. Readiness to feed
   D. Change of state to wakefulness

6. What would the most appropriate first intervention for this infant be?

   A. Call for an electroencephalogram (EEG)
   B. Administer early feedings
   C. Send serum glucose to the laboratory
   D. Give loading dose of phenobarbital

7. Neonatal seizures are most frequently characterized by:

   A. Tonic/clonic activity.
   B. Ability to be detected only by electroencephalogram (EEG).
   C. Subtle signs that may go unnoticed.
   D. Ability to be stopped with passive flexion.

8. A 3-day-old full-term baby with septic shock has a phenobarbital level of 12.5 μg/mL and is having breakthrough seizures. What would an appropriate initial step be?

A. Start phenytoin (Dilantin)
B. Re-bolus with phenobarbital
C. Continue same phenobarbital dose
D. Hold phenobarbital and obtain another measurement in 48 hours

9. A former 28-week-gestation premature infant is being treated with acetazolamide (Diamox) for post-hemorrhagic hydrocephalus. The nurse would expect to administer which of the following?

A. Calcium
B. Vitamin E
C. Magnesium
D. Sodium bicarbonate

10. When teaching the parents of a baby with a myelomeningocele, it is important to reinforce that the surgical repair will:

A. Improve leg movement.
B. Be needed for cosmetic reasons.
C. Not reverse sensorimotor deficits.
D. Not be painful due to decreased sensation.

11. A full-term infant has undergone myelomeningocele repair. Postoperatively, the nurse should evaluate the head circumference and fontanel for:

A. Potential for intraventricular hemorrhage (IVH).
B. Signs of hydrocephalus.
C. Signs of craniosynostosis.
D. Assurance of normal head growth.

12. Arnold-Chiari II malformation is most frequently associated with which condition?

A. Myelomeningocele
B. Dandy-Walker syndrome
C. Holoprosencephaly
D. Aqueductal stenosis

13. A 2-month-old infant is 2 days post VP shunt placement. The infant becomes irritable, with increased head circumference and bradycardia. What is the most likely reason for this?

A. Sepsis
B. Shunt blockage
C. Decompression of ventricles
D. New intracranial hemorrhage

14. An infant admitted with a subgaleal bleed may emergently need which intervention?

A. Electroencephalogram (EEG)
B. Lumbar tap
C. Head ultrasonogram
D. Packed red blood cell transfusion

15. Interventions for the infant who has experienced acute intraventricular hemorrhage include providing a quiet environment, elevating the head of the bed slightly, and positioning the infant:

A. Prone.
B. With neck flexed.
C. In slight Trendelenburg.
D. With head in the midline.

16. Periventricular echogenicity on a head ultrasonogram may be a sign of which condition?

A. Leukomalacia
B. TORCH infection
C. Subdural hemorrhage
D. Arteriovenous malformation

17. In evaluating an electroencephalogram (EEG) report of a term infant, which of the following would indicate a poor prognostic sign?

A. Low voltage
B. Poor differentiation of states
C. 60 cycle interference
D. Epileptiform activity

18. All of the following nursing interventions will help to prevent intraventricular hemorrhage except:

A. Avoid sedation
B. Slow infusion of hyperosmolar fluids
C. Avoid blood pressure swings
D. Maintain normal blood gas values

19. It is important to evaluate the baby whose status is post-treatment of meningitis for which condition?

A. Nerve palsies
B. Hearing loss

C. Encephalopathies

D. Central nervous system structural abnormalities

20. When administering fosphenytoin (Cerebyx), the nurse should know that:

A. It contains phosphorus.

B. It is an antidote to phenytoin (Dilantin).

C. It should be administered at an infusion rate <1.5 mg/kg/min.

D. It has different therapeutic levels than phenytoin (Dilantin).

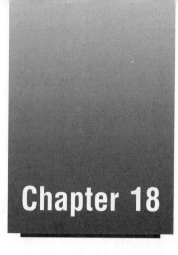

Chapter 18

Renal and Genitourinary Disorders

1. A post-renal etiology for acute renal failure is suggested by which of the following?

   A. Hypotension
   B. Perinatal asphyxia
   C. Posterior urethral valves
   D. Anuria following indomethacin administration

2. The accumulation and distention of the renal pelvis and calices due to obstruction of urine in the newborn would most likely be due to which of the following conditions?

   A. Ureteropelvic junction obstruction
   B. Prune-Belly syndrome
   C. Cystic kidney disease
   D. Urinary tract infection

3. Furosemide therapy can lead to development of which of the following conditions?

   A. Hyperkalemia
   B. Hyponatremia
   C. Hypercalcemia
   D. Hypokalemia

4. The most important objective in caring for the infant with hypertension is to:

   A. Monitor urine output and specific gravity.
   B. Restrict oral intake to limit total daily fluid intake.
   C. Assess daily weight to monitor for an inappropriate increase.
   D. Measure resting blood pressure with an appropriately sized blood pressure cuff.

5. When assessing an infant with an inguinal hernia, particular attention should be given to which of the following symptoms, which may indicate a complication due to the hernia?

   A. Positive transillumination of the hernia
   B. Vomiting
   C. Apnea and bradycardia
   D. Oliguria

Questions 6 and 7 refer to the following scenario: A full-term, small for gestational age infant presents with pulmonary hypoplasia with accompanying severe respiratory distress. Further evaluation reveals a bell-shaped chest, low-set ears, and wide-spaced eyes with epicanthal folds.

6. What is the most likely diagnosis?

   A. Potter syndrome
   B. VATER association
   C. Down syndrome
   D. Edwards syndrome

7. Which of the following would be the most useful tool to diagnose this infant's condition?

   A. Chromosome studies
   B. Echocardiogram
   C. Chest radiograph
   D. Renal ultrasonogram

8. A 3-day-old infant with a history of perinatal asphyxia is diagnosed with acute renal failure. Which of the following se-

rum indices is associated with this diagnosis?

	Creatinine	Sodium	Osmolality
A.	1.2 mg/dL	140 mEq/L	↑
B.	0.8 mg/dL	145 mEq/L	↓
C.	1.8 mg/dL	125 mEq/L	↓
D.	1.0 mg/dL	150 mEq/L	↑

9. Failure to void urine in the first 12 hours of life requires:

   A. Careful monitoring of urine output.
   B. A renal ultrasonogram to evaluate the kidneys.
   C. Measurement of serum electrolytes.
   D. Measurement of blood pressure.

10. Parents of an infant with a mild hypospadias ask the nurse what to expect for management of the infant until the condition is repaired. Accurate information to be provided includes:

    A. Avoidance of circumcision.
    B. Daily measuring of urine output upon discharge.
    C. Surgical repair will be performed during the neonatal period.
    D. A surgical repair that will be performed in several stages within the first few months of age.

Chapter 19

Genetics

1. Deoxyribonucleic acid (DNA) is organized into large macromolecular complexes, which are called:

    A. Genomes.
    B. Chromosomes.
    C. Nucleosomes.
    D. Autosomes.

2. An infant is born with a short, webbed neck, low-set ears, a broad nasal bridge, and coarctation of the aorta. These characteristics are clinical features of which condition?

    A. Trisomy 18
    B. Down syndrome
    C. Turner syndrome
    D. Trisomy 13

3. An infant is observed to have prominent epicanthal folds, a flat face, a protruding tongue, and a herniated umbilicus. What genetic disorder does this child likely have?

    A. Trisomy 18
    B. Trisomy 13
    C. Trisomy 21
    D. Turner syndrome X0

4. What are the clinical features of the VATER association?

    A. Abdominal mass, imperforate anus, myelodysplasia
    B. Abdominal mass, ventricular septal defect, single umbilical artery

    C. Anal atresia, vertebral abnormalities, cardiac anomalies
    D. Anal atresia, tracheoesophageal fistula, vertebral abnormalities

5. Loss of a chromosomal segment is called:

    A. Translocation.
    B. Deletion.
    C. Mosaicism.
    D. Nondisjunction.

6. An infant has been diagnosed with a genetic disorder. The mother of the infant does not exhibit the disorder but is a carrier. The mother's brother does have the disorder. This disorder is considered an:

    A. Autosomal recessive disorder.
    B. X-linked recessive disorder.
    C. X-linked dominant disorder.
    D. Autosomal dominant disorder.

7. A newborn female weighs 3.5 kg, has a prominent occiput and omphalocele, and has macroglossia. Laboratory tests reveal polycythemia and hypoglycemia. Which disorder does this infant most likely have?

    A. Beckwith-Wiedemann syndrome
    B. Turner syndrome
    C. Down syndrome
    D. Klinefelter syndrome

8. The parents of an infant with an autosomal dominant disorder ask the nurse what the chances are of giving birth to another baby with the same disorder. In

the response, the nurse should explain that:

A. All future babies born to the parents will have the disorder.
B. There is a 50% chance with each pregnancy of having another affected offspring.
C. If the baby is a girl, she will only be a carrier; if the baby is a boy, there is a 50% chance he will have the disorder.
D. If the baby is a boy, he will only be a carrier; if the baby is a girl, there is a 50% chance she will have the disorder.

9. Cleft lip with or without cleft palate is most commonly seen in what population?

A. Females
B. Males
C. American Indian population
D. American black population

10. An infant is born with an amputated hand due to amniotic bands. This defect is an example of which of the following?

A. Sequence
B. Malformation
C. Deformation
D. Disruption

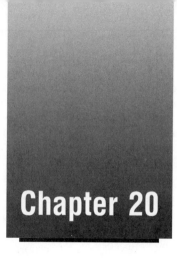

Chapter 20

Immunologic Disorders and Infections

1. Which of the following immunoglobulins is predominantly found in the mother's colostrum and breast-milk?

   A. IgA
   B. IgG
   C. IgE
   D. IgM

2. In infants who clinically respond to antimicrobial therapy, the C-reactive protein level is expected to:

   A. Decrease gradually.
   B. Fall rapidly.
   C. Peak within 12 hours of life.
   D. Return to normal in 2 to 3 days.

3. Initial report of a blood culture on a 1-day-old neonate reveals a "coagulase-negative" result. Which microorganism is most likely present?

   A. *Escherichia coli*
   B. Group B *Streptococcus*
   C. *Staphylococcus aureus*
   D. *Staphylococcus epidermidis*

4. Which intervention would be appropriate for a gentamicin serum peak of 13 µg/mL?

   A. Decrease dosage of drug
   B. Decrease dosing interval
   C. Discontinue drug immediately
   D. Maintain present dosage and interval

5. Which intrapartum electronic fetal monitoring finding would indicate the need to evaluate the newborn for the possibility of infection?

   A. Fetal tachycardia
   B. Loss of beat-to-beat variability
   C. Sinusoidal pattern
   D. Variable deceleration

6. A neonate is at least risk for associated varicella disease mortality if maternal varicella occurs when?

   A. Early in pregnancy
   B. 2 days after delivery
   C. 4 days before delivery
   D. 5 to 21 days before delivery

7. A 7-week-old female infant who was born at 34 weeks' gestation is being readmitted secondary to apnea. Her mother states that the infant has had a runny nose, coughing, and wheezing for the last 3 to 4 days. A chest radiograph shows bilateral symmetrical interstitial infiltrates. These symptoms are typically present in infants with which condition?

   A. Bronchopulmonary dysplasia
   B. Chlamydial pneumonia
   C. *Haemophilus* influenza
   D. Respiratory syncytial viral infection

8. Hepatosplenomegaly and direct hyperbilirubinemia in a neonate with intrauterine growth retardation is most likely indicative of which condition?

   A. Cytomegaloviral infection
   B. Human papillomaviral infection

C. *Listeria monocytogenes* infection
D. Maternal hepatitis infection

9. In addition to standard precautions, what step should be taken when caring for an infant who had been exposed to human immunodeficiency virus?

   A. Administer required childhood immunization at birth
   B. Cleanse infant's skin with antiseptic solution prior to any invasive procedure
   C. Give daily bath with antimicrobial agent
   D. Place infant in strict isolation

10. Strict isolation of neonates is required in which of the following cases?

   A. Neonates infected as a result of outbreaks of resistant organisms
   B. Neonates of mothers with active tuberculosis at time of birth
   C. Neonates of mothers with the human immunodeficiency virus
   D. Neonates with symptoms of congenital syphilis until antibiotic therapy has been administered for 24 hours

11. Which of the following vaccines should be administered subcutaneously?

   A. Diphtheria and tetanus toxoids with acellular pertussis vaccine
   B. *Haemophilus* B conjugate vaccine
   C. Hepatitis B vaccine
   D. Poliovirus vaccine inactivated

12. Which of the following statements is true about congenital syphilis?

   A. Infants asymptomatic at birth can develop stigmata of late congenital syphilis despite appropriate treatment in the neonatal period.
   B. Treatment of asymptomatic infected infants in the first 3 months of life is at this time not recommended.
   C. Uninfected infants with reactive serologic test for syphilis from transplacental transfer of maternal antibody should have a decrease in titer by 2 weeks of age.
   D. Yearly cerebrospinal fluid evaluation, in addition to serial nontreponemal titers, are recommended for infants with congenital neurosyphilis.

Questions 13 and 14 refer to the following scenario: A 980 g male infant is now 5 weeks old and receiving total parenteral nutrition and lipid emulsion through a central catheter. He has been previously treated with multiple antibiotics. Overnight, his condition deteriorates and he now presents with signs of respiratory distress, hypothermia, and lethargy.

13. A sepsis work-up on this infant will most likely reveal which of the following microorganisms?

   A. *Escherichia coli*
   B. *Malassezia furfur*
   C. *Klebsiella*
   D. *Listeria monocytogenes*

14. This infant should be further evaluated for possible complications, including which of the following?

   A. Central catheter occlusion
   B. Delayed response to antibiotics
   C. Hyperglycemia
   D. Hyperlipidemia

15. A 2000 g neonate presents with respiratory distress, apnea, and bradycardia at 8 hours of age. The result of a complete blood count reveals:

WBC	$6.5 \times 10^3/mm^3$
Segs	20%
Bands	10%
Lymphocytes	56%
Eosinophils	4%
Monocytes	7%
Basophils	3%
Platelets	198

These laboratory values indicate that the neonate has which of the following conditions?

   A. Leukocytosis
   B. Leukopenia
   C. Neutropenia
   D. Neutrophilia

Questions 16 and 17 refer to the following scenario: The complete blood cell count with differential of a 1-day-old neonate is reported as follows:

WBC	$7.8 \times 10^3/mm^3$
Segs	27%
Bands	18%
Lymphocytes	48%
Eosinophils	4%

Monocytes	2%
Basophils	1%
Platelets	187

16. This neonate's calculated immature-to-total neutrophil (I:T) ratio is:

   A. 0.40
   B. 0.55

C. 0.60
D. 0.66

17. What does the above I:T ratio indicate?

   A. A bacterial colonization
   B. An infection
   C. A right shift
   D. A neutropenia

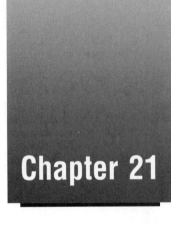

Chapter 21

Orthopedic Disorders

1. When performing a newborn assessment, the nurse recognizes which of the following factors as increasing the risk of developmental dysplasia of the hip (DDH)?

   A. African-American ethnicity
   B. Breech position
   C. Male gender
   D. Polyhydramnios

2. The parents of a newborn with developmental dysplasia of the hip (DDH) have been taught how to care for their baby in a Pavlik harness. The nurse recognizes that *further* clarification of teaching is needed when the parents:

   A. State the importance of maintaining the hip joint in abduction and flexion.
   B. State that reduction of the hip joint should occur within 2 to 3 weeks of splinting.
   C. Demonstrate how to remove the Pavlik harness daily to prevent contractures.
   D. Demonstrate how to bathe and diaper the infant in the Pavlik harness.

3. When caring for the infant with osteogenesis imperfecta (OI), an important nursing intervention is to:

   A. Treat the underlying pathologic cause of OI.
   B. Prepare the parents for normal growth and development.
   C. Educate the family regarding appropriate calcium and phosphorus intake to prevent any future fractures from occurring.
   D. Apply padded splints to the extremities to minimize the occurrence of new fractures.

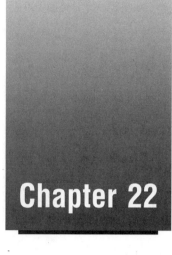

Chapter 22

Dermatologic Concerns

1. A 750 g infant is born at 26 weeks' gestation. When caring for the skin of this premature infant, the nurse should include which of the following measures?

   A. Daily bathing of the infant to prevent infection
   B. Use of a chemical solvent to remove tape or adhesives
   C. Provision of environmental humidity to decrease insensible water loss
   D. Use of alcohol to remove povidone-iodine after skin cleansing

2. Following the removal of tape or electrodes, a premature infant should be evaluated for visible damage secondary to which of the following characteristics of premature skin?

   A. Diminished cohesion between the dermis and epidermis
   B. Fewer layers of stratum corneum
   C. Less collagen present in the dermis
   D. Thinner layer of subcutaneous fat

3. A full-term neonate is diagnosed with epidermolysis bullosa. When developing a plan of care for this infant, the nurse should be aware that this condition:

   A. Is characterized by multiple hemangiomas.
   B. May result in death due to secondary infections.
   C. Rarely causes nutritional problems.
   D. Usually is associated with prematurity.

4. A male infant is born with congenital ichthyosis. When discussing his condition with his parents, the nurse explains that this disease is caused by:

   A. Absence of the epidermis.
   B. A genetic disorder.
   C. An infectious process.
   D. Severe zinc deficiency.

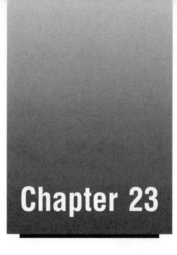

Chapter 23

Ophthalmologic Disorders

1. Which of the following infants has the highest risk for the development of retinopathy of prematurity (ROP)?

   A. 40 weeks' gestation with pneumothorax, in 100% oxygen by hood
   B. 36 weeks' gestation with mild respiratory distress syndrome (RDS), receiving oxygen by nasal cannula
   C. 32 weeks' gestation, weighing 1750 g, receiving phototherapy
   D. 27 weeks' gestation, weighing 950 g, requiring mechanical ventilation

2. A 26-week-gestation female infant has developed retinopathy of prematurity (ROP) at 6 weeks of age. When providing education to her parents, the nurse can best describe ROP as an arrest of normal vascular development of the retina, followed by:

   A. Lack of ocular development.
   B. Proliferation of abnormal blood vessels.
   C. Retinal detachment.
   D. Vitreous hemorrhage.

3. An infant with retinopathy of prematurity (ROP) had laser surgery 24 hours ago. The nurse should evaluate the infant for which of the following common postoperative complications?

   A. Arrhythmias
   B. Hypotension
   C. Infection
   D. Strabismus

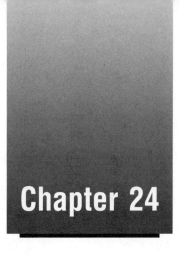

Chapter 24

Multisystem (Maternal-Fetal Complications, Hydrops, Pain, and Substance Abuse)

Maternal-Fetal Complications

1. A patient arrives for a routine prenatal visit. A review of her prenatal records reveals that her hematocrit at her initial visit was 25%. She was given a prescription for iron sulfate, 300 mg to take daily with a meal. Her repeat hematocrit today is 27%. The decision to maintain the current treatment plan or to initiate other interventions to further increase the hematocrit is based on the potential effects on the fetus. What are the likely effects?

   A. Normal growth/term delivery
   B. Macrosomia/post date delivery
   C. Hypoplastic lungs/post date delivery
   D. Low birth weight/preterm delivery

2. A patient with a 37-week gestation is admitted in active labor. She is visiting the area from another state and has no prenatal records available at this time. She states that her physician back home told her she had something called thrombocytopenia. Based on this information, what should the nurse assess the infant for?

   A. Fever
   B. Macrosomia

C. Hyperglycemia
D. Low birth weight

3. A 3-hour-old newborn infant born at 40 weeks' gestation is in the nursery. Her mother received 2 g magnesium sulfate ($MgSO_4$) for 48 hours prior to delivery for severe pregnancy-induced hypertension (PIH). What is/are anticipated intervention(s) based on knowledge of the possible effects of $MgSO_4$ on the newborn?

   A. Provide phototherapy, alternate formula and water feeding every 4 hours
   B. Give IV magnesium, check serum magnesium levels every 6 hours
   C. Give oxygen (O_2), gavage feedings
   D. Feed 30 mL formula every 2 hours

4. A patient is admitted to Labor & Delivery. She is 36 weeks' gestation, has elevated blood pressure, proteinuria, and epigastric pain. Laboratory analysis indicates HELLP syndrome. Doctor's orders are as follows:

   • Consent for C/S delivery
   • Loading dose of $MgSO_4$ 4 g IV over 30 minutes

- $MgSO_4$ @2 g/hr IV to follow
- 20 mL Bicitra PO
- Epidural anesthesia per anesthesiologist

What alteration in neonatal laboratory values would the nurse expect to see?

A. Polycythemia
B. Hypermagnesemia
C. Elevated WBCs
D. Hyponatremia

5. A patient presents in active labor with weeping chicken pox (varicella) lesions over her entire body. She says she "broke out" 2 days ago. The infant is born that day. Treatment for her infant after birth includes which of the following?

A. Room-in with mother, no isolation precautions
B. Open crib in the nursery, contact precautions
C. Room-in with mother after VZIG administered, contact and airborne precautions
D. Open crib in the nursery after VZIG administered, contact and airborne precautions

6. When caring for an infant prenatally exposed to group B streptococcus (GBS), the nurse should notify the physician if the infant exhibits which of the following signs/symptoms of GBS infection?

A. Hypothermia, poor feeding
B. Heart murmur, hypercalcemia
C. Anemia, pallor
D. Hyperglycemia, hyperthermia

7. A newborn is determined to be small for gestational age (SGA) at birth. When reviewing the mother's medical record, the nurse would expect to find which of the following?

A. Renal disease
B. Gestational diabetes
C. Previous macrosomia
D. Rh-positive blood group

8. A full-term infant is admitted to the nursery with a partial amputation of the right foot. The infant is otherwise normal and healthy. What is the most likely cause for this deformity?

A. Maternal rubella infection
B. Genetic defect

C. Maternal cytomegalovirus infection
D. Amniotic bands

9. Quantitative amniotic fluid volume assessment at 36 weeks' gestation reveals a decreased amniotic fluid volume. The infant should be assessed for which of the following conditions?

A. Down syndrome
B. Neural tube defects
C. Kidney disease
D. Tracheoesophageal fistula

10. Polyhydramnios might be associated with which of the following conditions of the infant?

A. Renal agenesis
B. Hypoplastic lungs
C. Congenital contractures
D. Anencephaly

11. A gravida 3 para 2 woman is admitted at term to the Labor & Delivery unit at 2 PM. She states she is here because she "broke her bag of waters" at around 2 AM. She states she took a shower, put on a perineal pad and went back to sleep. She had errands to run this morning and was waiting to go into labor before she came to the hospital. She has started having mild labor pains every 10 to 15 minutes. Temperature is 36.8° C (98.2° F); pulse, 76; respirations, 16; blood pressure, 116/72. Which laboratory data should be obtained on the newborn infant in the first few hours of life?

A. Chemistry panel
B. CBC with differential
C. Liver panel
D. Antibody screen

12. A pregnant patient at 37 weeks' gestation, who is visiting from out of state, is admitted to the hospital with complaints of fever and chills. Temperature is 39.4° C (103° F); pulse, 104; respirations, 22; blood pressure, 120/74. The patient gives a history of vaginal leaking for the past few days. Fern test confirms rupture of the amniotic membranes. Prenatal records are not available at this time. The infant is most at risk for which of the following?

A. Viral influenza
B. Hypoplastic lungs

C. Amniotic bands
D. Bacterial sepsis

13. A fetus in breech presentation is being delivered vaginally. During the delivery, the nurse is prepared for neonatal resuscitation knowing that in vaginal breech deliveries:

    A. The legs may get stuck.
    B. Meconium or amniotic fluid aspiration may occur.
    C. Lacerations of the maternal birth canal may occur.
    D. Developmental delay of the child may result.

14. A patient has been in second stage of labor for 2 hours, 10 minutes. Estimated fetal weight is 4000 g. What potential complication of delivery does the nurse anticipate?

    A. Umbilical cord prolapse
    B. HELLP syndrome
    C. Shoulder dystocia
    D. Breech delivery

15. A patient with a 36-week gestation is brought to Labor & Delivery from the emergency room for obstetric evaluation following a car accident. The patient's automobile was hit from behind and she was thrown forward into the steering wheel. She was wearing her seat belt. She currently complains of feeling weak and is experiencing severe abdominal pain. Physical examination of the patient reveals a stiff, board-like abdomen; no vaginal bleeding; blood pressure 98/60; pulse 120; fetal heart rate baseline 100 beats per minute with decreased variability; decelerations to 90 beats per minute noted after contractions; contraction pattern every minute lasting 30 to 45 seconds each (external monitor). Which of the following interventions for the newborn would the nurse expect to provide in the delivery room?

    A. Fluid resuscitation
    B. Narcan administration
    C. Normal newborn care
    D. Oxygen administration at 40%

16. The report on a woman in labor is that she is a gravida 10 para 8 spontaneous abortion 2; diet-controlled gestational diabetic. Estimated fetal weight is 4000 g.

While the patient is pushing, her blood pressure drops to 60/30 mm Hg and her pulse becomes rapid and thready. Delivery is accomplished via vacuum extractor. The placenta is delivered with the infant, and estimated blood loss is 1000 mL. For which of the following would the nurse assess the infant at birth?

    A. Diabetic ketoacidosis
    B. Hyperglycemia
    C. Hypovolemia
    D. Hypervolemia

17. A woman presents in labor with the following findings: gravida 3, para 2; 38 5/7 weeks pregnant by dates and ultrasonogram; amniotic membranes intact by history; vaginal examination findings, 4 cm dilated/50% effaced/floating; fetal presentation vertex; no vaginal bleeding; estimated fetal weight (EFW) 2500 g. Which of the following conditions is most likely to develop during the labor course of a patient with these assessment findings?

    A. Amniotic bands
    B. Umbilical cord prolapse
    C. Polyhydramnios
    D. Gestational diabetes

18. The assessment of a laboring patient who is 38 weeks' gestation includes:

    • 3 cm dilated, 100% effaced, 0 station
    • bright red vaginal bleeding
    • sharp, continuous abdominal pain
    • blood pressure 90/60, temperature 37° C (98.6° F), pulse 100, respirations 16
    • fetal strip: baseline tachycardia with decreased variability
    • prenatal record shows an ultrasonogram at 35 weeks that revealed an anterior placenta with no cervical margins

    What does this assessment suggest?

    A. Abruptio placenta
    B. Rh isoimmunization
    C. Placenta previa
    D. Shoulder dystocia

19. When caring for a labor patient with suspected abruptio placenta, which nursing action is most important to prepare for the delivery of the infant?

    A. Obtain patient's birth plan
    B. Preheat radiant warmer to 48.8° C (120° F)

C. Prepare vitamin K syringe and ophthalmic ointment

D. Turn on oxygen and suction

20. A pregnant woman has been diagnosed
with a total placenta previa. She has had
two episodes of vaginal bleeding, at 29
weeks' and 32 weeks' gestation. A cesarean section is performed at 34 weeks following a third episode of bleeding of
moderate amount. Which of the following
nursing actions will the nurse most likely
perform for this newborn within the first
hour?

A. Oral feeding with 2 ounces of formula

B. Blood pressure assessment

C. Head ultrasonogram

D. Admission bath

Hydrops

21. The birth of an infant with a prenatal diagnosis of nonimmune hydrops fetalis is imminent. In the delivery room, the nurse should be prepared for which of the following immediate complications?

    A. Hyperglycemia
    B. Kernicterus
    C. Seizures
    D. Severe respiratory distress

22. When reviewing the history of a neonate with nonimmune hydrops fetalis, which of the following is a common cause of the disorder?

    A. Fetal cardiac disorder
    B. Maternal substance abuse
    C. Oligohydramnios
    D. Rh isoimmunization

23. A nurse providing prenatal education instructs the client that maternal administration of Rho-gam (RhIG) during pregnancy decreases the incidence of hydrops fetalis caused by what condition?

    A. Maternal infection
    B. Premature birth
    C. Rh isoimmunization
    D. Twin-to-twin transfusion

Pain

24. Pain assessment and measurement in hospitalized preterm infants is best evaluated by:

    A. Crying and body movements.
    B. Heart rate, oxygen saturation, and facial expressions.
    C. Respiratory rate and blood pressure.
    D. A composite neonatal pain tool with established validity and reliability.

25. Which statement is *true* regarding the use of systemic opioids for pain management in infants?

    A. Postoperatively, infants with gastroschisis are at higher risk for respiratory depression.
    B. Opioid-induced cardiorespiratory side effects are common in neonates.
    C. Meperidine is preferred over morphine.
    D. Addiction to narcotics is a common clinical problem in infants.

26. A 5-day-old infant born at 26 weeks' gestation is being cared for in the neonatal intensive care unit (NICU). Planning for pain management following cardiac surgery should be based on the knowledge that:

    A. Preterm infants metabolize drugs in a similar fashion to children and adults.
    B. Newborns do not have the anatomical and functional components required for the perception of painful stimuli.
    C. Treatment of pain should be deferred until the certainty of pain is established through physiologic and behavioral measures.
    D. Preterm infants are more sensitive to pain than are term or older infants.

27. All of the following are true of the Premature Infant Pain Profile (PIPP) *except* that it:

    A. Takes into consideration contextual factors.
    B. Is a unidimensional approach to assessing preterm pain.
    C. Includes facial activity measures as indicators of pain.
    D. Uses an infant's baseline values to calculate scores for physiologic indicators.

28. Which of the following factors has been demonstrated to modify facial expressions of pain in neonates?

    A. Hunger
    B. Gender
    C. Behavioral state
    D. Environmental stress

29. Which of the following drugs is appropriate for pharmacologic management of severe pain in neonates?

    A. Morphine
    B. Midazolam
    C. Chloral hydrate
    D. Acetaminophen

30. Which of the following statements is *true* regarding pain assessment in infants?

    A. Pain responses and irritability/agitation behaviors are similar and cannot be distinguished from each other.
    B. Pain is a subjective experience that cannot be communicated by neonates.
    C. The frequency of painful procedures encountered in the neonatal intensive care unit (NICU) may impact subsequent behavioral responses to pain.
    D. Physiologic measures are sensitive and specific as indicators of pain in infants.

31. Clinical signs of opioid withdrawal in the neonate include all of the following *except*:

    A. Seizures
    B. Respiratory depression
    C. Projectile vomiting
    D. Watery stools

32. Assessing and managing pain in hospitalized preterm infants should be based on the knowledge that:

    A. Preterm infants have a similar capacity for recovery after acute procedure-induced pain as do full-term healthy infants.
    B. Behavioral responsiveness in preterm

neonates to noxious stimuli does not vary with postconceptional age.

C. Acute, episodic pain may lead to established or chronic pain.

D. Analgesics cannot be administered safely in preterm neonates, thus non-pharmacologic measures remain the preferred intervention for managing postoperative pain.

33. A former 28-week-gestation preterm infant, now 32 weeks of postconceptional age, is scheduled to have a heel stick performed at the same time that other caregiving activities are due. Which of the following interventions would be most appropriate?

A. Cluster the heel stick and caregiving activities to allow the infant to have a longer period of undisturbed sleep

B. Delay the caregiving activities until after the infant has had time to sufficiently recover from the heel stick procedure

C. Administer chloral hydrate to reduce the infant's pain and stress associated with the heel stick and caregiving activities

D. Administer morphine to reduce the infant's pain and stress associated with the heel stick and caregiving activities

34. A newborn infant weighing 4000 g had a circumcision procedure performed 2 hours earlier. The infant demonstrates increased wakefulness and irritability, increased heart rate, and a furrowed brow. What would appropriate management of this infant consist of?

A. Provide non-nutritive sucking opportunities using a sucrose pacifier

B. Administer 100 mg of acetaminophen by mouth

C. Administer chloral hydrate to enhance sleep and provide pain relief

D. Administer 0.4 mg morphine by intramuscular route

Substance Abuse

35. When anticipating the labor and delivery of a pregnant client who abuses cocaine, the nurse needs to be aware of which of the following potential complications?

    A. Abruptio placentae
    B. Placenta previa
    C. Postmaturity
    D. Prolonged labor

36. Which of the following characteristics would lead a nurse to suspect that a newborn was exposed to cocaine in utero?

    A. Facial anomalies and growth retardation
    B. Irritability and hypertonicity
    C. Lethargy and hypotonia
    D. Macrosomia and respiratory distress

37. An infant is born to a woman who abused cocaine during pregnancy. The mother admits to continuing occasional cocaine use while the infant is hospitalized. Appropriate nursing management related to the effects of perinatal cocaine exposure includes:

    A. Administering methadone as ordered.
    B. Encouraging frequent breast-feeding by the mother.
    C. Offering extra stimulation during routine care and feedings.
    D. Swaddling the infant and decreasing environmental stimuli.

38. When assessing neonates for congenital anomalies, the nurse should be aware that a drug with known teratogenic effects is which of the following?

    A. Alcohol
    B. Amphetamines
    C. Heroin
    D. Marijuana

39. The adolescent mother of an infant in the neonatal intensive care unit (NICU) tells the nurse that she drank beer every weekend during her pregnancy. She states, "I know I didn't drink enough to harm my baby." An appropriate intervention by the nurse is to:

    A. Tell her that consumption of hard liquor is more harmful than beer.
    B. Immediately inform her parents about her alcohol use.
    C. Discuss the potential effects of perinatal alcohol exposure on her infant's behavior.
    D. Reassure her that occasional ingestion of alcohol during pregnancy is not harmful.

40. When assessing an infant for signs of exposure to alcohol in utero, the nurse recognizes which of the following as the diagnostic criteria specific to fetal alcohol syndrome (FAS)?

    A. Cognitive problems and maternal drinking history
    B. Growth retardation, facial anomalies, central nervous system (CNS) dysfunction
    C. Hypertonicity and seizures
    D. Irritability, high-pitched cry, poor feeding

41. The mother of a newborn discloses to the neonatal intensive care unit (NICU) nurse that she smoked cigarettes during her pregnancy. She expresses concern about possible adverse effects on the infant. The nurse should educate her about the increased risk of which of the following conditions?

    A. Mental retardation
    B. Neonatal abstinence syndrome (NAS)
    C. Respiratory distress syndrome
    D. Sudden infant death syndrome (SIDS)

42. A woman smoked two packs of cigarettes per day during her pregnancy. The effect of nicotine on the placenta is most likely to result in which of the following infants?

    A. A 28-week-gestation infant who is small for gestational age
    B. A 36-week-gestation infant who is macrosomic
    C. A full-term infant who exhibits neonatal abstinence syndrome
    D. A post-term infant with meconium aspiration syndrome

43. A pregnant woman addicted to heroin is placed on methadone maintenance for the remainder of her pregnancy. An advantage to methadone maintenance versus continued heroin abuse during pregnancy is that:

    A. Repeated episodes of fetal withdrawal are prevented.
    B. Neonatal abstinence syndrome is prevented.
    C. Neonatal withdrawal occurs sooner.
    D. Neonatal withdrawal symptoms are less severe.

44. Perinatal exposure to heroin is associated with which of the following neonatal outcomes?

    A. Dysmorphic features
    B. Hypotonia and mental retardation
    C. Lower risk of respiratory distress syndrome
    D. Higher risk of intraventricular hemorrhage

45. A 2-day-old infant was born to a heroin-addicted mother at 36 weeks' gestation. The nurse caring for this infant demonstrates appropriate use of the Neonatal Abstinence Scoring System by:

    A. Determining a treatment plan based on a single score.
    B. Initiating pharmacologic treatment for a score of less than 8.
    C. Scoring the infant on a twice daily basis until symptoms subside.
    D. Trending withdrawal symptoms and evaluating treatment outcomes.

46. When planning an effective method to identify infants exposed to substance abuse during pregnancy, the nurse needs to:

    A. Initiate the Neonatal Abstinence Scoring System on all infants.
    B. Recognize that any infant may have been exposed to perinatal substance abuse.
    C. Obtain a urine drug screen on all infants.
    D. Classify only those infants of lower socioeconomic status as being at high risk.

SECTION
III

Professional Issues

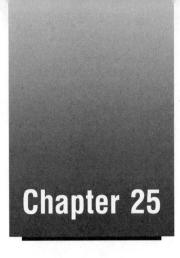

Chapter 25

Research

1. A well-written research problem statement

   • is written in the form of a question,
   • includes a description of the population to be sampled *and*

   A. Is written in the future tense.
   B. Includes the variables to be studied.
   C. Includes a description of the methods to be used.
   D. Includes a description of the outcomes.

2. Which of the following influences the questions that are asked, the data that are gathered, the methods used to gather the data, and the interpretation of the data?

   A. Results
   B. Subjects
   C. Assumptions
   D. Methods

3. A research hypothesis is:

   A. The purpose of the project.
   B. The overall plan of the project.
   C. A statement of the researcher's findings.
   D. A prediction of expected outcome.

4. The order of the phases in the research process is:

   A. Conceptual, empirical, design and planning, analytic, and dissemination.
   B. Conceptual, design and planning, analytic, empirical, and dissemination.
   C. Conceptual, design and planning, empirical, analytic, and dissemination.

   D. Design and planning, conceptual, analytic, empirical, and dissemination.

5. A neonatal nurse wants to explore a problem she notices in her practice. She has observed that on their first visit to the neonatal intensive care unit (NICU), mothers who have delivered their babies at the hospital where her NICU is located have a different anxiety level than mothers who have delivered their babies at a hospital 2 miles away. She decides to study the problem. The purpose of her study might be:

   A. To determine a way to facilitate mothers' first visit in the NICU.
   B. To determine which hospital has better informational brochures for mothers.
   C. To determine which nurses do a better job of orienting mothers to the NICU.
   D. To determine what medical diagnoses affect mothers' anxiety levels.

Questions 6 and 7 refer to the following scenario: A study that compared the effects of verbal and tactile stimulation on physiologic arousal in infants with congenital heart disease is reported in the literature.

6. What is the independent variable in this study?

   A. Tactile and verbal stimulation
   B. Physiologic arousal
   C. Congenital heart disease
   D. Vital signs

7. What is the dependent variable in this study?

   A. Tactile and verbal stimulation
   B. Physiologic arousal
   C. Congenital heart disease
   D. Vital signs

8. Which of the following data collection methods is *not* appropriate for qualitative research?

   A. Life histories
   B. Physiologic monitoring
   C. Semistructured interviews
   D. Participant observation

Questions 9 and 10 refer to the following scenario: A recent study compared the difference between saline and heparin in their effectiveness for maintaining the patency of 24-gauge peripheral intravenous catheters used for intermittent infusion. The study utilized rabbits as an animal model for neonates. The results indicated that the duration of catheter patency for the saline group was not significantly different than the duration of catheter patency for the heparin group.

9. What conclusion is evident in reviewing these results?

   A. Heparin is not necessary for maintaining the patency of 24-gauge peripheral intravenous catheter used intermittently in neonates.
   B. Rabbits are an effective animal model for studying neonatal intermittent intravenous catheter patency.
   C. It is safe to use saline instead of heparin to maintain peripheral intravenous catheters used for intermittent infusions.
   D. Normal saline is as effective as heparin in maintaining 24-gauge peripheral intravenous catheters for intermittent use in rabbits.

10. A recommendation for future research that would help neonatal nurses apply this information to their practice might include:

   A. Replicate the study with sheep.
   B. Replicate the study with humans.
   C. Replicate the study using central venous catheters.
   D. Replicate the study using 22-gauge catheters.

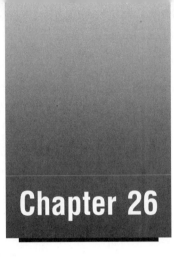

Chapter 26

Legal Issues in Neonatal Nursing

1. A nurse's note contains the following charting: "Apnea and bradycardia episodes increased over previous days. Now, most requiring stimulation. Color slightly pale, but no other signs of anemia present (HR, cap refill, BP all WNL). Theo level drawn as ordered. Results show level to be subtherapeutic (see flowsheet). Orders received and completed for a bolus of aminophylline and an increase in the maintenance doses (see MAR). Monitor infant for changes in breathing pattern."

   What does this nursing documentation reflect?

   A. Personal opinions of the nurse
   B. Nursing process
   C. Positive patient outcomes
   D. Quality of the nurse/physician relationship

2. Standards of Care are derived from all of the following *except*:

   A. Current professional literature
   B. Policies and procedures of an institution
   C. Personal practices
   D. State and federal regulations

3. Which of the following legal elements must be proven in a medical malpractice case?

   A. Duty, poor judgment, fault
   B. Poor judgment, intent, proximal cause, harm

   C. Intent, breach of duty, harm
   D. Duty, breach of duty, harm, proximal cause

4. "What a reasonable and prudent nurse would do under similar or same circumstances" defines which of the following?

   A. Standard of care
   B. Scope of practice
   C. Nursing process
   D. Practice guidelines

5. A nurse fails to perform an appropriate assessment on one of her patients, as outlined by hospital protocol. This breach of duty results in a negative outcome for the patient. Which legal condition is evident?

   A. Fault
   B. Harm
   C. Negligence
   D. Proximal cause

6. The nurse has documented: "1500-Electrolyte results reported from lab, $Na^+ = 121$. Dr. notified". This charting example:

   A. Removes the nurse from further responsibility.
   B. Demonstrates critical thinking.
   C. Provides incomplete documentation.
   D. Shows evidence of the nursing process.

7. A neonatologist has just spoken to a family concerning a procedure that she is about to perform on their infant. The neonatologist asks the nurse to be the witness on the consent form. The nurse's signa-

ture on the consent form means that the nurse:

A. Witnessed the information provided to the parents.
B. Verified the identity of the person signing the consent.
C. May be liable if something goes wrong.
D. Verified that informed consent occurred.

8. Per hospital policy, two nurses document that a new medication order has been transcribed and calculated correctly. Both nurses initialed the transcription. A medication error occurred and was traced back to an incorrect transcription. Who is responsible?

A. Only the nurse who gave the medication
B. Only the nurse who transcribed the order
C. No one, since hospital policy was followed
D. Both nurses who initialed the transcription

9. A registered nurse asks a nursing assistant to help with the following: gavage feed baby Jones after checking for residuals; bathe and weigh baby Smith; draw a heel stick CBC from baby Williams and; nipple feed baby Johnson. Which one of these requests should *not* have been delegated?

A. Checking for residuals and gavage feeding baby Jones
B. Bathing and weighing baby Smith
C. Drawing a heel stick CBC from baby Williams
D. Nipple feeding baby Johnson

10. A full-term, healthy newborn is lying prone in his bassinet in the newborn nursery. When he is turned over to have his diaper changed, he is discovered to be cyanotic, apneic, and pulseless. Extensive resuscitative efforts are futile and the infant is pronounced dead. SIDS is suspected in relation to the infant's sleeping position. A nurse with 25 years of newborn nursery experience was caring for the infant and stated "I don't know what the policy says, but I always put babies down on their stomachs. They're more comfortable that way." The nursery's policy on infant care is reviewed and states: "infants should be placed prone or side-lying to reduce the risk of aspiration should vomiting occur." The policy was last revised 5 years ago and reviewed 1 year ago. Based on this scenario, who is accountable for this outcome?

A. The nurse and the hospital
B. The nurse alone
C. No one
D. The hospital

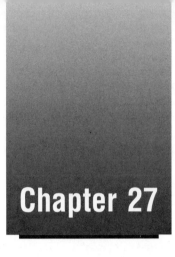

Chapter 27

Ethical Issues in Neonatal Nursing

1. An ethical dilemma is a situation requiring a choice between:

   A. Morally unreasonable alternatives.
   B. Difficult or immoral alternatives.
   C. Two morally acceptable, but opposing alternatives.
   D. Equally right or wrong alternatives.

2. Ethical frameworks have which of the following essential elements?

   A. Rights, outcomes, and goals
   B. Goals, duties, and rights
   C. Duties, obligations, and rights
   D. Principles, duties, and goals

3. Failing to tell parents the truth about their baby's prognosis violates what basic principle of health care ethics?

   A. Beneficence
   B. Role fidelity
   C. Confidentiality
   D. Veracity

4. Except in extraordinary circumstances, who is/are ultimately responsible for deciding what is in the best interests of a baby?

   A. Physicians
   B. Nurses
   C. Parents
   D. Lawyers

5. The best way to prevent ethical conflicts between parents and staff in the neonatal intensive care unit (NICU) is to focus on:

   A. Clear communication
   B. Patient care
   C. Saving lives
   D. Rapid diagnosis

6. When obtaining an informed consent for an infant going to surgery, the physician must discuss which of the following with the parents?

   A. The risks, benefits, and alternatives for surgery
   B. The pros and cons of caring for premature babies
   C. The risks and benefits of having a baby in the NICU
   D. The steps in the surgery preoperative check list

7. When more than one choice is appropriate, a paternalistic approach to selecting the best course of action would support:

   A. The parents making the decision without physicians.
   B. The physicians making the decision without parents.
   C. The nurses and parents deciding together.
   D. The physicians and parents deciding together.

8. An infant with ambiguous genitalia is chromosomally a boy, but anatomically a girl. The parents have given the baby a girl's name and confide in you that they believe she is a girl. The nurse believes the parents should know the truth, but

does not want to hurt them. What two principles are in conflict in this situation?

A. Veracity and paternalism
B. Nonmaleficence and beneficence
C. Autonomy and paternalism
D. Veracity and nonmaleficence

9. A nurse is caring for a baby with complex cardiac anomalies. On rounds, the physicians have expressed the opinion that the baby may survive, but that surgery has a high mortality rate. The physicians plan to offer the parents the option of surgery or comfort care with no aggressive intervention, which will mean certain death. The physicians have not yet spoken to the parents. The baby's parents express to the nurse their desire to learn about what options they have for treating their baby. They ask the nurse for assistance. What should the nurse recommend?

A. That they get a second opinion
B. That they hire a lawyer
C. That they contact the hospital ethics consultation service
D. That they speak with the physicians

10. A 24-week-gestation infant is now 2 weeks old. He has a grade III IVH and yeast in his blood. He remains on a ventilator with high settings, is not tolerating feedings, and requires pharmacologic support to maintain his blood pressure. The parents ask the physicians if they can stop treatment. The physicians admit the prognosis is dismal, but believe there is a chance the baby will survive. The physicians want to continue. The nurse helps to arrange a multidisciplinary discussion. After the discussion, the family still wishes to stop and the team is reluctant to do so. How should the nurse assist this family to resolve their conflict?

A. Help them find an alternative NICU.
B. Contact the hospital ethics consultation service.
C. Help them make funeral arrangements.
D. Contact the hospital chaplain.

SECTION
IV

Family Care

Chapter 28

Families in Crisis

1. The birth of a premature or sick infant and the death of an infant are events referred to as which of the following?

   A. Developmental stressors
   B. Situational stressors
   C. Maturational stressors
   D. Cultural stressors

2. Which of the following maternal behaviors is a predictor of poor parenting outcomes?

   A. Visits infrequently due to lack of transportation
   B. Worries about her competence as a mother
   C. Personalizes her infant's behavior as a failure of her ability to parent
   D. Exhibits a moderate to high anxiety level

3. Bonding is a gradual, reciprocal process that begins with which of the following?

   A. Acquaintance
   B. Attachment
   C. Birth
   D. Touching

4. Which term describe grief that occurs before an actual loss?

   A. Chronic grief
   B. Blocked grief
   C. Unresolved grief
   D. Anticipatory grief

5. When caring for parents experiencing a perinatal loss, the nurse should:

   A. Limit the number of family and friends with the parent.
   B. Discard mementos not taken by the parents at the time of infant death.
   C. Suggest that young siblings not be told of the infant's death until after the funeral.
   D. Encourage the family to see, hold, and spend time with their infant both before and after death.

6. An infant born at 24 weeks' gestation is intubated in the delivery room. The infant is pink with a heart rate of 152. The infant's mother is awake and understands that the infant is critically ill. Which of the following interventions would be most appropriate?

   A. Tell the mother the baby is very tiny and rush the baby to the neonatal intensive care unit (NICU).
   B. Transport the baby to the NICU then return to the mother's room to discuss parent visitation guidelines.
   C. Briefly show the infant to the mother and allow her to touch the infant, even if only for a few moments, before going to the NICU.
   D. Tell the mother's nurse to call the NICU before she brings the mother for her first visit.

Questions 7 and 8 refer to the following scenario: Crystal, a 15-year-old, recently delivered a son at 26 weeks' gestation. Her 16-year-old boyfriend John is the infant's father. They both live at home with their parents, who accompany them during visits to the

NICU. Their parents do not want them to get married. Crystal and John do not want either of their parents telling them what to do or helping them with childcare.

7. Crystal and John's reactions are not un-usual because, consistent with their age, they:

   A. Have the ability to foresee that they will be able to care for their baby and finish school without help from their parents.
   B. May be trying to take on adult respon-sibilities while feeling they are being treated as children.
   C. Are capable of thinking abstractly and anticipating future problems.
   D. Are capable of problem solving and decision making without help from adults.

8. The best way to respond to the conflict between Crystal and John and their par-ents is to:

   A. Make a referral to the local Children Services Bureau and let them decide what is best for Crystal, John, and their infant.
   B. Tell their parents to let Crystal and John make their own decisions.
   C. Assist Crystal and John in defining their roles with their own parents by helping them learn how to talk with their parents.
   D. Reassure Crystal and John they are capable of caring for their infant with-out help from their parents.

Questions 9 and 10 refer to the following scenario: Twin boys are delivered at 26 weeks' gestation. On the fourth day of life, twin A suffers a massive grade IV intraven-tricular hemorrhage. The infant's condition deteriorates and on the seventh day of life the mother and father decide to withdraw life support measures. Twin A dies in his parent's arms. Twin B remains in serious but stable condition. One week later, the mother re-mains tearful and talks constantly to the NICU nurses about the loss of twin A. The father returns to work and rarely speaks of twin A during his visits to the NICU.

9. The nurse caring for these parents should recognize that this couple is experiencing which of the following?

   A. Incongruent grieving
   B. Congruent grieving
   C. Abnormal grieving
   D. Anticipatory grieving

10. Which of the following interventions would be most helpful in facilitating the parents' grief?

    A. Wait for the parents to mention twin A before you make any comments
    B. Openly acknowledge the pain of their loss
    C. Leave the parents alone at twin B's bedside during visits
    D. Reassure the parents their sense of loss will eventually go away

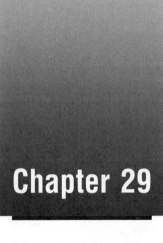

Chapter 29

Transition of the High-Risk Neonate to Home

1. When does transition planning for discharge home begin?

   A. One week after admission
   B. One week before discharge
   C. At admission
   D. The day before discharge

2. Nursing strategies to plan for the transition home include all of the following *except*:

   A. Evaluating the need for home care services
   B. Utilizing highly structured, rigid protocols of care
   C. Sequencing of education to meet parent learning needs
   D. Modeling infant care interventions

3. Case-managed care is a model of care that:

   A. Focuses on costs and outcomes rather than the needs of neonates and their families.
   B. Advocates primarily for the institution instead of for neonates and their families.
   C. Does not allow for variations in the anticipated progress of neonates and families.
   D. Utilizes clinical pathways and/or case managers to coordinate care and discharge of neonates and their families.

4. An infant born at 26 weeks' gestation is now 2 months old and is still hospitalized in the special care nursery. Which of the following immunizations should the nurse administer?

   A. HBV, IPV, HiB
   B. DTP, OPV, HiB
   C. DTP, OPV, HBV
   D. DTaP, IPV, HiB

5. A health care trend that affects transitional planning involves:

   A. The lack of legislative initiatives regarding access to care.
   B. The lack of involvement from reimbursement sources.
   C. The recognition of the parent(s) as the best person(s) to care for the infant.
   D. The recognition that employees of home care technology programs are the best providers of infant care in the home.

Questions 6, 7, and 8 refer to the following scenario: A 26 6/7th weeks' gestation, 960 g infant was born to a 40-year-old gravida 1, para 1 mother. After a 68-day stay in the neonatal intensive care unit (NICU), the now 36 5/7th weeks' gestational age infant will be discharged home on oxygen, theophylline, and an apnea monitor with twice weekly visits from a home care nurse. The infant's mother expresses fear about managing the oxygen at home and does not want to take her baby home until "everything is normal."

6. The nurse caring for this family should recognize that the mother:

A. May have fears about assuming responsibility for her infant's care at home.
B. Has not bonded adequately with her infant.
C. Really does not want to take her infant home.
D. Is overwhelmed and will not be able to care for her infant at home.

7. When preparing this mother for discharge, the nurse should:

A. Tell the mother not to worry, that it is the responsibility of the home care nurse to manage the infant's oxygen at home.
B. Educate and involve the mother in the daily care of her infant.
C. Reassure the mother that eventually everything will be "normal."
D. Refer the mother to social services for failure to bond with her infant.

8. Which of the following screening tests does this infant need prior to discharge?

A. Eye examination, hearing screen, and bilirubin level
B. Eye examination, car seat safety observation, and bilirubin level
C. Eye examination, hearing screen, and car seat safety observation
D. Hearing screen, bilirubin level, and car seat safety observation

9. What is the most important parameter to monitor during a car seat safety observation?

A. The infant's position
B. The infant's temperature
C. The amount of sleep/wake time
D. The presence of apnea, bradycardia, and oxygen desaturations

10. Which of the following demonstrates effective transition planning?

A. The lack of infant readmission to the hospital within 30 days
B. The lack of parent telephone call backs to the neonatal intensive care unit (NICU) after discharge
C. The failure to achieve outcome goals/discharge criteria by target dates
D. The decreased number of community resources needed in the home

Chapter 30

Follow-Up and Outcome in Premature Infants

1. Which of the following is the most important objective in caring for a patient with chronic lung disease?

   A. Maintain diuretics
   B. Increase caloric intake
   C. Rotate bronchodilators
   D. Maintain appropriate oxygen saturation

2. The parents of a 700 g infant ask the nurse what the future intelligence of their infant is likely to be. In the response, the nurse indicates that what percent of infants with a birth weight less than 750 g have an intelligence quotient (IQ) greater than 85?

   A. 20%
   B. 45%
   C. 65%
   D. 80%

3. The parents of a premature infant ask the nurse when their infant should receive immunizations. The nurse explains that the infant should receive the diphtheria-tetanus-pertussis and poliomyelitis vaccines when?

   A. At 2 months of adjusted age
   B. At 2 months of chronologic age
   C. At the first outpatient office visit
   D. Just prior to discharge from the neonatal intensive care unit (NICU)

4. A bright-eyed 6-month adjusted age infant smiles, laughs, and blinks during developmental assessment. However, visual tracking and object permanence were not demonstrated. What condition should be suspected?

   A. Myopia
   B. Color blindness
   C. Cortical blindness
   D. Attachment disorder

5. A 3-month adjusted age infant demonstrates symptoms of arching back during feeding, irritability, feeding problems, vomiting, and poor weight gain. What condition is suspected?

   A. Colic
   B. Seizures
   C. Formula allergy
   D. Gastroesophageal reflux

6. A 27-week-gestation infant is born on February 4, 1999. How old is the infant on 10/3/1999?

   A. 4 months adjusted age
   B. 4 months chronologic age
   C. 5 months adjusted age
   D. 5 months chronologic age

7. A former 30-week-gestation infant evaluated at 6 months of adjusted age has growth measurements less than the 5th percentile. Which activity would be most appropriate to do first?

   A. Contact Community Health office
   B. Evaluate for gastroesophageal reflux

C. Instruct mother on need for high-calorie diet

D. Plot growth and compare to previous examination findings

8. Adjusted age should be used when plotting a preterm infant's growth up until what age?

A. 1 year
B. 1 1/2 years
C. 2 1/2 years
D. 5 years

9. The following were noted during the developmental evaluation of a 24-month adjusted age infant:

- Says "mama", "d" for dog, "b" for ball
- Has difficulty finding pictures that are named
- Ignores mother
- Points and grunts for items desired

On the basis of these activities, the most appropriate additional evaluation would include which of the following:

A. Hearing evaluation
B. Infant personality inventory
C. Psychosocial home evaluation
D. Magnetic resonance imaging (MRI) of brain

10. A 6-month-old infant born at 28 weeks' gestation has hypertonic lower extremities with increased deep tendon reflexes. Movement of the upper extremities and face is normal. Which type of neuromuscular condition may be suspected?

A. Diplegia
B. Athetosis
C. Hemiplegia
D. Transient dystonia

SECTION
V

Answers to Core Review Questions

Section I
General Assessment and Management

CHAPTER 1
ASSESSMENT OF FETAL WELL-BEING

1. (**D**) Alpha-fetoprotein (AFP) concentration levels of the maternal serum triple screen may indicate the presence of open neural tube defects. The levels would be increased in this situation. Levels may also be increased with multiple gestation, and if the pregnancy is not dated accurately. The AFP concentration levels would be decreased in a fetus with Down syndrome.

References: Kendig, S., and Barron, M. L.: Antenatal care and risk assessment strategies. *In* Simpson, K. R., and Creehan, P. A. (Eds.): *Perinatal Nursing.* Philadelphia, Lippincott, 1996, p. 88.
Landry, N.: Uncomplicated antepartum, intrapartum and postpartum care. *In* Deacon, J., and O'Neill, P. (Eds.): *Core Curriculum for Neonatal Intensive Care Nursing,* 2nd ed. Philadelphia, W. B. Saunders, 1999, p. 2.
Olds, S. B., London, M. L., and Lafewig, P. A.: *Maternal-Newborn Nursing,* 6th ed. Upper Saddle River, New Jersey, Prentice Hall Health, 2000.

2. (**B**) A biophysical profile score of 2/10 strongly suggests chronic asphyxia and necessitates immediate delivery regardless of gestational age.

References: Landry, N.: Uncomplicated antepartum, intrapartum and postpartum care. *In* Deacon, J., O'Neill, P. (Eds.): *Core Curriculum for Neonatal Intensive Care Nursing,* 2nd ed. Philadelphia, W. B. Saunders, 1999, p. 2.
Olds, S. B., London, M. L., and Lafewig, P. A.: *Maternal Newborn Nursing,* 6th ed. Upper Saddle River, New Jersey, Prentice Hall Health, 2000.

3. (**B**) Fetal biparietal diameter measurements are most accurate in the second trimester. This is frequently the time that gestational age by ultrasonogram is established. Crown-rump length measurements are usually done in the first trimester, when relatively few women present for prenatal care.

References: Landry, N.: Uncomplicated antepartum, intrapartum and postpartum care. *In* Deacon, J., and O'Neill, P. (Eds.): *Core Curriculum for Neonatal Intensive Care Nursing,* 2nd ed. Philadelphia, W. B. Saunders, 1999, p. 2.
Olds, S. B., London, M. L., and Lafewig, P. A.: *Maternal Newborn Nursing,* 6th ed. Upper Saddle River, New Jersey, Prentice Hall Health, 2000, p. 444.
O'Neill, P., et al: Maternal factors affecting the newborn. *In* Thureen, P. J., et al. (Eds.): *Assessment and Care of

the Well Newborn. Philadelphia, W. B. Saunders, 1999, p. 7.

4. (**B**) All of the tests are used to determine fetal lung maturation. Only the PG test is documented as accurate in the pregnant diabetic patient.

References: Jasper, M. L.: Antepartum fetal assessment. *In* Mattson, S., Smith, J. (Eds.): *Core Curriculum for Maternal-Newborn Nursing,* 2nd ed. Philadelphia, W. B. Saunders, 2000, p. 127.
Landry, N.: Uncomplicated antepartum, intrapartum, and postpartum care. *In* Deacon, J., and O'Neill, P. (Eds.): *Core Curriculum for Neonatal Intensive Care Nursing,* 2nd ed. Philadelphia, W. B. Saunders, 1999, p. 2.

5. (**D**) A nearly flat or flat baseline is a nonreassuring pattern associated with poor or absent variability. This is among fetal heart rate (FHR) patterns reported to be associated with an increased incidence of fetal compromise.

Reference: Landry, N.: Uncomplicated antepartum, intrapartum and postpartum care. *In* Deacon, J., and O'Neill, P. (Eds.): *Core Curriculum for Neonatal Intensive Care Nursing,* 2nd ed. Philadelphia, W. B. Saunders, 1999, p. 2.

6. (**A**) Late decelerations are characterized by a symmetric fall in the fetal heart rate (FHR), beginning at or after the peak of the uterine contraction and returning to baseline only after the contraction has ended.

Reference: Landry, N.: Uncomplicated antepartum, intrapartum and postpartum care. *In* Deacon, J., and O'Neill, P. (Eds.): *Core Curriculum for Neonatal Intensive Care Nursing,* 2nd ed. Philadelphia, W. B. Saunders, 1999, p. 2.

7. (**D**) Fetal baseline tachycardia is characterized by a heart rate above 160 bpm. This may be a nonreassuring sign in a term fetus. The most common cause of fetal tachycardia at term is maternal fever. Another cause is fetal hypoxia.

Reference: Landry, N.: Uncomplicated antepartum, intrapartum and postpartum care. *In* Deacon, J., and O'Neil, P. (Eds.): *Core Curriculum for Neonatal Intensive Care Nursing,* 2nd ed. Philadelphia, W. B. Saunders, 1999, p. 2.

8. (**C**) Potential fetal side effects of terbutaline tocolysis are an increase in maternal and fetal heart rate and a subsequent decrease in fetal heart rate (FHR) variability. $MgSO_4$ tocolysis may cause a decrease in FHR variability and either no change or a transient decrease in FHR baseline. Pro-

longed ruptured amniotic membranes are associated with amnionitis and a subsequent increase in the FHR baseline due to maternal fever. However, this patient has intact amniotic membranes and no maternal fever.

References: Broussard, A.: Antepartum-intrapartum complications. *In* Deacon, J., and O'Neill, P. (Eds.): *Core Curriculum for Neonatal Intensive Care Nursing,* 2nd ed. Philadelphia, W. B. Saunders, 1999, p. 18.
Olds, S. B., London, M. L., and Lafewig, P. A.: *Maternal-Newborn Nursing,* 6th ed. Upper Saddle River, New Jersey, Prentice Hall Health, 2000.

9. **(B)** Maternal hypotension is a complication of epidural anesthesia. Hypotension can cause a decrease in blood flow to the placenta leading to decreased oxygen to the fetus.

Reference: Broussard, A. B.: Antepartum-intrapartum complications. *In* Deacon, J., and O'Neill, P. (Eds.): *Core Curriculum for Neonatal Intensive Care Nursing,* 2nd ed. Philadelphia, W. B. Saunders, 1999, p. 18.

10. **(D)** The infant has a cephalohematoma, most likely related to the forceps-assisted delivery. The infant is most likely to develop hyperbilirubinemia as a result of the increased number of red blood cells that must be broken down as the cephalohematoma resolves. There is no evidence of further birth trauma, based on the assessment findings.

References: Olds, S. B., London, M. L., and Lafewig, P. A.: *Maternal-Newborn Nursing,* 6th ed. Upper Saddle River, New Jersey: Prentice Hall Health, 2000.
Smith, K.: Normal childbirth. *In* Mattson, S., and Smith, J. (Eds.): *Core Curriculum for Maternal-Newborn Nursing,* 2nd ed. Philadelphia, W. B. Saunders, 2000, p. 241.

CHAPTER 2
ADAPTATION TO EXTRAUTERINE LIFE

1. **(A)** The Apgar score provides an assessment of the infant's transition to extrauterine life, but the decision to initiate resuscitation is not delayed until determination of the score. Research evidence has demonstrated that Apgar scores alone are not predictive of perinatal asphyxia or eventual outcome.

References: Bakewell-Sachs, S., Shaw, V., and Tashman, A.: *Assessment of Risk in the Term Newborn.* White Plains, N.Y.: March of Dimes Birth Defects Foundation, 1997, p. 18.
Ballard, R.: Resuscitation in the delivery room. *In* Taeusch, H., and Ballard, R. (Eds.): *Avery's Diseases of the Newborn,* 7th ed. Philadelphia, W. B. Saunders, 1998, p. 319.

Letko, M.: Understanding the APGAR score. *JOGNN 25:* 299, 1996.

2. **(C)** Perinatal asphyxia has been used inconsistently and, based on long-term outcomes, inaccurately as a diagnosis. The Committee on Maternal-Fetal Medicine and Fetus and Newborn of the American College of Obstetricians and Gynecologists (ACOG) and the American Academy of Pediatrics (AAP) defined four essential criteria, all of which must be present for perinatal asphyxia:

Profound acidemia (pH <7.00) on umbilical artery sampl
Apgar score of 0–3 for > 5 minutes
Clinical neurologic sequelae in the immediate neonatal period
Clinical evidence of multiorgan system dysfunction in the immediate neonatal period

Reference: Bakewell-Sachs, S., Shaw, V., and Tashman, A.: *Assessment of Risk in the Term Newborn.* White Plains, N.Y.: March of Dimes Birth Defects Foundation, 1997, p. 19.

3. **(D)** The mother/parent(s) needs uninterrupted time with the newborn during the alert state following birth to interact with and "claim" the infant. To do this, the mother needs to indicate when she is ready.

References: Niermeyer, S., Clarke, S.: Delivery room care. *In* Merenstein, G., and Gardner, S.: *Handbook of Neonatal Intensive Care,* 4th ed. St. Louis, C. V. Mosby, 1998, p. 46.
Klaus, M., and Kennell, J.: Care of the mother, father and infant. *In* Fanaroff, A. A., and Martin, R. J. (Eds.): *Neonatal-Perinatal Medicine: Diseases of Fetus and Infant,* 6th ed. St. Louis, C. V. Mosby, 1997, p. 548.

4. **(B)** Shunting of blood through the foramen ovale directs blood with the highest oxygen content to the coronary arteries and brain while the ductus arteriosus directs deoxygenated blood toward the placenta.

References: Bakewell-Sachs, S., Shaw, V., and Tashman, A.: *Assessment of Risk in the Term Newborn.* White Plains, N.Y., March of Dimes Birth Defects Foundation, 1997, p. 16.
Zahka, K. G., and Patel, C. R.: Cardiovascular problems of the neonate. *In* Fanaroff, A. A., and Martin, R. J. (Eds.): *Neonatal-Perinatal Medicine: Diseases of the Fetus and Infant,* 6th ed. St. Louis, C. V. Mosby, 1997, p. 1158.

5. **(D)** When low-resistance placental circulation is removed, increased systemic vascular resistance results. Initiation of respi-

ration decreases pulmonary vascular resistance. These changes alter pressure changes within the heart and result in decreased systemic venous return, which closes the ductus venosus. The left atrial pressure rises, closing the foramen ovale. Decreasing pulmonary vascular resistance and increased oxygenation lead to closure of the ductus arteriosus.

References: Bakewell-Sachs, S., Shaw, V., and Tashman, A.: *Assessment of Risk in the Term Newborn.* White Plains, N.Y., March of Dime Birth Defects Foundation, 1997, p. 16.
Zahka, K. G., and Patel, C. R.: Cardiovascular problems of the neonate. *In* Fanaroff, A. A., and Martin, R. J. (Eds.): *Neonatal-Perinatal Medicine: Diseases of the Fetus and Infant*, 6th ed. St. Louis, C. V. Mosby, 1997, p. 1158.

6. **(D)** The newborn infant responds to illness or stress by "turning off" reactions. Early signs of distress or illness tend to be subtle. Illness is suspected when the infant is hypotonic, feeds poorly, or is difficult to arouse or bring to an alert state.

Reference: Lepley, C. J., Gardner, S. L., Lubchenco, L. O.: Initial nursery care. *In* Merenstein, G., and Gardner, S. (Eds.): *Handbook of Neonatal Intensive Care*, 4th ed. St. Louis, C. V. Mosby, 1998, p. 70.

7. **(A)** Essential elements of nursing care include recognition of newborns at risk, and initial and ongoing assessments to facilitate early identification of infection. Newborn clinical signs may present rapidly within the first 12 to 24 hours of life.

References: Bakewell-Sachs, S., Shaw, V., and Tashman, A.: *Assessment of Risk in the Term Newborn.* White Plains, N.Y., March of Dimes Birth Defects Foundation, 1997, p. 61.
Merenstein, G., Adams, K., Weisman, L. E.: Infection in the neonate. *In* Merenstein, G., and Gardner, S. (Eds.): *Handbook of Neonatal Intensive Care*, 4th ed. St. Louis, C. V. Mosby, 1998, p. 413.

8. **(C)** TTN is thought to be the probable cause of delayed clearance of lung fluid. The population most likely to experience TTN is full-term infants born by cesarean section or having experienced some sort of perinatal hypoxic stress. Either of these events would result in increased protein concentration in lung fluid, preventing transfer of fluid into pulmonary circulation.

Reference: Hansen, T., Corbet, A.: Disorders of the transition. *In* Taeusch, H., and Ballard, R. (Eds.): *Avery's Diseases of the Newborn*, 7th ed. Philadelphia, W. B. Saunders, 1998, p. 602.

9. **(B)** The prevention of neonatal hepatitis depends on prompt administration of immune globulin and hepatitis B vaccine. HVIG administration is recommended within 12 hours of delivery and vaccine in the first week of life for all neonates at risk.

Reference: Cowles, T., Gonik, B.: Perinatal infections. *In* Fanaroff, A. A., and Martin, R. J. (Eds.): *Neonatal-Perinatal Medicine: Diseases of the Fetus and Infant*, 6th ed. St. Louis: C. V. Mosby, 1997, p. 327.

10. **(D)** With the recent discovery of the newborn's ability to interact and breast-feed when the baby is not removed from the mother during the first hour for eye prophylaxis, vitamin K injection, or bathing, care protocols for the first hour of life are changing. If the infant is healthy, parent(s) and the baby should have a period of time alone in a comfortable and quiet atmosphere. The infant may receive eye prophylaxis by 1 hour of age after allowing parent(s) initial contact and time.

References: Bakewell-Sachs, S., Shaw, V., and Tashman, A.: *Assessment of Risk in the Term Newborn.* White Plains, N. Y., March of Dimes Birth Defects Foundation, 1997, p. 54.
Wetzel, R. C.: Anesthesia for premature infants. *In* Fanaroff, A. A., and Martin, R. J. (Eds.): *Neonatal-Perinatal Medicine: Diseases of Fetus and Infant*, 6th ed. St. Louis, C. V. Mosby, 1997, p. 525.

11. **(A)** Respiratory depression is not uncommon when a narcotic has been administered to the mother within 4 hours of delivery. Neonatal depression related to the drug without overlying asphyxia usually requires only ventilation. Naloxone is effective to antagonize the respiratory depression if the narcotic agent was administered within 4 hours of birth. The effect of the narcotic may outlast the effect of naloxone, requiring a repeated dose. Naloxone should never be given to a narcotic-addicted mother because of the potential for infant withdrawal. Verification of drug history prior to administration of naloxone may prevent this situation.

References: Bakewell-Sachs, S., Shaw, V., and Tashman, A.: *Assessment of Risk in the Term Newborn.* White Plains, N.Y., March of Dimes Birth Defects Foundation, 1997, p. 21.
Bloom, R. S.: Delivery room resuscitation of the newborn. *In* Fanaroff, A. A., and Martin, R. J. (Eds.): *Neonatal-Perinatal Medicine: Diseases of Fetus and Infant*, 6th ed. St. Louis, C. V. Mosby, 1997, p. 376.

CHAPTER 3
NEONATAL RESUSCITATION

1. (**D**) Evaluation occurs throughout the entire process of resuscitation after each action so that a decision can be made as to what further actions are needed.

Reference: Bloom, R. S., and Cropley, C.: *Textbook of Neonatal Resuscitation*, 3rd ed.: Dallas, American Heart Association, 1994, p. 1.

2. (**B**) Adequate preparation of equipment and personnel are required for all deliveries. In the case of an anticipated difficult resuscitation, having a team that can work together effectively and is dedicated to the infant is especially important. Without the team, protocols and equipment cannot effectively be utilized.

Reference: Bloom, R. S., and Cropley, C.: *Textbook of Neonatal Resuscitation*, 3rd ed.: Dallas, American Heart Association, 1994, p. 1.

3. (**D**) Because this infant is not vigorous, intubation and tracheal suctioning are needed to remove as much meconium as possible prior to stimulating the baby and beginning positive-pressure ventilation. Stimulation or PPV prior to removal of thick particulate meconium from the trachea can result in the advancement of meconium plugs further into the bronchioles.

Reference: American Heart Association: Neonatal resuscitation. *Circulation 2000*, 102(suppl I):I–343.

4. (**B**) The ratio of ventilations to compressions is 1:3. For every one ventilation, three compressions occur. In a 1-minute period, 30 ventilations and 90 compressions, or 120 events, will occur.

References: Bloom, R. S., and Cropley, C.: *Textbook of Neonatal Resuscitation*, 3rd ed.: Dallas, American Heart Association, 1994, p. 4.
Harrell, H.: Neonatal Delivery Room Resuscitation. *In* Deacon, J., and O'Neill, P. (Eds.): *Core Curriculum for Neonatal Intensive Care Nursing*, 2nd ed.: Philadelphia, W. B. Saunders, 1999, p. 111.

5. (**A**) The neonatal resuscitation guidelines state that the indication for epinephrine is when the heart rate remains below 60 beats per minute despite a minimum of 30 seconds of adequate ventilation with 100% oxygen and chest compressions.

The dosage range is 0.1 to 0.3 mL/kg of 1:10,000 epinephrine given either ETT (diluted) or IV. There are insufficient data to support the use of high-dose epinephrine.

Reference: American Heart Association: Neonatal resuscitation. *Circulation 2000*, 102(suppl I):I–343.

6. (**B**) Based on the given history, the patient may have likely experienced a placenta abruptio. In this case, fetal blood loss and resulting hypovolemia or shock can be expected. Volume expanders increase the neonate's circulating blood volume to correct hypovolemia and facilitate tissue perfusion.

References: Bloom, R. S., and Cropley, C.: *Textbook of Neonatal Resuscitation*, 3rd ed.: Dallas, American Heart Association, 1994, p. 6.
Harrell, H.: Neonatal Delivery Room Resuscitation. *In* Deacon, J., and O'Neill, P. (Eds.): *Core Curriculum for Neonatal Intensive Care Nursing*, 2nd ed.: Philadelphia, W. B. Saunders, 1999, p. 112.

7. (**C**) The signs and symptoms experienced by the infant are most consistent with a diaphragmatic hernia. Persistent central cyanosis is an indication for ventilatory assistance. To prevent the intestinal distension and further compression of the lungs caused by bag and mask ventilation, direct ventilation of the lungs with an endotracheal tube is necessary.

References: Bloom, R. S., and Cropley, C.: *Textbook of Neonatal Resuscitation*, 3rd ed.: Dallas, American Heart Association, 1994, p. 3B.
Harrell, H.: Neonatal Delivery Room Resuscitation. *In* Deacon, J., O'Neill, P. (Eds.): *Core Curriculum for Neonatal Intensive Care Nursing*, 2nd ed.: Philadelphia, W. B. Saunders, 1999, p. 113.

8. (**D**) The clinical picture is suggestive of an infant with hydrops fetalis. To allow adequate expansion of the lungs during the resuscitation, a thoracentesis may be needed to remove excess fluid from the thoracic cavity. Although a double volume exchange may be necessary later in the infant's course, it would not be the first priority in the delivery room. An umbilical venous catheter would be placed rather than a percutaneous central catheter.

Reference: Watson, R.: Gastrointestinal disorders. *In* Deacon, J., and O'Neill, P. (Eds.): *Core Curriculum for Neonatal Intensive Care Nursing*, 2nd ed.: Philadelphia, W. B. Saunders, 1999, p. 290.

9. (**A**) Hypoxia results from a lack of oxygen availability to the fetal tissues. Fetal hypoxia and acidosis results in secondary apnea, which cannot be resolved with normal stimulation, bradycardia, decreased blood pressure, and perfusion.

References: Bloom, R. S., and Cropley, C.: *Textbook of Neonatal Resuscitation*, 3rd ed.: Dallas, American Heart Association, 1994, p. 1.
Harrell, H.: Neonatal delivery room resuscitation. *In* Deacon, J., and O'Neill, P. (Eds.): *Core Curriculum for Neonatal Intensive Care Nursing*, 2nd ed.: Philadelphia, W. B. Saunders, 1999, p. 103.

10. (**C**) Respiratory distress immediately after birth and cyanosis when quiet is indicative of bilateral choanal atresia because of the blockage of the primary airway, the nose.

References: Bloom, R. S., and Cropley, C.: *Textbook of Neonatal Resuscitation*, 3rd ed.: Dallas, American Heart Association, 1994, p. 3B.
Harrell, H.: Neonatal delivery room resuscitation. *In* Deacon, J., and O'Neill, P. (Eds.): *Core Curriculum for Neonatal Intensive Care Nursing*, 2nd ed.: Philadelphia, W. B. Saunders, 1999, p. 114.

CHAPTER 4
PHYSICAL ASSESSMENT

1. (**C**) The normal heart rate for a newborn ranges between 80 and 160 bpm. Even though a healthy term neonate rarely may have a heart rate as low as 70 bpm, this is not considered the low end of normal. Neonates cannot tolerate a heart rate consistently higher than 200 bpm for an extended period of time.

Reference: Vargo, L.: The basics of neonatal EKG interpretation. *Neonatal Network* 17(8):7, 1998.

2. (**D**) A constant feature of RDS is the early onset of clinical signs of the disease, within the first 6 hours of delivery. Inadequate observation may lead to the impression of a symptom-free period of several hours. The uncomplicated clinical course is characterized by a progressive worsening of symptoms with a peak severity by days 2 to 3 and onset of recovery by 72 hours.

Reference: Martin, R. J., and Fanaroff, A. A.: The respiratory distress syndrome and its management. *In* Fanaroff, A. A., and Martin, R. J. (Eds.): *Neonatal-Perinatal Medicine: Diseases of the Fetus and Infant*, 6th ed. St. Louis, Mosby, 1997, p. 1018.

3. (**D**) Because the ductus arteriosus generally enters the aorta after the origin of the right subclavian and carotid arteries, blood arriving at these two sites will be well oxygenated, whereas blood samples from the left subclavian artery and aorta will be less oxygenated. Thus preductal gases can be obtained from the right radial artery, and postductal gases can be drawn through the left radial artery, descending aorta, or any lower extremity artery. Alternatively, placement of two transcutaneous PO_2 electrodes (one on the right upper chest and the other on the abdomen) or two pulse oximeters (one on the right hand and the other on the left hand or either foot) accomplishes the same effect in differentiating preductal and postductal oxygen saturation.

Reference: Carlo, W. A.: Assessment of pulmonary function. *In* Fanaroff, A. A., and Martin, R. J. (Eds.): *Neonatal-Perinatal Medicine: Diseases of the Fetus and Infant*, 6th ed. St. Louis, Mosby, 1997, p. 1009.

4. (**B**) Maternal estrogen can result in engorged and enlarged breasts in the newborn that secrete a white substance known as "witch's milk."

Reference: Askin, D. F.: Chest and lungs assessment. *In* Tappero, E. P., and Honeyfield, M. E.: *Physical Assessment of the Newborn: A Comprehensive Approach to the Art of Physical Examination*, 2nd ed. Santa Rosa, CA, NICU INK, 1996, p. 67.

5. (**A**) Simple VSD is the single most common congenital heart malformation, accounting for about 20 to 25% of all cases of congenital heart disease.

Reference: Lott, J. W.: Assessment and management of cardiovascular dysfunction. *In* Kenner, C., Lott, J. W., and Flandermeyer, A. A.: *Comprehensive Neonatal Nursing: A Physiologic Perspective*. Philadelphia, W. B. Saunders, 1998, p. 306.

6. (**C**) Hypertrophic cardiomyopathy is a condition often associated with macrosomic infants of diabetic mothers as a consequence of fetal insulin stimulation. Increases in myocardial nuclei, cell number, and fiber occur, resulting in septal hypertrophy with decreased left ventricular function and left ventricular outflow obstruction.

Reference: Suevo, D.: The infant of the diabetic mother. *Neonatal Network* 16(5):22, 1997.

7. (**B**) In cyanotic heart disease, PaO_2 increases very little from values obtained while breathing ambient room air compared with values during 100% oxygen

administration. However, there is usually a very significant increase in PaO_2 when oxygen is administered to an infant with lung disease.

Reference: Wolfe, R. R., Boucek, M., Schaffer, M., and Wiggins, J. W.: Cardiovascular diseases. *In* Hay, W. W., Groothius, J. R., Hayward, A. R., and Levin, M. J. (Eds.): *Current Pediatric Diagnosis & Treatments*, 13th ed. Stamford, CT, Appleton & Lange, 1997, p. 474.

8. **(B)** During fetal circulation, the right ventricle pumps against the higher pressure (constricted pulmonary artery.) After birth, blood is no longer diverted from pulmonary circulation through the ductus arteriosus. The highest pressure is now in the aorta. This must be overcome for the left ventricle to eject blood.

Reference: Wolfe, R. R., Boucek, M., Schaffer, M., and Wiggins, J. W.: Cardiovascular diseases. *In* Hay, W. W., Groothius, J. R., Hayward, A. R., and Levin, M. J. (Eds.): *Current Pediatric Diagnosis & Treatments*, 13th ed. Stamford, CT, Appleton & Lange, 1997, p. 474.

9. **(B)** A "caput" is characterized by hemorrhagic edema of the scalp and muscles; it is most pronounced at birth, giving a "cone-shaped" appearance to the head. It resolves in 2 to 3 days.

Reference: Moe, P. G., Seay, A. R.: Neurologic and muscular disorders. *In* Hay, W. W., Groothius, J. R., Hayward, A. R., and Levin, M. J. (Eds.): *Current Pediatric Diagnosis & Treatments*, 13th ed. Stamford, CT, Appleton & Lange, 1997, p. 631.

10. **(B)** The ductus arteriosus closes primarily in response to increased arterial oxygen concentration. Decreased prostaglandin E_1 and an increase in acetylcholine and bradykinin also contribute to ductal closure. Functional ductal closure normally occurs by about 15 hours of life. Patency of the ductus arteriosus in a healthy term infant beyond 24 hours of life is considered a patent ductus arteriosus.

Reference: Lott, J. W.: Assessment and management of cardiovascular dysfunction. *In* Kenner, C., Lott, J. W., and Flandermeyer, A. A. (Eds.): *Comprehensive Neonatal Nursing: A Physiologic Perspective*, 2nd ed. Philadelphia, W. B. Saunders, 1998, p. 306.

11. **(D)** Newborns can see, respond to changes in light, and fixate on objects. The newborn's visual acuity is estimated in the range of 20/400. By 2 to 3 years of age, visual acuity is 20/30 to 20/20.

Reference: Olitsky, S. E., and Nelson, L. B.: Disorders of the eye: growth and development. *In* Behrman, R. E., Kliegman, R. M., and Jenson, H. B. (Eds.): *Nelson Textbook of Pediatrics*, 16th ed. Philadelphia, W. B. Saunders, 2000, p. 1895.

12. **(A)** The initial sign of retinoblastoma in the majority of infants is a white pupillary reflex instead of the red reflex.

Reference: Olitsky, S. E., and Nelson, L. B.: Disorders of the eye: disorders of the retina and vitreous. *In* Behrman, R. E., Kliegman, R. M., and Jenson, H. B. (Eds.): *Nelson Textbook of Pediatrics*, 16th ed. Philadelphia, W. B. Saunders, 2000, p. 1925.

13. **(A)** Microcephaly is defined as a head circumference that measures 2 standard deviations below the mean for age, sex, and race and is caused by poor brain growth. The sutures are often closed because of the lack of brain growth. Hydranencephaly is a complete absence of cerebral hemispheres. Cranioschisis is the failure of the skull to close. Aqueductal stenosis can result in hydrocephalus and would not be associated with a smaller than normal head circumference.

Reference: DeMyer, W.: Microcephaly, micrencephaly, megalocephaly, and megalencephaly. *In* Swaiman, K. F., and Ashwal, S. (Eds.): *Pediatric Neurology: Principles & Practice*, 3rd ed. St. Louis, Mosby, 1999, p. 301.

14. **(A)** A cephalohematoma is an accumulation of blood under the periosteum of the skull. It is caused by injury to the periosteum during labor. It can occur with vaginal or cesarean section deliveries.

Reference: Mangurten, H. H.: Birth injuries. *In* Fanaroff, A. A., Martin, R. J. (Eds.): *Neonatal-Perinatal Medicine: Diseases of the Fetus and Infant*, 6th ed. St. Louis, Mosby, 1997, p. 425.

15. **(C)** Primary craniosynostosis results from premature fusion of one or more cranial sutures. Failure of the skull to close, cranioschisis, is associated with anencephaly. Craniosclerosis is a thickening of the skull.

Reference: Ashwal, S.: Congenital structural defects. *In* Swaiman, K. F., Ashwal, S. (Eds.): *Pediatric Neurology: Principles & Practice*, 3rd ed. St. Louis, Mosby, 1999, p. 234.

16. **(D)** Unilateral vocal cord paralysis may be a consequence of excessive traction on the head during breech delivery or lateral traction with forceps in a cephalic presentation. An infant with unilateral vocal

cord paralysis is often asymptomatic at rest but exhibits hoarseness and mild inspiratory stridor when crying. An infant with bilateral vocal cord paralysis typically has more severe respiratory distress. Choanal atresia is associated with respiratory distress at rest and no hoarseness or stridor. Subglottic mass is associated with stridor even at rest.

Reference: Mangurten, H. H.: Birth injuries. *In* Fanaroff, A. A., Martin, R. J. (Eds.): *Neonatal-Perinatal Medicine: Diseases of the Fetus and Infant*, 6th ed. St. Louis, Mosby, 1997, p. 425.

17. **(C)** Pierre-Robin syndrome is caused by a single prenatal onset defect in development: mandibular hypoplasia. The tongue is relatively small for the oral cavity. The tongue drops back, blocking closure of the posterior palatal shelves, causing a U-shaped cleft palate.

Reference: Hudgins, L., and Cassidy, S. B.: Congenital anomalies. *In* Fanaroff, A. A., and Martin, R. S. (Eds.): *Neonatal-Perinatal Medicine: Diseases of the Fetus and Infant*, 6th ed. St. Louis, Mosby, 1997, p. 455.

18. **(A)** The description of the lesions is that of milia, a transient and benign lesion found in 40% of term newborns. Milia are epidermal cysts caused by accumulation of sebaceous gland secretions. Milia resolve within the first few weeks of life.

Reference: Witt, C.: Skin assessment. *In* Tappero, E. P., and Honeyfield, M. E.: *Physical Assessment of the Newborn: A Comprehensive Approach to the Art of Physical Examination*, 2nd ed, Santa Rosa, Calif., NICU INK, 1996, p. 39.

19. **(B)** Injury to the fifth and sixth cervical roots may follow a breech presentation with the arms extended over the head; excessive traction on the shoulder in the delivery of the head may result in stretching of the plexus. Brachial palsy may result.

Reference: Mangurten, H. H.: Birth injuries. *In* Fanaroff, A. A., Martin, R. J. (Eds.): *Neonatal-Perinatal Medicine: Diseases of the Fetus and Infant*, 6th ed. St. Louis, Mosby, 1997, p. 425.

20. **(C)** Redundant skin/webbing of the neck can be found with Noonan, trisomy 21, and Turner syndromes.

Reference: Jones, K. L.: *Smith's Recognizable Patterns of Human Malformation*, 5th ed. Philadelphia, W. B. Saunders, 1996.

21. **(B)** Fracture of the clavicles is the most common fracture associated with delivery. An infant with shoulder dystocia is at increased risk of fracturing the clavicle. A radiograph is the most appropriate diagnostic tool.

Reference: Butler, J.: Assessment and management of musculoskeletal dysfunction. *In* Kenner, C., Lott, J. W., and Flandermeyer, A. A. (Eds.): *Comprehensive Neonatal Nursing: A Physiologic Perspective*, 2nd ed. Philadelphia, W. B. Saunders, 1998, p. 608.

22. **(D)** Erythema toxicum is a benign, self-limited eruption that occurs in 50% of all full-term infants. The cause is unknown. Miliaria is characterized by clear, thin vesicles. Nevus simplex, or stork bite, is an irregularly shaped pink macule composed of dilated and distended capillaries. Pustular melanosis starts as vesiculopustular lesions, rupturing 12 to 48 hours after birth and leaving small pigmented macules.

References: Sahn, E. E., and Esterly, N. B.: The skin. *In* Fanaroff, A. A., and Martin, R. J. (Eds.): *Neonatal-Perinatal Medicine: Diseases of the Fetus and Infant*, 6th ed. St. Louis, Mosby, 1997, p. 1637.
Witt, C.: Skin assessment. *In* Tappero, E. P., Honeyfield, M. E. (Eds): *Physical Assessment of the Newborn: A Comprehensive Approach to the Art of Physical Examination*, 2nd ed. Santa Rosa, Calif., NICU INK, 1996, p. 39.

23. **(B)** Dubowitz scoring system is accurate to ± 2 weeks. It uses physical and neurologic criteria to estimate gestation age.

Reference: Katz, K., and Nishioka, E.: Neonatal assessment. *In* Kenner, C., Lott, J. W., and Flandermeyer, A. A. (Eds.): *Comprehensive Neonatal Nursing: A Physiologic Perspective*, 2nd ed. Philadelphia, W. B. Saunders, 1998, p. 223.

24. **(C)** The discoloration is due to meconium staining. The fetus passes meconium in response to intrauterine stress. Meconium in the amniotic fluid stains the umbilical cord and fetus, notably the skin and nails.

Reference: Miller, M. J., Fanaroff, A. A., and Martin, R. J.: Respiratory disorders in preterm and term infants. *In* Fanaroff, A. A., and Martin, R. J. (Eds.): *Neonatal-Perinatal Medicine: Diseases of the Fetus and Infant*, 6th ed. St. Louis, Mosby 1997, p. 1040.

25. **(C)** The Barlow test is performed to determine developmental dysplasia of the hips. It is performed by stabilizing the pelvis with one hand, then flexing and adducting the opposite hip while applying posterior force.

Reference: Thompson, G. H., Scoles, P. V.: Bone and joint disorders: The hip. *In* Behrman, R. E., Kliegman, R.

M., and Jenson, H. B. (Eds.): *Nelson Textbook of Pediatrics*, 16th ed. Philadelphia, W. B. Saunders, 2000, p. 2077.

26. **(B)** Spontaneous pneumothorax occurs in 1% of all deliveries. Clinical manifestations include an increase in respiratory rate, grunting, pallor, cyanosis, and decreased breath sounds on the affected side.

Reference: Miller, M. J., Fanaroff, A. A., and Martin, R. J.: Respiratory disorders in preterm and term infants. *In* Fanaroff, A. A., and Martin, R. J. (Eds.): *Neonatal-Perinatal Medicine: Diseases of the Fetus and Infant*, 6th ed. St. Louis, Mosby, 1997, p. 1040.

27. **(B)** Cryptorchidism occurs when one or both testes fail to descend into the scrotum. The testes will not develop and then will atrophy, causing infertility. Patients have a 20 to 44% increased risk of developing a malignant testicular tumor, and inguinal hernias always accompany true undescended testes.

Reference: Elder, J. S.: Urologic disorders in infants and children: Disorders and anomalies of the scrotal contents. *In* Behrman, R. E., Kliegman, R. M., and Jenson, H. B. (Eds.): *Nelson Textbook of Pediatrics*, 16th ed. Philadelphia, W. B. Saunders, 2000, p. 1650.

28. **(A)** Brachial palsy is seen most often in labor ending in traumatic delivery and large babies prone to stretching injuries of the brachial plexus. The infant with upper arm paralysis holds the affected arm adducted and internally rotated, with extension at the elbow, pronation of the forearm, and flexion of the wrist.

Reference: Tappero, E. P.: Musculoskeletal system assessment. *In* Tappero, E. P., Honeyfield, M. E. (Eds.): *Physical Assessment of the Newborn: A Comprehensive Approach to the Art of Physical Examination*, 2nd ed. Santa Rosa, Calif., NICU INK, 1996, p. 117.

29. **(D)** Trigeminal-cranial nerve V supplies the jaw muscles and is responsible for the sensory innervation of the face. The three divisions of this nerve are mandibular, maxillary, and ophthalmic. Opening the mouth and observing for jaw deviation assesses the motor component of cranial nerve V. Masseter strength, also part of cranial nerve V function, is tested by placing a gloved finger in the mouth and evaluating the biting portion of the suck. Touching the lashes with a cotton ball tests the sensory component of cranial-nerve V, not the motor component. Introducing a light into the peripheral visual field is a test used for the optic-cranial nerve II and has nothing to do with V.

Reference: Carey, B. E.: Neurologic assessment. *In* Tappero, E. P., and Honeyfield, M. E. (Eds.): *Physical Assessment of the Newborn: A Comprehensive Approach to the Art of Physical Examination*, 2nd ed. Santa Rosa, Calif., NICU INK, 1996, p. 137.

30. **(C)** Micrognathia (small jaw) may present a serious airway problem if a normal-size tongue is too large to fit in an abnormally small mandible, leading to airway obstruction. Micrognathia is frequently seen in Pierre-Robin, Treacher-Collins, and de Lange syndromes. Infants with Down syndrome or trisomy 21 have normal-size mandibles but have protuberant tongues. The potential for airway obstruction is of a different nature than in children with the other three syndromes.

Reference: Buschbach, D.: Physical assessment of the newborn infant. *In* Deacon, J., and O'Neill, P. (Eds.): *Core Curriculum for Neonatal Intensive Care Nursing*, 2nd ed. Philadelphia, W. B. Saunders, 1999, p. 74.

31. **(B)** Epstein's pearls are small, white inclusion cysts commonly found on the hard and soft palates and on the gum margins. They usually disappear a few weeks after birth. A respiratory infection may cause periods of apnea, but not necessarily loud, noisy breathing. Cleft palate does not cause noisy breathing or apnea. Newborns are obligate nose breathers. The classic way to assess choanal atresia is to have a baby breathe against a cold, flat object to assess nares patency. If the nares are patent, the cold object should get foggy with exhalation.

Reference: Buschbach, D.: Physical assessment of the newborn infant. *In* Deacon, J., O'Neill, P. (Eds.): *Core Curriculum for Neonatal Intensive Care Nursing*, 2nd ed. Philadelphia, W. B. Saunders, 1999, p. 74.

32. **(C)** Neither the Ortolani maneuver nor the Barlow maneuver rely on an audible "clunk," but rather on a palpable "clunk." These tests are for assessment of dislocated hip and unstable hip, respectively. The Barlow maneuver uses adduction with downward pressure. The Ortolani maneuver uses abduction. Choice C is correct because it uses the word "palpable," and the correct motion (abduction) is matched with the correct maneuver.

Reference: Buschbach, D.: Physical assessment of the newborn infant. *In* Deacon, J., O'Neill, P. (Eds.): *Core*

Curriculum for Neonatal Intensive Care Nursing, 2nd ed. Philadelphia, W. B. Saunders, 1999, p. 74.

33. **(D)** "Crackles" is the preferred term for what used to be called rales. Crackles are classified as fine, moderate, or coarse. Rhonchi are more musical in quality than crackles and have a lower pitch than wheezes. Vesicular breath sounds are normal breath sounds. Stridor is a high-pitched sound heard on inspiration or expiration and usually indicates airway obstruction.

Reference: Askin, D. F.: Chest and lungs assessment. *In* Tappero, E. P., and Honeyfield, M. E. (Eds.): *Physical Assessment of the Newborn: A Comprehensive Approach to the Art of Physical Examination*, 2nd ed. Santa Rosa, Calif., NICU INK, 1996, p. 67.

34. **(D)** Milia and Epstein pearls (oral milia) are of no concern and resolve during the first few weeks of life. Harlequin color change is of no pathologic significance. Circumoral cyanosis may be present during the first 12 to 24 hours after birth. Circumoral cyanosis lasting longer than 24 hours should be investigated.

Reference: Witt, C.: Skin assessment. *In* Tappero, E. P., Honeyfield, M. E. (Eds.): *Physical Assessment of the Newborn: A Comprehensive Approach to the Art of Physical Examination*, 2nd ed. Santa Rosa, Calif., NICU INK, 1996, p. 167.

35. **(D)** An imaginary line drawn across the canthi is a standard way to assess ear position. Ears that are lower than an imaginary line drawn across the canthi are considered "low-set."

Reference: Bodurtha, J.: Assessment of the newborn with dysmorphic features. *Neonatal Network* 18:27, 1999.

36. **(D)** TTN typically presents as respiratory distress in term infants or preterm infants who are close to term. Prominent perihilar streaking is the characteristic finding that may represent engorgement of the periarterial lymphatics that participate in the clearance of alveolar fluid. The preferred explanation for the clinical features is delayed resorption of fetal lung fluid; thus it is seen more commonly after cesarean section, because the infant's thorax is not subjected to the same pressures as when delivery takes place vaginally.

Reference: Miller, M. J., Fanaroff, A. A., and Martin, R. J.: Respiratory disorders in preterm and term infants. *In* Fanaroff, A. A., and Martin, R. J. (Eds.): *Neonatal-Perinatal Medicine: Diseases of the Fetus and Infant*, 6th ed. St. Louis, Mosby, 1997, p. 1040.

37. **(C)** The urine output for this infant is 5 mL/kg/hr. The excessive urine output and dilute urine should alert the nurse to the possibility of antidiuretic hormone (ADH) deficiency. In a neonate with suspected ADH deficiency, vomiting or fever secondary to dehydration in the presence of high urine output (>4 mL/kg/day) warrants the measurement of serum and urine electrolytes and osmolarity.

Reference: Dorton, A. M.: The pituitary gland: embryology, physiology and pathophysiology. *Neonatal Network* 19(2):9, 2000.

38. **(D)** Hypoparathyroidism leads to impaired parathyroid hormone (PTH) release, which leads to hypocalcemia. Hypocalcemia impairs normal cardiac function, decreasing cardiac contractility. This results in poor perfusion, tachycardia, and hypotension. Prolonged bleeding from intravenous line sites or heel stick puncture sites occurs because of the role calcium has in the clotting process.

Reference: Steffensrud, S.: Parathyroids: The forgotten glands. *Neonatal Network* 19(1):9, 2000.

39. **(D)** Evaluation of muscle tone involves assessing passive and active tone. Active tone correlates with postural tone and is best evaluated by grasping the newborn's hands and pulling him slowly from the supine to the sitting position. Placing a newborn supine and turning his head to one side should elicit the tonic neck reflex. Holding the newborn upright and allowing the soles of his feet to touch a flat surface should elicit the stepping reflex. Stimulating the palmar surface of the newborn's hand will elicit the palmar grasp reflex.

Reference: Carey, B. E.: Neurologic assessment. *In* Tappero, E. P., and Honeyfield, M. E. (Eds.): *Physical Assessment of the Newborn: A Comprehensive Approach to the Art of Physical Examination*, 2nd ed. Santa Rosa, Calif., NICU INK, 1996, p. 137.

40. **(D)** Exposure to maternal hormones can stimulate a vaginal discharge that may be a creamy white or blood-tinged color.

Reference: Cavaliere, T. A.: Genitourinary assessment. *In* Tappero, E. P., and Honeyfield, M. E. (Eds.): *Physical Assessment of the Newborn: A Comprehensive Approach to the Art of Physical Examination*, 2nd ed. Santa Rosa, Calif., NICU INK, 1996, p. 103.

41. **(A)** The normal anterior fontanel measures 4 to 5 cm across. A very large ante-

rior fontanel is associated with hypothyroidism. Down syndrome is associated with defect in the parietal bone (third fontanel). Neither intraventricular hemorrhage nor intracranial arteriovenous malformation is associated with a large anterior fontanel.

Reference: Johnson, C. B.: Head, eyes, ears, nose, mouth, and neck assessment. *In* Tappero, E. P., Honeyfield, M. E. (Eds.): *Physical Assessment of the Newborn: A Comprehensive Approach to the Art of Physical Examination*, 2nd ed. Santa Rosa, Calif., NICU INK, 1996, p. 53.

42. **(B)** A port-wine nevus that follows the area of the trigeminal nerve may indicate Sturge-Weber syndrome. This syndrome is associated with glaucoma, mental retardation, and seizures. Kasabach-Merritt and Klippel-Trenaunay-Weber syndromes are both associated with a cavernous hemangioma.

Reference: Witt, C.: Skin assessment. *In* Tappero, E. P., and Honeyfield, M. E. (Eds.): *Physical Assessment of the Newborn: A Comprehensive Approach to the Art of Physical Examination*, 2nd ed. Santa Rosa, Calif., NICU INK, 1996, p. 39.

CHAPTER 5
GESTATIONAL AGE ASSESSMENT

1. **(A)** Small for gestational age (SGA) infants have limited fat and glycogen stores and are therefore at risk for hypoglycemia and hypothermia. Because of these limited reserves, SGA infants are more likely to experience fetal distress, which may result in intrauterine meconium passage and subsequent meconium aspiration.

Reference: Dodd, V.: Gestational age assessment. *Neonatal Network* 15:27, 1996.

2. **(B)** The 28-week-gestation infant has a thinner epidermal skin layer. As a result, the skin is translucent and pink or red owing to visible capillaries. Additionally, the premature infant lacks subcutaneous fat, resulting in visible veins through the skin. Lanugo decreases in amount with gestation and is expected to cover a significant portion of the body at 28 weeks. Testes are not in the upper scrotum until approximately 36 weeks' gestation and rugae begin to form around 28 weeks. Plantar creases appear at approximately 32 weeks.

References: Dodd, V.: Gestational age assessment. *Neonatal Network* 15:27, 1996.
Katz, K., Nishioka, E.: Neonatal assessment. *In* Kenner,

C., Lott, J. W., and Flandermeyer, A. A. (Eds.): *Comprehensive Neonatal Nursing: A Physiologic Perspective*, 2nd ed. Philadelphia, W. B. Saunders, p. 223, 1998.

3. **(D)** Gestational age and whether the infant's development is appropriate for that age have significant impact on neonatal outcome. By comparing development (weight, head circumference, length) to gestational age, infants can be classified as being average for gestational age, small for gestational age, or large for gestational age. Neonatal morbidities have been identified for each classification.

Reference: Katz, K., Nishioka, E.: Neonatal assessment. *In* Kenner, C., Lott, J. W., and Flandermeyer, A. A. (Eds.): *Comprehensive Neonatal Nursing: A Physiologic Perspective, 2nd ed*. Philadelphia, W. B. Saunders, 1998, p. 223.

4. **(C)** A neonatal morbidity associated with large for gestational age (LGA) is being an infant of a diabetic mother (IDM). Common problems associated with IDMs include hypoglycemia, respiratory distress syndrome, hypocalcemia, hypomagnesemia, and hyperbilirubinemia. All LGA infants should be assessed for hypoglycemia.

References: Gamblian, V., Bivens, K., Burton, K. S., Kistler, C. H., Kleeman, T. A., and Prows, C.: Assessment and management of endocrine dysfunction. *In* Kenner, C., Lott, J. W., and Flandermeyer, A. A. (Eds.): *Comprehensive Neonatal Nursing: A Physiologic Perspective*, 2nd ed. Philadelphia, W. B. Saunders, 1998, p. 476.
Katz, K., Nishioka, E.: Neonatal assessment. *In* Kenner, C., Lott, J. W., and Flandermeyer, A. A. (Eds.): *Comprehensive Neonatal Nursing: A Physiologic Perspective*, 2nd ed.. Philadelphia, W. B. Saunders, 1998, p. 223.

5. **(D)** An infant of any gestational age who is larger than the 90% of infants of the same age is considered large for gestational age. Standardized graphs for newborn size based on gestational age indicate the 10th percentile or below as small for gestational age, the 90th percentile and above as large for gestational age, and the area in between as appropriate for gestational age.

References: Dodd, V.: Gestational age assessment. *Neonatal Network* 15:27, 1996.
Katz, K., and Nishioka, E.: Neonatal assessment. *In* Kenner, C., Lott, J. W., Flandermeyer, A. A. (Eds.): *Comprehensive Neonatal Nursing*, 2nd ed. Philadelphia, W. B. Saunders, 1998, p. 223.

6. **(B)** This infant is full-term and small for gestational age (SGA). The SGA infant is at risk for hypoglycemia, meconium aspiration, congenital infections, congeni-

tal anomalies, temperature instability, and polycythemia.

Reference: Buschbach, D.: Physical assessment of the newborn infant. *In* Deacon, J., and O'Neill, P. (Eds.): *Core Curriculum for Neonatal Intensive Care Nursing,* 2nd ed. Philadelphia, W. B. Saunders, 1999, p. 74.

7. **(D)** These characteristics are consistent with those of a full-term infant. The full-term infant has thick skin in which veins are difficult to see, a breast bud of 5 to 10 mm, and ears that are formed and have instant recoil.

Reference: Katz, K., and Nishioka, E.: Neonatal assessment. *In* Kenner, C., Lott, J. W., and Flandermeyer, A. A. (Eds.): *Comprehensive Neonatal Nursing: A Physiologic Perspective,* 2nd ed. Philadelphia, W. B. Saunders, 1998, p. 223.

8. **(D)** A full-term infant is an infant who has completed 37 weeks of gestation. Ninety percent of infants born at 38 weeks' gestation have a birth weight greater than approximately 2400 grams. This infant is small for gestational age.

Reference: Katz, K., and Nishioka, E.: Neonatal assessment. *In* Kenner, C., Lott, J. W., and Flandermeyer, A. A. (Eds.): *Comprehensive Neonatal Nursing: A Physiologic Perspective,* 2nd ed. Philadelphia, W. B. Saunders, 1998, p. 223.

9. **(A)** A simplified version of the Dubowitz scoring examination, the Ballard examination assesses six physical and six neuromuscular characteristics.

Reference: Katz, K., and Nishioka, E.: Neonatal assessment. *In* Kenner, C., Lott, J. W., and Flandermeyer, A. A. (Eds.): *Comprehensive Neonatal Nursing: A Physiologic Perspective,* 2nd ed. Philadelphia, W. B. Saunders, 1998, p. 223.

10. **(A)** Alpha-fetoprotein levels in amniotic fluid are measured primarily to identify fetal anomalies. Elevated levels are associated with neural tube defects; low levels have been associated with Down syndrome. Gestational age must be known for accurate interpretation of alpha-fetoprotein levels.

Reference: Kenner, C., Hilse, M. A., and Hetteberg, C.: Human genetics. *In* Kenner, C., Lott, J. W., and Flandermeyer, A. A. (Eds.): *Comprehensive Neonatal Nursing: A Physiologic Perspective,* 2nd ed. Philadelphia, W. B. Saunders, 1998, p. 87.

11. **(C)** The square window sign evaluates joint mobility and is performed by flexing the infant's hand to the forearm. The degree of wrist flexion is then measured.

Reference: Katz, K., Nishioka, E.: Neonatal assessment. *In* Kenner, C., Lott, J. W., and Flandermeyer, A. A.

(Eds.): *Comprehensive Neonatal Nursing: A Physiologic Perspective,* 2nd ed. Philadelphia, W. B. Saunders, 1998, p. 223.

12. **(B)** Resting posture, arm recoil, scarf sign, leg recoil, arm recoil, head lag, and ventral suspension are all components of the Dubowitz scoring examination, which evaluates muscle tone. Muscle tone increases with gestational age.

Reference: Katz, K., and Nishioka, E.: Neonatal assessment. *In* Kenner, C., Lott, J. W., and Flandermeyer, A. A. (Eds.): *Comprehensive Neonatal Nursing: A Physiologic Perspective,* 2nd ed. Philadelphia, W. B. Saunders, 1998, p. 223.

13. **(C)** Neonatal and maternal conditions can affect the gestational age assessment examination findings. When a large discrepancy exists between maternal dates and the examination results, the infant should be re-evaluated again after 24 hours.

Reference: Katz, K., Nishioka, E.: Neonatal assessment. *In* Kenner, C., Lott, J. W., and Flandermeyer, A. A. (Eds.): *Comprehensive Neonatal Nursing: A Physiologic Perspective,* 2nd ed. Philadelphia, W. B. Saunders, 1998, p. 223.

14. **(A)** For infants less than 26 weeks of gestational age, the New Ballard Score has been shown to be most reliable when the examination is performed before 12 hours of age.

Reference: Ballard, J. L., Khoury, J. C., Wedig, K., Wang, L., and Eilers-Walsman, M. B.: New Ballard Score, expanded to include extremely premature infants. *J Pediatrics* 119:417, 1991.

15. **(B)** Infants with asymmetric growth restriction are usually below the 10th percentile for only weight. Infants with symmetric growth restriction have delays in weight, length, and head circumference. These infants have suffered from a longer and earlier growth restriction. Additionally, decreased head circumference indicates decreased brain growth. There is a more frequent association of viral diseases and chromosomal anomalies in the symmetric group.

Reference: Dodd, V.: Gestational age assessment. *Neonatal Network* 15:27, 1996.

16. **(D)** The arm recoil is performed by flexing the arms at the elbows for 5 seconds, then extending the arms to the infant's side, then releasing the arms. Full-term infants will quickly return their arms to the flexed position. Premature infants react with a range of responses, from no flexion to relaxed and little flexion.

Reference: Katz, K., and Nishioka, E.: Neonatal assessment. *In* Kenner, C., Lott, J. W., and Flandermeyer, A. A. (Eds.): *Comprehensive Neonatal Nursing: A Physiologic Perspective,* 2nd ed. Philadelphia, W. B. Saunders, 1998, p. 223.

17. **(C)** Plantar creases over the entire sole are not evident until term. Resistance of the arm to being pulled to the opposite side of the body is also not seen until near term. The skin of a very premature infant, for example, 28 weeks, would be expected to be gelatinous with visible veins. Of the characteristics listed, the finding most consistent with a 32-week-gestation infant would be the ear characteristics, which is well formed yet not thick or stiff.

Reference: Katz, K., Nishioka, E.: Neonatal assessment. *In* Kenner, C., Lott, J. W., and Flandermeyer, A. A. (Eds.): *Comprehensive Neonatal Nursing: A Physiologic Perspective,* 2nd ed. Philadelphia, W. B. Saunders, 1998, p. 223.

18. **(C)** Fentanyl is an analgesic and sedative and thus may influence an infant's posture and muscle tone.

Reference: Dodd, V.: Gestational age assessment. *Neonatal Network* 15(1):127, 1996.

19. **(C)** Because this infant is small for gestational age in all three measurements, this infant has symmetric growth restriction. These infants have experienced an earlier or longer growth deficit than asymmetrically growth restricted infants. Congenital viral infections and congenital anomalies are included in the causes of symmetric growth restriction.

Reference: Dodd, V.: Gestational age assessment. *Neonatal Network* 15(1):27, 1996.

20. **(D)** The term, healthy neonate displays a flexed posture, indicating good muscle tone. Preterm neonates have a relaxed posture. Hypertonicity or hypotonicity may be indicative of many other problems.

Reference: Katz, K., and Nishioka, E.: Neonatal assessment. *In* Kenner, C., Lott, J. W., and Flandermeyer, A. A. (Eds.): *Comprehensive Neonatal Nursing,* 2nd ed. Philadelphia, W. B. Saunders, 1998, p. 223.

21. **(D)** Recall of the date of LMP is accurate in 75 to 85% of women. Utilizing Nägele's rule with the date of LMP allows an approximate calculation of gestational age.

Reference: Katz, K., and Nishioka, E.: Neonatal assessment. *In* Kenner, C., Lott, J. W., and Flandermeyer, A. A. (Eds.): *Comprehensive Neonatal Nursing,* 2nd ed. Philadelphia, W. B. Saunders, 1998, p. 223.

22. **(D)** The preterm neonate lacks subcutaneous fat, and blood vessels are evident over the chest and abdomen. The rest are attributes of a term neonate.

Reference: Katz, K., and Nishioka, E.: Neonatal assessment. *In* Kenner, C., Lott, J. W., and Flandermeyer, A. A. (Eds.): *Comprehensive Neonatal Nursing,* 2nd ed. Philadelphia, W. B. Saunders, 1998, p. 223.

23. **(B)** The angle of the square window decreases with increasing gestational age.

Reference: Buschbach, D.: Physical assessment of the newborn infant. *In* Deacon, J., O'Neill, P. (Eds.): *Core Curriculum for Neonatal Intensive Care Nursing,* 2nd ed. Philadelphia, W. B. Saunders, 1999, p. 74.

24. **(A)** At 36 weeks' gestation, an infant has a thick layer of vernix over the entire body. As the gestation increases, the fetus' continuous exposure to amniotic fluid decreases the amount of vernix until only the vernix within the skinfolds remains.

Reference: Katz, K., and Nishioka, E.: Neonatal assessment. *In* Kenner, C., Lott, J. W., and Flandermeyer, A. A. (Eds.): *Comprehensive Neonatal Nursing,* 2nd ed. Philadelphia, W. B. Saunders, 1998, p. 223.

25. **(D)** The post-term infant who has been exposed to amniotic fluid for a prolonged period of time will develop desquamation at the ankles and wrists and possibly of the palms of the hands and soles of the feet. All of the other findings are consistent with a preterm infant.

Reference: Gardner, S., Lepley, C., and Lubchenco, L.: Initial nursery care. *In* Gardner, S., Merenstein, G. (Eds.): *Handbook of Neonatal Care,* 4th ed. St. Louis, Mosby-YearBook, 1998, p. 76.

26. **(D)** Congenital infection typically results in a neonate who is small for gestational age (SGA). Birth trauma occurs from complications of the large neonate trying to move through the birth passage; asphyxia is frequently caused by the trauma of this birth process. Hypoglycemia can be due to gestational diabetes leading to a large neonate, but does occur in LGA infants without maternal diabetes.

Reference: Buschbach, D.: Physical assessment of the newborn infant. *In* Deacon, J., and O'Neill, P. (Eds.): *Core Curriculum for Neonatal Intensive Care Nursing,* 2nd ed. Philadelphia, W. B. Saunders, 1999, p. 74.

27. **(C)** At 23 weeks' gestation, the neonate's skin will be sticky, friable, and transparent with **no** lanugo. The rest of the findings are all characteristic of a very low birth weight (VLBW) neonate.

Reference: Buschbach, D.: Physical assessment of the newborn infant. *In* Deacon, J., and O'Neill, P. (Eds.): *Core Curriculum for Neonatal Intensive Care Nursing*, 2nd ed. Philadelphia, W. B. Saunders, 1999, p. 74.

28. **(D)** This infant is large for gestational age (LGA). Large infants who have difficulty in passing through the birth canal can have damage to their cervical or brachial plexus due to stretching during delivery. Asymmetrical movement of the upper extremities is consistent with peripheral nerve damage.

References: Buschbach, D.: Physical assessment of the newborn infant. *In* Deacon, J., and O'Neill, P. (Eds.): *Core Curriculum for Neonatal Intensive Care Nursing*, 2nd ed. Philadelphia, W. B. Saunders, 1999, p. 74.
McCulloch, M.: Neurologic disorders. *In* Deacon, J., and O'Neill, P. (Eds.): *Core Curriculum for Neonatal Intensive Care Nursing*, 2nd ed. Philadelphia, W. B. Saunders, 1999, p. 474.

29. **(D)** Maternal chronic hypertension predisposes the neonate to intrauterine growth retardation secondary to decreased placental blood flow. There can also be premature placental aging or placental infarction.

Reference: Broussard, A.: Antepartum-intrapartum complications. *In* Deacon, J., and O'Neill, P. (Eds.): *Core Curriculum for Neonatal Intensive Care Nursing*, 2nd ed. Philadelphia, W. B. Saunders, 1999, p. 18.

30. **(A)** The Ballard examination (Ballard Maturational Score) was refined and expanded to include assessment of extremely premature infants (<26 weeks' gestation). This revised gestational age assessment tool is the New Ballard Score.

Reference: Ballard, J. L., Khoury, J. C., Wedig, K., Wang, L., and Eilers-Walsman, M. B.: New Ballard Score, expanded to include extremely premature infants. *J Pediatrics* 119:417, 1991.

31. **(A)** The skin of the extremely premature infant is sticky, transparent, and without any lanugo. The premature infant has smooth skin with visible veins, the term infant has thick skin with few visible veins, and the post-term infant has skin like parchment.

References: Ballard, J. L., Khoury, J. C., Wedig, K., Wang, L., and Eilers-Walsman, M. B.: New Ballard Score, expanded to include extremely premature infants. *J Pediatrics* 119:417, 1991.
Dodd, V.: Gestational age assessment. *Neonatal Network* 15:27, 1996.

32. **(D)** Eyelid separation was included in the New Ballard Score because separation normally occurs toward the end of gestation. Eyelid separation is scored as either loosely fused (closed, but able to open with gentle traction) or tightly fused.

Reference: Ballard, J. L., Khoury, J. C., Wedig, K., Wang, L., and Eilers-Walsman, M. B.: New Ballard Score, expanded to include extremely premature infants. *J Pediatrics* 119:417, 1991.

CHAPTER 6
THERMOREGULATION

1. **(C)** A Servocontrolled warmer/incubator can generate excess heat, causing hyperthermia if the probe is malfunctioning or becomes detached from the infant's skin.

References: Chatson, K., Fant, M., Cloherty, J.: Temperature control. *In* Cloherty, J., and Stark, A. (Eds.): *Manual of Neonatal Care*, 4th ed. Philadelphia, Lippincott-Raven Publishers, 1998, p. 139.
Perlstein, P. H.: Physical environment. *In* Fanaroff, A. A., and Martin, R. J. (Eds.): *Neonatal-Perinatal Medicine: Diseases of the Fetus and Infant*, 6th ed. St. Louis, C. V. Mosby, 1997, p. 481.

2. **(A)** Hypermetabolism requires an energy source and can quickly deplete glycogen stores. Evaporative heat loss can lead to dehydration.

Reference: Blake, W. W., Murray, J. A.: Heat balance. *In* Merenstein, G., and Gardner, S. (Eds.): *Handbook of Neonatal Intensive Care*, 4th ed. St. Louis, C. V. Mosby, 1998, p. 100.
Amlung, S.: Neonatal thermoregulation. *In* Kenner, C., Lott, J., and Flandermeyer, A. (Eds.): *Comprehensive Neonatal Nursing: A Physiologic Perspective*, 2nd ed. Philadelphia, W. B. Saunders, 1998, p. 207.

3. **(D)** The physiologically competent infant will respond to overheating from a hot environment through heat-losing mechanisms such as vasodilation and evaporative heat loss due to tachypnea and sweating. Hyperactivity and irritability are typical responses to overheating. The skin will be warmer than the core temperature.

Reference: Perlstein, P. H.: Physical environment. *In* Fanaroff, A. A., and Martin, R. J. (Eds.): *Neonatal-Perinatal Medicine: Diseases of the Fetus and Infant*, 6th ed. St. Louis, C. V. Mosby, 1997, p. 481.

4. **(B)** The neonatal head represents one fifth of the body surface and is a source of significant heat loss in the infant. The brain's heat production is 55% of total metabolic heat production in the newborn.

Reference: Perlstein, P. H.: Physical environment. *In* Fanaroff, A. A., and Martin, R. J. (Eds.): *Neonatal-Perina-*

tal Medicine: Diseases of the Fetus and Infant, 6th ed. St. Louis, C. V. Mosby, 1997, p. 481.

5. **(A)** Because the infant's head surface is the greatest source of heat loss, and the infant emerges from a wet, warm environment into a dry, cooler environment, evaporative heat loss potential is great. Heat loss will continue until the infant is dried, wrapped with the head covered (blanket or insulated fabric head covering), and placed with the mother or placed in a preheated warmer.

Reference: Perlstein, P. H.: Physical environment. *In* Fanaroff, A. A., and Martin, R. J. (Eds.): *Neonatal-Perinatal Medicine: Diseases of the Fetus and Infant*, 6th ed. St. Louis, C. V. Mosby, 1997, p. 481.

6. **(C)** A heat-gaining environment exists only if the infant begins to get warm; warming the air temperature higher than the infant's temperature is inadequate. The goal is to produce an environment in which the infant is rewarmed by the heat actually generated by the infant.

Reference: Perlstein, P. H.: Physical environment. *In* Fanaroff, A. A., and Martin, R. J. (Eds.): *Neonatal-Perinatal Medicine: Diseases of the Fetus and Infant*, 6th ed. St. Louis, C. V. Mosby, 1997, p. 481.

7. **(A)** Skin temperature can vary widely. Appropriate placement is over the liver, between the umbilicus and pubis, but not over areas of brown adipose tissue (brown fat) or poorly vasoreactive areas like extremities, bony prominences, or excoriated areas.

Reference: Perlstein, P. H.: Physical environment. *In* Fanaroff, A. A., and Martin, R. J. (Eds.): *Neonatal-Perinatal Medicine: Diseases of the Fetus and Infant*, 6th ed. St. Louis, C. V. Mosby, 1997, p. 481.

8. **(B)** Thermal instability often occurs in a septic infant, but there is no proven basis to identify hypothermia as a sign of sepsis. Profound sepsis produces shock and vasodilation that can increase heat loss and suppress the infant's normal homeothermic reactions.

Reference: Perlstein, P. H.: Physical environment. *In* Fanaroff, A. A., and Martin, R. J. (Eds.): *Neonatal-Perinatal Medicine: Diseases of the Fetus and Infant*, 6th ed. St. Louis, C. V. Mosby, 1997, p. 481.

9. **(B)** The infant's weight is 5% of the adult's, whereas its body surface is 15% of the adult's, increasing the surface-to-body ratio of the infant.

Reference: Bakewell-Sachs, S., Shaw, V., and Tashman, A.: *Assessment of Risk in the Term Newborn.* White Plains, N.Y., March of Dimes Birth Defects Foundation, 1997, p. 32.

10. **(D)** Nonshivering thermogenesis (NST) is initiated by release of norepinephrine in response to cold stress. The end-point of this metabolic process is lysis of brown fat for heat production. Inhibiting norepinephrine's physiologic effect decreases the potential for heat production by NST.

References: Blake, W. W., and Murray, J. A.: Heat balance. *In* Merenstein, G., and Gardner, S. (Eds.): *Handbook of Neonatal Intensive Care*, 4th ed. St. Louis, C. V. Mosby, 1998, p. 100.
Amlung, S.: Neonatal thermoregulation. *In* Kenner, C., Lott, J., and Flandermeyer, A. (Eds.): *Comprehensive Neonatal Nursing: A Physiologic Perspective*, 2nd ed. Philadelphia, W. B. Saunders, 1998, p. 207.

11. **(D)** Brown fat is distributed in the well-perfused upper thorax, paraspinal areas, and perirenal area.

Reference: Perlstein, P. H.: Physical environment. *In* Fanaroff, A. A., and Martin, R. J. (Eds.): *Neonatal-Perinatal Medicine: Diseases of the Fetus and Infant*, 6th ed. St. Louis, C. V. Mosby, 1997, p. 481.

12. **(D)** Brown fat begins to develop at 26 to 30 weeks' gestation. Decreased brown fat stores in preterm infants limit thermoregulatory potential and are usually depleted in response to heat-losing events in the first hours and days of life.

Reference: Baumgart, S.: Temperature regulation of the premature infant. *In* Taeusch, H., and Ballard, R. (Eds.): *Avery's Diseases of the Newborn*, 7th ed. Philadelphia, W. B. Saunders, 1998, p. 367.

13. **(D)** In a thermoneutral state, an infant is neither gaining nor losing heat, oxygen consumption is minimal, and the core-to-skin gradient is small ($\pm$ 0.5° C).

References: Chatson, K., Fant, M., and Cloherty, J.: *In* Cloherty, J. and Stark, A. (Eds.): *Manual of Neonatal Care*, 4th ed. Philadelphia, Lippincott-Raven Publishers, 1998, p. 139.
Perlstein, P. H.: Physical environment. *In* Fanaroff, A. A., and Martin, R. J. (Eds.): *Neonatal-Perinatal Medicine: Diseases of the Fetus and Infant*, 6th ed. St. Louis, C. V. Mosby, 1997, p. 481.

14. **(C)** An increased metabolic rate complicates the course for immature/compromised infants by increased oxygen consumption. Stressed infants may be unable to provide enough oxygen, and heat production converts to an anaerobic process

resulting in oxygen debt and lactic acidosis.

References: Baumgart, S.: Temperature regulation of the premature infant. *In* Taeusch, H., and Ballard, R. (Eds.): *Avery's Diseases of the Newborn*, 7th ed. Philadelphia, W. B. Saunders, 1998, p. 367.
Perlstein, P. H.: Physical environment. *In* Fanaroff, A. A., and Martin, R. J. (Eds.): *Neonatal-Perinatal Medicine: Diseases of the Fetus and Infant*, 6th ed. St. Louis, C. V. Mosby, 1997, p. 481.

15. **(C)** Raising humidity in the incubator increases the water vapor pressure and decreases fluid and heat loss by evaporation.

References: Lund, C., Kuller, J., Lane, A., Wright-Lott, J., and Raines, D.: Neonatal skin care: the scientific basis for practice. *J Obstet Gynecol Neonatal Nurs* 28(3):241, 1999.
Perlstein, P. H.: Physical environment. *In* Fanaroff, A. A., and Martin, R. J. (Eds.): *Neonatal-Perinatal Medicine: Diseases of the Fetus and Infant*, 6th ed. St. Louis, C. V. Mosby, 1997, p. 481.

16. **(B)** Heat is dissipated to the skin surface through blood, conducted from the body surface to surrounding air (boundary layer), and diffused to moving air particles. The air temperature and air flow in an enclosed incubator are not homogeneous. The air temperature is modified by air flow (associated with wind chill factor introduced by a circulating fan).

References: Bakewell-Sachs, S., Shaw, V., and Tashman, A.: *Assessment of Risk in the Term Newborn*. White Plains, N.Y., March of Dimes Birth Defects Foundation, 1997, p. 32.
Perlstein, P. H.: Physical environment. *In* Fanaroff, A. A., and Martin, R. J. (Eds.): *Neonatal-Perinatal Medicine: Diseases of the Fetus and Infant*, 6th ed. St. Louis, C. V. Mosby, 1997, p. 481.

17. **(A)** Infants lose heat to cooler incubator walls. Infants will gain heat when a heat source, such as a lamp, traps heat in the incubator, resulting in a "greenhouse" effect.

Reference: Perlstein, P. H.: Physical environment. *In* Fanaroff, A. A., and Martin, R. J. (Eds.): *Neonatal-Perinatal Medicine: Diseases of the Fetus and Infant*, 6th ed. St. Louis, C. V. Mosby, 1997, p. 481.

18. **(D)** Conduction describes the transfer of heat between contacting solid objects of different temperatures. The rate at which heat is transferred is proportional to the size of the internal gradient.

Reference: Perlstein, P. H.: Physical environment. *In* Fanaroff, A. A., and Martin, R. J. (Eds.): *Neonatal-Perinatal Medicine: Diseases of the Fetus and Infant*, 6th ed. St. Louis, C. V. Mosby, 1997, p. 481.

19. **(C)** Thermal receptors in the skin, with the trigeminal area of the face being the most sensitive, are mediators of the hypothalmic response to cold stress or temperature change. Stimulation of these receptors initially leads to heat-conserving responses such as peripheral vasoconstriction, which manifests as acrocyanosis.

Reference: Blake, W. W., and Murray, J.: Heat balance. *In* Merenstein, G., and Gardner, S. (Eds.): *Handbook of Neonatal Intensive Care*, 4th ed. St. Louis, Mosby, 1998, p. 100.

20. **(B)** Little variation in physiologic parameters, including thermoregulation, has been demonstrated in studies of kangaroo care. Both average for gestational age (AGA) and small for gestational age (SGA) infants experience a beneficial warming and stable skin and core temperatures when held skin-to-skin. Mothers exhibit thermal synchrony with the infants so their body temperatures increase and decrease to maintain the infants' thermal neutrality.

References: Blake, W. W., and Murray, J. A.: Heat balance. *In* Merenstein, G., and Gardner, S. (Eds.): *Handbook of Neonatal Intensive Care*, 4th ed. St. Louis, C. V. Mosby, 1998, p. 100.
Legault, M., and Goulet, C.: Comparison of kangaroo care and traditional methods of removing preterm infants from incubators. *J Obstet Gynecol Neonatal Nurs* 24(6):503, 1995.

21. **(D)** The AWHONN research utilization project to test research-based protocols for thermoregulation established that the infant is eligible to begin the process of weaning from an incubator to an open crib when:

The infant weighs approximately 1500 g
The infant has 5 consistent days of weight gain
Apnea and bradycardia episodes have stabilized
Nutrition is enteral
The infant is medically stable
The infant does not require assisted ventilation

Reference: Medoff-Cooper, B.: Transition of the preterm infant to an open crib. *J Obstet Gynecol Neonatal Nurs* 23(4):329, 1994.

CHAPTER 7
FLUIDS AND ELECTROLYTES

1. **(A)** In the diuretic phase, urine output is increased up to 7 mL/kg/hr, insensible

water loss (IWL) remains high, and body weight decreases 1 to 3% per day. Urinary sodium loss natriuresis accompanies diuresis.

Reference: Cloherty, J. P., and Stark, A. R.: *Manual of Neonatal Care*, 4th ed. Philadelphia, Lippincott-Raven, 1998, p. 87.

2. **(B)** Poor skin keratinization, high skin water content, decreased amount of subcutaneous fat, and a large surface area to mass ratio predisposes the preterm infant to high evaporative losses. This infant has lost 16% of his birth weight. The maximum amount an infant should lose is 10 to 15% of the birth weight. In this case, the fluids are too low for the losses. The humidity is set too low to minimize insensible water loss.

Reference: Sequin, J.: Relative humidity under radiant warmers: influence of humidifier and ambient relative humidity. *Am J Perinatol* 14:515, 1997.

3. **(D)** Improved renal function in the days after birth from increased glomerular filtration rate (GFR) will affect the excretion of medications administered. Antidiuretic hormone (ADH) is released from the posterior pituitary.

Reference: Cloherty, J. P., and Stark, A. R.: *Manual of Neonatal Care*, 4th ed. Philadelphia, Lippincott-Raven, 1998, p. 591.

4. **(C)** Edema is the abnormal accumulation of extracellular fluid (ECF) within the interstitial spaces and may be caused by increased hydrostatic pressure within the capillaries, increased capillary permeability, or low colloid osmotic pressure.

Reference: Stokowski, L. C.: Metabolic disorders. *In* Deacon, J., and O'Neill, P. (Eds.): *Core Curriculum for Neonatal Intensive Care Nursing*, 2nd ed. Philadelphia, W. B. Saunders, 1999, p. 326.

5. **(A)** The laboratory results indicate that this infant is hyponatremic (Na <130 mEq/L). A chronic hyponatremic state is corrected gradually with sodium chloride within 48 to 72 hours to prevent injury to brain cells. Although the serum potassium is normal, the increased CO_2 (normal 14–27 mEq/L) suggests there is an intracellular depletion of potassium. KC1 supplementation is indicated to treat the intracellular depletion of potassium.

Reference: Modi, N.: Hyponatremia in the newborn. *Arch Dis Child Fetal Neonatal Ed* 78:F84, 1998.

6. **(A)** Hyponatremia may be asymptomatic, but apnea irritability, twitching, or seizures occur if Na^+ drops acutely or falls to less than 115 mEq/L.

Reference: Modi, N.: Hyponatremia in the newborn. *Arch Dis Child Fetal Neonatal Ed* 78:F84, 1998.

7. **(A)** The infant is being placed to breast but the intake is too low, as noted by only two wet diapers per day. The infant is portraying the symptomatology of hypernatremia.

Reference: Molteni, K. H.: Initial management of hypernatremic dehydration in the breast-fed infant. *Clin Pediatrics* 33:731, 1994.

8. **(D)** Hypokalemia potentiates digitalis toxicity, which can cause first-degree heart block.

Reference: Young, T. E., and Mangum, O. B.: *Neofax: A Manual of Drugs Used in Neonatal Care*, 13th ed. Raleigh, Acorn Publishing, 2000, p. 13.

9. **(C)** Metabolic acidosis will shift potassium out of the cells. Glomerular filtration rate (GFR) is decreased and the normal post-natal shift of potassium is from intracellular compartment to extracellular compartment. A traumatic premature birth will cause endogenous release of potassium from tissue destruction, hypoperfusion, and bruising.

Reference: Lorenz, J. M., Kleinman, L. I., and Markarian, K.: Potassium metabolism in extremely low birth weight infants in the first week of life. *J Pediatrics* 131:82, 1997.

10. **(D)** Phototherapy and increased environmental temperature will increase insensible water loss (IWL). Increasing fluid administration does not influence IWL. Use of an incubator can decrease IWL by as much as 50% compared with a radiant warmer.

Reference: Oh, W.: Fluid and electrolyte management. *In* Fanaroff, A. A., and Martin, R. J. (Eds.): *Neonatal-Perinatal Medicine: Diseases of the Fetus and Infant*, 6th ed. St. Louis, Mosby, 1997, p. 622.

11. **(D)** The laboratory findings indicate hyperkalemia. Glucose/insulin infusions increase cellular uptake of potassium. Kayexalate binds with potassium and eliminates it from the body. Calcium gluconate stabilizes the cell membrane, protecting cell membranes against the effect of hyperkalemia. Sodium chloride does not decrease serum potassium.

Reference: Lorenz, J. M., Kleinman, L. I., and Markarian, K.: Potassium metabolism in extremely low birth weight infants in the first week of life. *J Pediatrics* 131:82, 1997.

12. **(D)** Hyperkalemia manifests with ventricular tachycardia, peaked T waves, and a widened QRS. Hypercalcemia manifests with hypotonia, weakness irritability, and poor feeding. Hypokalemia manifests with flattened T waves, prominent U waves, ST depression, hypotonia, and abdominal distention. The main clinical finding of hypocalcemia is jitteriness and seizures.

References: Demarini, S., Mimouni, F. B., and Tsang, R. C.: Disorders of calcium, phosphorus, and magnesium metabolism. *In* Fanaroff, A. A., and Martin, R. J. (Eds.): *Neonatal-Perinatal Medicine: Diseases of the Fetus and Infant*, 6th ed. St. Louis, Mosby, 1997, p. 1463.
Tsang, R. C., Demarini, S., and Rath, L. L.: Fluids, electrolytes, vitamins, and trace minerals: basis of ingestion, digestion, elimination, and metabolism. *In* Kenner, C., Lott, J. W., and Flandermeyer, A. A. (Eds.): *Comprehensive Neonatal Nursing: A Physiologic Perspective*, 2nd ed. Philadelphia, W. B. Saunders, 1998, p. 336.

13. **(D)** Calcium chloride is used generally during cardiopulmonary resuscitation. When calcium gluconate is administered, the patient should be monitored and the administration should be on a syringe pump for 20 to 30 minutes. There have been reports of intestinal necrosis and liver necrosis when a calcium infusion has been given via umbilical catheter.

Reference: Young, T. E., and Mangum, O. B.: *Neofax: A Manual of Drugs Used in Neonatal Care*, 13th ed. Raleigh, Acorn Publishing, 2000, p. 196.

14. **(B)** Trisomy 13, trisomy 18, and Down syndromes are not associated with hypocalcemia. DiGeorge syndrome is absence of the thymus and parathyroid glands.

Reference: Cloherty, J. P., and Stark, A. R.: *Manual of Neonatal Care*, 4th ed. Philadelphia, Lippincott-Raven, 1998, p. 83.

15. **(B)** A dose of 70 mL/kg/day for an 865 g infant equals 2.5 mL/hr (70 mL/day × 0.865 kg ÷ 24 h). This rate provides 3.6 mg/kg/min of glucose (75 mg glucose/mL × 2.5 mL/hr ÷ 60 min/hr ÷ 0.865 kg). The minimal amount of glucose to be administered to maintain homeostasis is 4 mg/kg/min to prevent hypoglycemia.

Reference: Stokowski, L. C.: Metabolic disorders. *In* Deacon, J., and O'Neill, P. (Eds): *Core Curriculum for Neo-*

natal Intensive Care Nursing, 2nd ed. Philadelphia, W. B. Saunders, 1999, p. 326.

16. **(B)** Water is the most abundant component of the body. At birth, total body water accounts for approximately 75% of body weight and extracellular fluid accounts for approximately 40% of total body weight in full-term infants. Total body water and extracellular fluid increase with decreasing gestational age. Total body water accounts for approximately 83% of body weight and extracellular fluid accounts for approximately 5% of body weight in the preterm infant born at 32 weeks' gestation.

References: Oh, W.: Fluid and electrolyte management. *In* Fanaroff, A. A., and Martin, R. J. (Eds.): *Neonatal-Perinatal Medicine: Diseases of the Fetus and Infant*, 6th ed. St. Louis, Mosby, 1997, p. 622.
Tsang, R. C., Demarini, S., and Rath, L. L.: Fluids, electrolytes, vitamins, and trace minerals: basis of ingestion, digestion, elimination, and metabolism. *In* Kenner, C., Lott, J. W., and Flandermeyer, A. A. (Eds.): *Comprehensive Neonatal Nursing: A Physiologic Perspective*, 2nd ed. Philadelphia, W. B. Saunders, 1998, p. 336.

17. **(D)** This infant's urine output is 6.9 mL/kg/hr (160 mL ÷ 24 h ÷ 0.965 kg). In the diuretic phase, urine output is increased up to 7 mL/kg/hr, IWL remains high and body weight decreases 1 to 3% per day.

Reference: Cloherty, J. P., and Stark, A. R.: *Manual of Neonatal Care*, 4th ed. Philadelphia, Lippincott-Raven, 1998, p. 87.

18. **(A)** IV fluids/day = 93.6 mL (3.9 mL/hr × 24 hr). PO fluids/day = 96 mL (12 mL × 8 feedings/day). Total daily fluids = 189.6 mL (93.6 mL × 96 mL). Daily fluids/kg = 150 mL/kg/day (189.6 ÷ 1.265 kg).

Reference: Cloherty, J. P., and Stark, A. R.: *Manual of Neonatal Care*, 4th ed. Philadelphia, Lippincott-Raven, 1998, p. 87.

19. **(D)** Generally if an infant fails to respond to therapy for hypocalcemia, the correlating problem is hypomagnesemia.

Reference: Cloherty, J. P., and Stark, A. R.: *Manual of Neonatal Care*, 4th ed. Philadelphia, Lippincott-Raven, 1998, p. 719.

20. **(C)** Diagnostic test for metabolic bone disease will indicate a normal calcium, low phosphorus, and high alkaline phosphatase level.

Reference: Cloherty, J. P., and Stark, A. R.: *Manual of Neonatal Care*, 4th ed. Philadelphia, Lippincott-Raven, 1998, p. 553.

21. **(A)** The laboratory results and clinical presentation of the infant are consistent with hypocalcemia. Normal serum results for fullterm infants are: Na^+ 135–145 mEq/L, K^+ 3.8–6 mEq/L, Ca^+ (<1 week) 7–12 mg/dl, Cl^- 96–109 mEq/L.

References: Cloherty, J. P., and Stark, A. R.: *Manual of Neonatal Care*, 4th ed. Philadelphia, Lippincott-Raven, 1998, p. 553.
Zenk, K., Sills, J. H., and Koeppel, R. M.: *Neonatal Medications and Nutrition: A Comprehensive Guide.* Santa Rosa, CA, NICU Ink, 1999.

CHAPTER 8
NUTRITION AND FEEDING

1. **(B)** Erythropoietin is used to stimulate the production of red blood cells from the bone marrow. Increasing erythropoiesis in preterm infants already low in iron stores requires additional iron supplementation.

Reference: Shannon, K. M., Keith, J. F., Mentzer, W. C., Ehrenkranz, R. A., et al.: Recombinant human erythropoietin stimulates erythropoiesis and reduces erythrocyte transfusions in very low birth weight preterm infants. *Pediatrics* 95(1):1, 1995.

2. **(C)** Portagen is a specialized formula designed for infants who cannot efficiently digest or absorb conventional dietary fat or have certain lymphatic anomalies. Common indications are infants with fatty acid metabolism defects and those with persistent chylothorax. Soy-based formulas are indicated for infants with IgE-mediated reaction to cow's milk protein. Portagen is not indicated for infants with feeding intolerance or renal insufficiency.

Reference: American Academy of Pediatrics Committee on Nutrition: *Pediatric Nutrition Handbook*, 4th ed. Elk Grove Village, Ill., The Academy, 1998.

3. **(B)** Preterm infants fed human milk have a lower rate of a variety of infections, including necrotizing enterocolitis and urinary tract infections. Although the preferred enteral feeding, breast-milk requires fortification to adequately supply the preterm infant's need for protein, calcium, phosphorus, and calories. Additionally, the nutritional value of breast-milk changes during lactation.

Reference: El-Mohandes, A. E., Picard, M. B., Simmens, S., et al.: Use of human milk in the intensive care

nursery decreases the incidence of nosocomial sepsis. *J Perinatol* 17:130, 1997.
Schanler, R. J.: Human milk fortification for premature infants. *Am J Clin Nutrit* 64:249, 1996.

4. **(C)** Elevated sodium, chloride, and blood urea nitrogen (BUN) levels are indicative of dehydration. In addition, interpreting these electrolyte values in conjunction with physical assessment findings (gelatinous skin) and insensible water losses (radiant warmer and phototherapy) makes dehydration the most likely condition. Fluid volume overload presents with diluted chemistry panel results. An elevated creatinine level often accompanies renal failure.

Reference: Oh, W.: Fluid and electrolyte management. *In* Fanaroff, A. A., and Martin, R. J. (Eds.): *Neonatal-Perinatal Medicine, Diseases of the Fetus and Infant*, 6th ed. St. Louis, Mosby-Year Book, 1997, p. 622.

5. **(D)** Calcium and other important substances (such as iron) are passed on to the fetus during the third trimester. Therefore, infants at this gestational age have low stores of calcium. The occurrence of early hypocalcemia in the preterm infant may be as high as 90%. Providing calcium early after birth assists in preventing the development of hypocalcemia.

Reference: Denne, S. C., Clark, S. E., Poindexter, B. B., et al.: Nutrition and metabolism in the high risk neonate. *In* Fanaroff, A. A., and Martin, R. J. (Eds.): *Neonatal-Perinatal Medicine, Diseases of the Fetus and Infant*, 6th ed. St. Louis, Mosby-Year Book, 1997, p. 601.

6. **(C)** Owing to this infant's gestational age, premature skin, and additional fluid losses (phototherapy and radiant warmer use), higher fluid volumes are required to maintain normovolemia. Frequent chemistry panels in addition to close monitoring of vital signs are required to carefully evaluate the fluid status. Premature infants are unable to adequately filter urine even in dehydration states. Maintaining a moderately high relative humidity (35–40%) will decrease insensible water loss (IWL). If humidity is decreased, IWL will increase.

Reference: Oh, W.: Fluids, electrolytes and acid-base homeostasis. *In* Fanaroff, A. A., and Martin, R. J. (Eds.): *Neonatal-Perinatal Medicine, Diseases of the Fetus and Infant*, 6th ed. St. Louis, Mosby-Year Book, 1997, p. 622.

7. **(D)** This infant's acute deterioration is a result of a pleural effusion from an infil-

trated PICC. A pneumothorax would reveal air in the pleural space on radiograph and pneumonia most often reveals consolidation on radiograph. Sepsis could be likely; however, the chest radiographic results are most consistent with a pleural effusion.

Reference: Fioravanti, J., Buzzard, C., and Harris, J.: Pericardial effusion and tamponade as a result of percutaneous silastic catheter use. *Neonatal Network* 17(5):39, 1998.

8. (**A**) Vitamin E stores are low in the premature newborn and rapid growth rates require vitamin E supplementation. Vitamin E is fat soluble and is an antioxidant that is absorbed greater from human milk than from formulas.

Reference: American Academy of Pediatrics Committee on Nutrition: *Pediatric Nutrition Handbook*, 4th ed. Elk Grove Village, Ill., The Academy, 1998.

9. (**C**) Pregestimil is a protein-hydrolysate based formula that is used for infants with malabsorption problems caused by gastrointestinal or hepatobiliary disease. Infants with these problems often have direct hyperbilirubinemia.

Reference: American Academy of Pediatrics Committee on Nutrition: *Pediatric Nutrition Handbook*, 4th ed. Elk Grove Village, Ill., The Academy, 1998.

10. (**C**) Healthy newborns require 100 to 120 kcal/kg/day for adequate growth and development.

Reference: American Academy of Pediatrics Committee on Nutrition: *Pediatric Nutrition Handbook*, 4th ed. Elk Grove Village, Ill., The Academy, 1998.

11. (**D**) Reducing substance in the stool is indicative of excessive sugar content often associated with carbohydrate malabsorption. However, the presence of reducing substance in the stool must be correlated with other signs of malabsorption, such as loose or diarrheal stools and poor weight gain. Although associated with early signs of necrotizing enterocolitis, a positive reducing substance in the stool is not diagnostic and must be evaluated in conjunction with other physical assessment findings.

Reference: American Academy of Pediatrics Committee on Nutrition: *Pediatric Nutrition Handbook*, 4th ed. Elk Grove Village, Ill., The Academy, 1998.

12. (**B**) Similac PM 60/40 is a cow's milk–based formula that has a low phosphorus content and low renal solute load. It is indicated for use in patients with renal insufficiency and infants with hypoparathyroidism.

Reference: American Academy of Pediatrics Committee on Nutrition: *Pediatric Nutrition Handbook*, 4th ed. Elk Grove Village, Ill., The Academy, 1998.

13. (**A**) The presence of bile-stained aspirates, regardless of amount, is never normal and the infant should not be fed until a full evaluation has been done by the physician. Prompt recognition, aggressive monitoring, and early treatment are the mainstays in preventing necrotizing enterocolitis.

Reference: La Gamma, E. F., and Browne, L. E.: Feeding practices for infants weighing less than 1500 g at birth and the pathogenesis of necrotizing enterocolitis. *Clin Perinatol* 21(2):271, 1994.

14. (**C**) The main limiting factor in providing enteral nutrition to preterm infants is gastrointestinal motility. Although gastric capacity is small in preterm infants and gastroesophageal reflux (GER) common, continuous feedings can be used to establish enteral feedings and minimize the symptoms of GER. Unless there is malabsorption syndrome or other intestinal disease, absorption from the gastrointestinal tract of preterm newborns is not altered.

Reference: Berseth, C.: Gastrointestinal motility in the neonate. *Clin Perinatol* 23:179, 1996.

15. (**C**) An elevated alkaline phosphatase level, although nonspecific, is associated with bone demineralization. Hepatobiliary disease also presents with an elevated alkaline phosphatase. Alkaline phosphatase levels in conjunction with calcium and phosphorus should be monitored at routine intervals to assess bone mineralization status and additional calcium and phosphorus supplementation added if levels are elevated.

Reference: Frentner, S.: Metabolic bone disease. *Central Lines* 11(1):4, 1995.

16. (**D**) Total parenteral nutrition (TPN) is associated with cholestasis and cholestatic jaundice, infection, and hyper- and hypoglycemia. Although frequently used as supportive therapy for necrotizing enterocolitis, TPN has not necessarily been associated with the incidence of necrotizing enterocolitis.

Reference: Briones, E., and Iber, F.: Liver and biliary tract changes and injury associated with total parenteral nutrition: Pathogenesis and prevention. *J Am Coll Nutrit* 14(3):219, 1995.

17. **(C)** Early minimal feeding of the premature newborn is associated with improved calcium and phosphorus retention. Other benefits include higher serum calcium and lower alkaline phosphatase levels and shorter intestinal transit times. Early minimal feeding was not associated with an increased incidence of necrotizing enterocolitis.

Reference: Schanler, R. J., Schulman, R. J., Lau, C., et al.: Feeding strategies for premature infants: randomized trial of gastrointestinal priming and tube feeding method. *Pediatrics* 103:434, 1999.

18. **(C)** Carnitine is an essential nutrient for fat metabolism and the production of energy and is present in sufficient quantities in formula and human milk. Owing to poor stores, possible lack of necessary enzymes to synthesize carnitine, and NPO status, the preterm infant is carnitine deficient. This deficiency may lead to increased apnea and bradycardia, failure to thrive, and decreased muscle tone. Infants not being fed enterally are carnitine deficient and require supplementation via total parenteral nutrition.

Reference: Borum, P.: Carnitine in neonatal nutrition. *J Child Neurol* 10(2):2S25, 1995.

19. **(D)** Intravenous lipid administration is associated with many morbidities, including alteration in leukocyte function. Other morbidities include decreased pulmonary diffusion of gases, hyperphospholipidemia, decrease in peripheral oxygenation, and displacement of bound bilirubin by free fatty acids.

Reference: Heird, W.: Amino acid and energy needs of pediatric patients receiving parenteral nutrition. *Pediatric Nutrition* 42(4):765, 1995.

20. **(D)** Preterm infant formulas differ from term infant formulas in many ways. The preterm infant formula provides increased calcium and phosphorus, increased medium chain triglycerides as a fat source, reduced amount of lactose, and increased protein content. These modifications are to enhance the digestability and absorption of nutrients for infants with immature gut function.

Reference: Ernst, J., and Gross, S.: Types and methods of

feeding for infants. *In* Polin, R., and Fox, W. (Eds.): *Fetal and Neonatal Physiology*, 2nd ed. Philadelphia, W. B. Saunders, 1998, p. 363.

21. **(C)** Soy-based formulas are indicated for infants with IgE-mediated reaction to cow's milk protein, for those with lactase deficiency or galactosemia. It is not indicated for infants with bloody stools without further investigation of etiology or for feeding intolerance. Soy-based formulas are not recommended for infants less than 1800 grams because of an increased risk of osteopenia.

Reference: American Academy of Pediatrics Committee on Nutrition: *Pediatric Nutrition Handbook*, 4th ed. Elk Grove Village, Ill., The Academy, 1998.

CHAPTER 9
DEVELOPMENTAL CARE

1. **(A)** The synactive theory of development describes how infants interact and respond with the environment in an attempt to achieve homeostasis. There are five hierarchical subsystems to the theory: autonomic or physiologic, motor, state, attention or interactional, and self-regulation. Behavioral organization occurs when an infant can respond to environmental stimuli with a balance among the subsystems.

References: Koch, S.: Developmental support in the neonatal intensive care unit. *In* Deacon, J., and O'Neill, P. (Eds.): *Core Curriculum for Neonatal Intensive Care Nursing*, 2nd ed. Philadelphia, W. B. Saunders, 1999, p. 522.
Vergara, E.: Understanding newborn infant behavior: neonatal stability. *In Foundations for Practice in the Neonatal Intensive Care Unit and Early Intervention: A Self-Guided Practice Manual*, vol. 1. Rockville, MD., The American Occupational Therapy Association, 1993, p. 23.

2. **(B)** Paced feedings create shortened sucking bursts, which allow the infant to pause, swallow, and breathe. Longer feeding periods would tire the infant out. The number of gavage feedings can be determined when the infant's ability to nipple feed is assessed. Increasing the rate at which the liquid comes from the nipple would allow a large volume of formula to flow without much sucking effort and may overwhelm the infant's ability to swallow quickly enough to prevent choking.

References: Koch, S.: Developmental support in the neonatal intensive care unit. *In* Deacon, J., and O'Neill,

P. (Eds.): *Core Curriculum for Neonatal Intensive Care Nursing*, 2nd ed. Philadelphia, W. B. Saunders, 1999, p. 522.

Vergara, E.: Feeding. *In Foundations for Practice in the Neonatal Intensive Care Unit and Early Intervention: A Self-Guided Practice Manual*, vol. 1. Rockville, MD, The American Occupational Therapy Association, 1993, p. 171.

Wolf, L. S., and Glass, R. P.: Therapeutic treatment strategies for infant feeding dysfunction. *In Feeding and Swallowing Disorders in Infancy: Assessment and Management*. Tucson, AZ, Therapy Skill Builders, 1992, p. 207.

3. **(A)** Developmental care revolves around the relationship that is built between the caregiver and the infant. The relationship develops from the caregiver's learning to observe an infant's behavior and interpret his responses to stimuli and respond appropriately. Developmental care is more than following a protocol of tasks or creating a certain "environment." It is best achieved by creating an individualized care plan that constantly adapts to the infant's state, taking into account his environmental, social, and clinical needs.

References: Koch, S.: Developmental support in the neonatal intensive care unit. *In* Deacon, J., and O'Neill, P. (Eds.): *Core Curriculum for Neonatal Intensive Care Nursing*, 2nd ed. Philadelphia, W. B. Saunders, 1999, p. 522.

VandenBerg, K. A.: Basic principles of developmental caregiving. *Neonatal Network* 16(7):69, 1997.

4. **(D)** Based on the hierarchical relationship of the subsystems in the synactive theory of development, if an infant is already showing signs of decompensation or disorganization (as evidenced by time-out signals), the infant's physiologic stability may be compromised if the offending stimulus is not removed.

References: Koch, S.: Developmental support in the neonatal intensive care unit. *In* Deacon, J., and O'Neill, P. (Eds.): *Core Curriculum for Neonatal Intensive Care Nursing*, 2nd ed. Philadelphia, W. B. Saunders, 1999, p. 522.

VandenBerg, K. A.: Behaviorally supportive care for the extremely premature infant. *In* Gunderson, L. P., and Kenner, C. (Eds.): *Care of the 24–25 Week Gestational Age Infant: Small Baby Protocol*. Petaluma, CA, NICU INK, 1995, p. 129.

Vergara, E.: Understanding newborn infant behavior: neonatal stability. *In Foundations for Practice in the Neonatal Intensive Care Unit and Early Intervention: A Self-Guided Practice Manual*, vol. 1. Rockville, MD, The American Occupational Therapy Association, 1993, p. 23.

5. **(B)** Interacting with an infant who is in or near a sleep state should be avoided, if at all possible. Sleep disruption may

interfere with neuron maturation and growth hormone secretion, which could affect growth and development. Trying to elicit interaction with an infant in an active alert state may be difficult because the motor activity can interfere and actually compete with the intended interaction. The quiet alert state is most appropriate for interacting with an infant. In this state, the infant is best able to focus on, and respond to, stimuli.

References: Gardner, S. L., and Lubchenco, L. O.: The neonate and the environment: impact on development. *In* Merenstein, G. B., and Gardner, S. L. (Eds.): *Handbook of Neonatal Intensive Care*, 4th ed. St. Louis, Mosby-Year Book, 1998, p. 197.

Vergara, E.: Preterm infant development. *In Foundations for Practice in the Neonatal Intensive Care Unit and Early Intervention: A Self-Guided Practice Manual*, vol. 1. Rockville, MD, The American Occupational Therapy Association, 1993, p. 41.

6. **(C)** Efficient feeding can best occur when a number of variables are developed. These variables include mature rooting, sucking, and swallowing reflexes; sucking pads; flexor tone; coordination of swallowing and breathing; and appropriate alertness.

References: Koch, S.: Developmental support in the neonatal intensive care unit. *In* Deacon, J., and O'Neill, P. (Eds.): *Core Curriculum for Neonatal Intensive Care Nursing*, 2nd ed. Philadelphia, W. B. Saunders, 1999, p. 522.

Vergara, E.: Feeding. *In Foundations for Practice in the Neonatal Intensive Care Unit and Early Intervention: A Self-Guided Practice Manual*, vol. 1. Rockville, MD, The American Occupational Therapy Association, 1993, p. 171.

7. **(C)** Several variables may have an influence over oral feeding readiness. The infant's overall medical condition and weight gain pattern should be reviewed. Oral-motor control should be assessed because of its primary importance to oral feeding. Head control is a developmental milestone that usually occurs between 0 and 3 months of age and it is not necessary for oral feeding readiness.

References: Koch, S.: Developmental support in the neonatal intensive care unit. *In* Deacon, J., and O'Neill, P. (Eds.): *Core Curriculum for Neonatal Intensive Care Nursing*, 2nd ed. Philadelphia, W. B. Saunders, 1999, p. 522.

Vergara, E.: Feeding. *In Foundations for Practice in the Neonatal Intensive Care Unit and Early Intervention: A Self-Guided Practice Manual*, vol. 1. Rockville, MD, The American Occupational Therapy Association, 1993, p. 171.

Wolf, L. S., and Glass, R. P.: Therapeutic treatment strategies for infant feeding dysfunction. *In Feeding and Swallowing Disorders in Infancy: Assessment and Management*. Tucson, AZ, Therapy Skill Builders, 1992, p. 207.

8. **(A)** Nutritive suck has two parts: suction and expression. The objective is nutritional intake. It occurs at a rate of one suck per second with a low suck-to-swallow ratio (1–3:1). Non-nutritive suck (NNS) only contains suction. There is no expression of nutritional liquid but it may satisfy the infant's sucking desire. NNS has a rate of two sucks per second and a 6:1 or 8:1 suck/swallow ratio. Preterm sucking patterns have a short sucking burst, with only 3 to 5 sucks before pausing. In preterm infants, the sucking rhythm may be stronger than the breathing rhythm, leading to apnea. A dysfunctional suck disrupts the feeding process because of abnormal tongue and jaw movements.

References: Palmer, M. M.: Identification and management of the transitional suck pattern in premature infants. *J Perinatal Neonatal Nursing* 7(1):66, 1993.
Vergara, E.: Feeding. *In Foundations for Practice in the Neonatal Intensive Care Unit and Early Intervention: A Self-Guided Practice Manual*, vol. 1. Rockville, MD, The American Occupational Therapy Association, 1993, p. 171.
Wolf, L. S., and Glass, R. P.: Functional anatomy and physiology of the suck/swallow/breathe triad. *In Feeding and Swallowing Disorders in Infancy: assessment and management*. Tucson, AZ, Therapy Skill Builders, 1992, p. 3.

9. **(B)** Although each infant must be assessed individually, most are able to coordinate sucking, swallowing, and breathing by 32 to 34 weeks of corrected gestational age. This coordination occurs as a result of the myelinization of the medulla.

References: Koch, S.: Developmental support in the neonatal intensive care unit. *In Deacon, J., and O'Neill, P. (Eds.): Core Curriculum for Neonatal Intensive Care Nursing*, 2nd ed. Philadelphia, W. B. Saunders, 1999, p. 522.
Palmer, M. M.: Identification and management of the transitional suck pattern in premature infants. *J Perinatal Neonatal Nursing* 7(1):66, 1993.
Vergara, E.: Preterm infant development. *In Foundations for Practice in the Neonatal Intensive Care Unit and Early Intervention: A Self-guided Practice Manual*, vol. 1. Rockville, MD, The American Occupational Therapy Association, 1993, p. 41.

10. **(A)** The infant shows signs of decompensation from overstimulation during the nursing intervention. Providing contain-

ment, either manually through "tuck" or with positioning devices, will provide comfort to the infant and allow him to engage his own self-regulating behaviors. Touching the infant while talking to him, playing music, and changing his environment to rock him may provide too much stimulation to an infant who is already stressed.

References: Koch, S.: Developmental support in the neonatal intensive care unit. *In Deacon, J., and O'Neill, P. (Eds.): Core Curriculum for Neonatal Intensive Care Nursing*, 2nd ed. Philadelphia, W. B. Saunders, 1999, p. 522.
Wyly, M. V., and Allen, J.: Optimizing the NICU environment for newborns. *In Stress and Coping in the Neonatal Intensive Care Unit*, part II. Tucson, AZ, Communication Skill Builders, 1990, p. 7.

11. **(D)** Self-regulating behaviors are ways in which an infant attempts to manage his own stress levels. Self-regulating behaviors of infants include finger or pacifier sucking, hand clasping or grasping, hand-to-mouth positioning, covering their eyes or ears with their hands, and placing themselves up against the side of the bed to facilitate self-containment.

References: Koch, S.: Developmental support in the neonatal intensive care unit. *In Deacon, J., and O'Neill, P. (Eds.): Core Curriculum for Neonatal Intensive Care Nursing*, 2nd ed. Philadelphia, W. B. Saunders, 1999, p. 522.
Wyly, M. V., and Allen, J.: Optimizing the NICU environment for newborns. *In Stress and Coping in the Neonatal Intensive Care Unit*, part II. Tucson, AZ, Communication Skill Builders, 1990, p. 7.

12. **(C)** Moving to the side or bottom of the bed to make contact with walls is a way of maintaining organization control through containment. If the infant is not given "boundaries," he will expend energy trying to find his own. The use of blanket rolls or nesting devices can provide containment for the infant.

References: Koch, S.: Developmental support in the neonatal intensive care unit. *In Deacon, J., and O'Neill, P. (Eds.): Core Curriculum for Neonatal Intensive Care Nursing*, 2nd ed. Philadelphia, W. B. Saunders, 1999, p. 522.
Wyly, M. V., and Allen, J.: Optimizing the NICU environment for newborns. *In Stress and Coping in the Neonatal Intensive Care Unit*, part II. Tucson, AZ, Communication Skill Builders, 1990, p. 7.

13. **(D)** Feeding the infant more often with a smaller volume would not help a poor weight gain problem. This intervention is helpful for the infant who tires before

finishing the ordered volume. Infants with poor oral motor tone need cheek and jaw support during a feeding. Paced feedings assist those infants with an uncoordinated suck/swallow/breathing pattern.

References: Koch, S.: Developmental support in the neonatal intensive care unit. *In* Deacon, J., and O'Neill, P. (Eds.): *Core Curriculum for Neonatal Intensive Care Nursing,* 2nd ed. Philadelphia, W. B. Saunders, 1999, p. 522.
Vergara, E.: Feeding. *In Foundations for Practice in the Neonatal Intensive Care Unit and Early Intervention: A Self-guided Practice Manual,* vol. 1. Rockville, MD, The American Occupational Therapy Association, 1993, p. 171.
Wolf, L. S., and Glass, R. P.: Therapeutic treatment strategies for infant feeding dysfunction. *In Feeding and Swallowing Disorders in Infancy: Assessment and Management.* Tucson, AZ, Therapy Skill Builders, 1992, p. 207.

14. **(C)** Stress in NICU infants can be reduced through careful observation and understanding of their behaviors. Interventions for the infants should be individualized to accommodate the infants' behavioral needs. Parents should be taught about how infants respond to the environment and how, in turn, they can respond to the infants. There are many ways the parents can participate in developmental care, and their input should always be encouraged.

References: Gardner, S. L., and Lubchenco, L. O.: The neonate and the environment: impact on development. *In* Merenstein, G. B., and Gardner, S. L. (Eds.): *Handbook of Neonatal Intensive Care,* 4th ed. St. Louis, Mosby-Year Book, 1998, p. 197.
Koch, S.: Developmental support in the neonatal intensive care unit. *In* Deacon, J., and O'Neill, P. (Eds.): *Core Curriculum for Neonatal Intensive Care Nursing,* 2nd ed. Philadelphia, W. B. Saunders, 1999, p. 522.
VandenBerg, K. A.: Basic principles of developmental caregiving. *Neonatal Network* 16(7):69, 1997.

15. **(B)** Improper prone positioning can result in extension of the extremities and external rotation of the hips. The prone position improves ventilation by increasing the stability of the chest wall and allowing greater excursion of the chest wall. Because the prone position is comfortable and calming to infants, it increases their time in quiet sleep and decreases their energy use.

References: Gardner, S. L., and Lubchenco, L. O.: The neonate and the environment: Impact on development. *In* Merenstein, G. B., and Gardner, S. L. (Eds.): *Handbook of Neonatal Intensive Care,* 4th ed. St. Louis, Mosby-Year Book, 1998, p. 197.

Koch, S.: Developmental support in the neonatal intensive care unit. *In* Deacon, J., and O'Neill, P. (Eds.): *Core Curriculum for Neonatal Intensive Care Nursing,* 2nd ed. Philadelphia, W. B. Saunders, 1999, p. 522.
Vergara, E.: Positioning. *In Foundations for Practice in the Neonatal Intensive Care Unit and Early Intervention: A Self-guided Practice Manual,* vol. 1. Rockville, MD, The American Occupational Therapy Association, 1993, p. 143.

16. **(C)** Stress reactions that result from overstimulation can be avoided by watching an infant's signals. Care activities should be carefully scrutinized to identify those that may be modified, or eliminated, that work against the infant's current state or behavioral capability. To truly respect the infant's developmental status, care activities should not be performed based on the clock (i.e., on a schedule) but rather on cue from the infant.

References: VandenBerg, K. A.: Basic principles of developmental caregiving. *Neonatal Network* 16(7):69, 1997.
Vergara, E.: Understanding newborn infant behavior: neonatal stability. *In Foundations for Practice in the Neonatal Intensive Care Unit and Early Intervention: A Self-guided Practice Manual,* vol. 1. Rockville, MD, The American Occupational Therapy Association, 1993, p. 23.

17. **(D)** Two sets of behaviors have been described in relation to an infant's organization. Avoidance behaviors are displayed when an infant is disorganized or under stress. These behaviors are also known as "time-out" signals. "Approach signals" is the term given to a group of behaviors that may be seen in an infant who is calm and alert and most likely to be capable of responding to interaction.

References: Koch, S.: Developmental support in the neonatal intensive care unit. *In* Deacon, J., and O'Neill, P. (Eds.): *Core Curriculum for Neonatal Intensive Care Nursing,* 2nd ed. Philadelphia, W. B. Saunders, 1999, p. 522.
Vergara, E.: Understanding newborn infant behavior: neonatal stability. *In Foundations for Practice in the Neonatal Intensive Care Unit and Early Intervention: A Self-guided Practice Manual,* vol. 1. Rockville, MD, The American Occupational Therapy Association, 1993, p. 23.
Wyly, M. V., and Allen, J.: Optimizing the NICU environment for newborns. *In Stress and Coping in the Neonatal Intensive Care Unit,* part II. Tucson, AZ, Communication Skill Builders, 1990, p. 7.

18. **(B)** If at all possible, a sleeping infant should not be awakened. If it is necessary to awaken the infant, as gentle a method as possible should be used. Nurses should educate parents on their infant's behavioral states and cues. Parental

involvement should never be discouraged, but if the interaction is inappropriate, parents should be given alternatives. Because infants spend so much time asleep, parents need to be taught activities that they can do even while their infant is asleep.

References: Koch, S.: Developmental support in the neonatal intensive care unit. *In* Deacon, J., and O'Neill, P. (Eds.): *Core Curriculum for Neonatal Intensive Care Nursing,* 2nd ed. Philadelphia, W. B. Saunders, 1999, p. 522.
Vergara, E.: Preterm infant development. *In Foundations for Practice in the Neonatal Intensive Care Unit and Early Intervention: A Self-guided Practice Manual,* vol. 1. Rockville, MD, The American Occupational Therapy Association, 1993, p. 41.
Wyly, M. V., and Allen, J.: Optimizing the NICU environment for newborns. *In Stress and Coping in the Neonatal Intensive Care Unit,* part II. Tucson, AZ, Communication Skill Builders, 1990, p. 7.

19. **(C)** Although the parent could come back and visit at another time, it is quite possible that the infant will be sleeping then as well. The parent needs an activity that she or he can do while the infant is asleep, since waking the infant is not preferred. Hand encircling of the infant will give warmth, passive touch, and the smell of the parent.

References: Koch, S.: Developmental support in the neonatal intensive care unit. *In* Deacon, J., and O'Neill, P. (Eds.): *Core Curriculum for Neonatal Intensive Care Nursing,* 2nd ed. Philadelphia, W. B. Saunders, 1999, p. 522.
Vergara, E.: Preterm infant development. *In Foundations for Practice in the Neonatal Intensive Care Unit and Early Intervention: A Self-guided Practice Manual,* vol. 1. Rockville, MD, The American Occupational Therapy Association, 1993, p. 41.
Wyly, M. V., and Allen, J.: Optimizing the NICU environment for newborns. *In Stress and Coping in the Neonatal Intensive Care Unit,* part II. Tucson, AZ, Communication Skill Builders, 1990, p. 7.

20. **(D)** Increased environmental noise levels are a stressor to infants in the NICU. The intensity and duration of sound exposure must be considered when evaluating environmental noises and their effects on infants. Both intermittent, high-pitched noises (such as machine alarms) and monotonous, low-pitched sounds (such as incubator motors) have been demonstrated to have deleterious effects on infants' responses to sound. The AAP has stated that the maximum safe level for decibels in the NICU is 58. A normal speaking voice is between 50 and 60 decibels. Machine alarms can range from 60

to 90 decibels. Closing a plastic porthole door can create noise levels of greater than 100 decibels.

References: Gardner, S. L., and Lubchenco, L. O.: The neonate and the environment: impact on development. *In* Merenstein, G. B., Gardner, S. L. (Eds.): *Handbook of Neonatal Intensive Care,* 4th ed. St. Louis, Mosby-Year Book, 1998, p. 197.
Koch, S.: Developmental support in the neonatal intensive care unit. *In* Deacon, J., and O'Neill, P. (Eds.): *Core Curriculum for Neonatal Intensive Care Nursing,* 2nd ed. Philadelphia, W. B. Saunders, 1999, p. 522.
Wyly, M. V., and Allen, J.: Optimizing the NICU Environment for Newborns. *In Stress and Coping in the Neonatal Intensive Care Unit,* part II. Tucson, AZ, Communication Skill Builders, 1990, p. 7.

21. **(C)** Infants in the NICU are exposed to bright lights from a variety of sources. They are often thrust from a dimmed environment into one of extreme brightness, such as when an examination light is turned on or an incubator cover is taken off. This sudden exposure to light can cause physiologic instability (decreased oxygenation, increased apnea, and bradycardia). Light in the NICU is present 24 hours a day. It usually does not follow a day/night, cycled pattern. Constant light exposure disrupts circadian rhythms and sleeping patterns. Reduced levels of lighting help infants become more alert and capable of engaging in social interactions.

References: Gardner, S. L., and Lubchenco, L. O.: The neonate and the environment: impact on development. *In* Merenstein, G. B., and Gardner, S. L. (Eds.): *Handbook of Neonatal Intensive Care,* 4th ed. St. Louis, Mosby-Year Book, 1998, p. 197.
Wyly, M. V., and Allen, J.: Optimizing the NICU environment for newborns. *In Stress and Coping in the Neonatal Intensive Care Unit,* part II. Tucson, AZ, Communication Skill Builders, 1990, p. 7.

CHAPTER 10
RADIOGRAPHIC EVALUATION

1. **(C)** Respiratory distress syndrome is characterized by a reticulogranular pattern with air bronchogram and diffuse alveolar infiltrates.

Reference: Hedlund, G. L., Griscom, T., Cleveland, R. H., et al.: Respiratory system. *In* Kirks, D. R. (Ed.): *Practical Pediatric Imaging: Diagnostic Radiology of Infants and Children,* 3rd ed. Philadelphia, Lippincott-Raven, 1998, p. 619.

2. **(D)** Pulmonary interstitial emphysema is alveolar overdistention due to assisted ventilation visualized as small cyst-like radiolucencies which may be bilateral,

unilateral, or localized in a diffuse pattern.

Reference: Deacon, J.: Radiologic evaluation of the newborn infant. *In* Deacon, J., and O'Neill, P. (Eds.): *Core Curriculum for Neonatal Intensive Care Nursing,* 2nd ed. Philadelphia, W. B. Saunders, 1999, p. 673.

3. **(D)** A normal lung pattern with mild infiltrates and overexpanded lung may be seen in some mild cases. Bilateral asymmetric areas of atelectasis, hyperaeration with flattened hemidiaphragms with possible atelectasis, is the generalized picture of meconium aspiration syndrome.

Reference: Hedlund, G. L., Griscom, T., Cleveland, R. H., et al.: Respiratory system. *In* Kirks, D. R. (Ed.): *Practical Pediatric Imaging: Diagnostic Radiology of Infants and Children,* 3rd ed. Philadelphia, Lippincott-Raven, 1998, p. 619.

4. **(D)** The classic radiograph of a pneumomediastinum features an irregular gas collection, with air outlining the undersurface of the thymus gland.

Reference: Swischuk, L. E., and John, S. D.: *Differential Diagnosis in Pediatric Radiology,* 2nd ed. Baltimore, Williams & Wilkins, 1995.

5. **(B)** This describes a pneumothorax in a mildly symptomatic infant. The primary intervention would be to supply oxygen to the infant secondary to low saturation. A chest tube may be indicated at a later time, but there is no sign of mediastinal shift or of acute distress.

Reference: Swischuk, L. E., and John, S. D.: *Differential Diagnosis in Pediatric Radiology,* 2nd ed. Baltimore, Williams & Wilkins, 1995.

6. **(D)** A full-term infant in acute distress with a scaphoid abdomen and apnea is indicative of a diaphragmatic hernia. Bag-valve-mask ventilation would fill the bowel with air, causing obstruction of the ventilation of the lung, which is not affected.

Reference: Hedlund, G. L., Griscom, T., Cleveland, R. H., et al.: Respiratory system. *In* Kirks, D. R. (Ed.): *Practical Pediatric Imaging: Diagnostic Radiology of Infants and Children,* 3rd ed. Philadelphia, Lippincott-Raven, 1998, p. 619.

7. **(A)** The appropriate position for an umbilical arterial catheter is either at a low placement between the third and fourth lumbar vertebrae, or at a high placement between the sixth through tenth thoracic vertebrae. An umbilical artery catheter tip

at the eleventh thoracic vertebrae is too low for a high placement and too high for a low placement. The catheter should be pulled back so that the tip is at the third to fourth lumbar vertebrae.

Reference: Short-Bartlett, S. C.: Arterial catheterization. *In* Taeusch, W. H., Christiansen, R. O., and Buescher, E. S. (Eds.): *Pediatric and Neonatal Tests and Procedures.* Philadelphia, W. B. Saunders, 1996, p. 165.

8. **(A)** This is indicative of duodenal atresia, as it presents with vomiting episodes in the first hours of life. With stenosis, vomiting may present at variable times. This is correlated with Down syndrome in 33% of infants.

Reference: Swischuk, L. E., and John, S. D.: *Differential Diagnosis in Pediatric Radiology,* 2nd ed. Baltimore, Williams & Wilkins, 1995.

9. **(C)** This radiograph is indicative of necrotizing enterocolitis, and the infant should remain on NPO status with a nasogastric tube to suction and closely followed with repeat radiographs to evaluate for perforation.

Reference: Buonomo, C., Taylor, G. A., and Share, J. C.: Gastrointestinal tract. *In* Kirks, D. R. (Ed.): *Practical Pediatric Imaging: Diagnostic Radiology of Infants and Children.* Philadelphia, Lippincott-Raven, 1998, p. 821.

10. **(A)** Relative to a midline and neutral position of the head, an endotracheal tube (ETT) can move up or down in the trachea and with head flexion, extension, and rotation. When the head is rotated or extended, the ETT advances further down the trachea. When the head is flexed, the ETT moves higher in the trachea. The optimal position for head position is midline and neutral.

References: Hedlund, G. L., Griscom, T., Cleveland, R. H., et al.: Respiratory system. *In* Kirks, D. R. (Ed.): *Practical Pediatric Imaging: Diagnostic Radiology of Infants and Children,* 3rd ed. Philadelphia, Lippincott-Raven, 1998, p. 619.
Quinn, W., Sandifer, L., and Goldsmith, J. P.: Pulmonary care. *In* Goldsmith, J. P., and Karotkin, E. H. (Eds.): *Assisted Ventilation of the Neonate,* 3rd ed. Philadelphia, W. B. Saunders, 1996, p. 101.

CHAPTER 11
PHARMACOLOGY

1. **(C)** Dopamine stimulates both α (alpha) and β (beta) adrenergic receptors as well as dopaminergic receptors. Isoproterenol stimulates β_1 and β_2 receptors, resulting in relaxation of bronchial smooth muscle

while increasing heart rate and contractility. Albuterol relaxes bronchial smooth muscle by acting on β₂ receptors with little effect on heart rate. Methylprednisolone is an anti-inflammatory agent used in the treatment of hematologic, allergic, inflammatory, neoplastic, and autoimmune conditions.

References: Martin, R. G.: Pharmacology in neonatal care. In Deacon, J., and O'Neill, P. (Eds.): Core Curriculum for Neonatal Intensive Care Nursing, 2nd ed. Philadelphia, W. B. Saunders, 1999, p. 652.
Taketomo, C. K., Hodding, J. H., and Kraus, D. M.: Pediatric Dosage Handbook, 6th ed. Cleveland, Lexi-Comp, Inc., 1999.

2. **(A)** All items are adverse reactions of the drug. However, apnea appearing during the first hour of drug infusion occurs in 10 to 12% of neonates with congenital heart defects. Clinicians deciding to utilize alprostadil must be prepared to intubate and mechanically ventilate the infant. Careful monitoring for apnea or respiratory depression is mandatory. In some institutions, elective intubation occurs prior to initiation of the medication.

Reference: Taketomo, C. K., Hodding, J. H., and Kraus, D. M.: Pediatric Dosage Handbook, 6th ed. Cleveland, Lexi-Comp, Inc., 1999.

3. **(C)** Only unbound drugs can be distributed to active receptor sites. Therefore, the more of a drug that is bound to protein, the less is available for the desired drug effect.

Reference: Martin, R. G.: Pharmacology in neonatal care. In Deacon, J., and O'Neill, P. (Eds.): Core Curriculum for Neonatal Intensive Care Nursing, 2nd ed. Philadelphia, W. B. Saunders, 1999, p. 652.

4. **(B)** A variety of specific transport systems cross the placental exchange surface, including all of the above. Research demonstrates that simple diffusion is the most common method.

Reference: Evans, M. I., Reichler, A., Isada, N. B., Pryde, P. G., and Johnson, M. P.: Fetal metabolic and hormonal defects. In Spitzer, A. R. (Ed.): Intensive Care of the Fetus and Neonate. St. Louis, Mosby, 1996, p. 157.

5. **(B)** Infants with fetal hydantoin syndrome present with a variety of abnormalities. Most notable are digit and nail hypoplasia, unusual facies, and growth and mental deficiencies. Additional craniofacial defects are common. Phenobarbital withdrawal symptoms (restlessness,

hypertonicity, diarrhea, vomiting, poor suck) and seizures present at 3 to 7 days after birth due to the long half-life of the drug.

References: Beckman, D. A., and Brent, R. L.: The effects of maternal drugs on the developing fetus. In Avery, G. B., Fletcher, M. A., and MacDonald, M. G. (Eds.): Neonatology: Pathophysiology and Management of the Newborn, 5th ed. Philadelphia, Lippincott, Williams & Wilkins, 1999, p. 209.
Jones, K. L.: Smith's Recognizable Patterns of Human Malformation, 5th ed. Philadelphia, W. B. Saunders, 1997.
Ostrea, E. M., Jr., Posecion, J. E., and Villanueva, E. T.: The infant of the drug-dependent mother. In Avery, G. B., Fletcher, M. A., and MacDonald, M. G. (Eds.): Neonatology: Pathophysiology and Management of the Newborn, 5th ed. Philadelphia, Lippincott, Williams & Wilkins, 1999, p. 1407.

6. **(C)** The loss of electrolytes is a common side effect of loop diuretic therapy. Loss of potassium can result in digoxin toxicity.

References: Martin, R. G.: Pharmacology in neonatal care. In Deacon, J., and O'Neill, P. (Eds.): Core Curriculum for Neonatal Intensive Care Nursing, 2nd ed. Philadelphia, W. B. Saunders, 1999, p. 652.
Taketomo, C. K., Hodding, J. H., and Kraus, D. M.: Pediatric Dosage Handbook, 6th ed. Cleveland, Lexi-Comp, Inc., 1999.

7. **(D)** Women presenting with no prenatal care and a history of sexually transmitted diseases are suspect for illicit drug usage. Almost all narcotic drugs ingested by the pregnant addict cross the placenta and enter fetal circulation. Naloxone is an opiate antagonist. Its administration blocks opiate receptor sites and may result in acute withdrawal manifested by immediate bradycardia, hypertension, breathing abnormalities, increased movement and tone, and desynchronized electrocortical activity.

References: Hurt, H.: Substance use during pregnancy. In Spitzer, A. R. (Ed.): Intensive Care of the Fetus and Neonate. St. Louis, Mosby, 1996, p. 257.
Ostrea, E. M., Jr., Posecion, J. E., and Villanueva, E. T.: The infant of the drug-dependent mother. In Avery, G. B., Fletcher, M. A., and MacDonald, M. G. (Eds.): Neonatology: Pathophysiology and Management of the Newborn, 5th ed. Philadelphia, Lippincott, Williams & Wilkins, 1999, p. 1407.

8. **(D)** Care of an infant presenting with hydrops fetalis is complex, and survival is approximately 25%. Fluid management is an important aspect of care. The volume of water-soluble drug distribution changes rapidly as the extracellular fluid levels increase while total body water

content decreases in the first few days of life. Diuretics assist in eliminating excessextracellular water. Water excretion is also altered by the glomerular filtration rate (a combination of volume, cardiac output, blood pressure, and gestational age). Fluid intake should be limited. Serum chemistries should be monitored closely. Gentamicin levels should be checked when steady state is near or has been reached (dose 3–5), not at 1 week of life. Ototoxicity is a concern when furosemide and gentamicin are given concurrently but usually does not present on day 1 of life.

References: Martin, R. G.: Pharmacology in neonatal care. *In* Deacon, J., and O'Neill, P. (Eds.): *Core Curriculum for Neonatal Intensive Care Nursing,* 2nd ed. Philadelphia, W. B. Saunders, 1999, p. 652.
Phibbs, R.: Hydrops fetalis. *In* Spitzer, A. R. (Ed.): *Intensive Care of the Fetus and Neonate.* St. Louis, Mosby, 1996, p. 149.

9. (**A**) Fentanyl can cause respiratory depression, hypotension, and chest wall rigidity. This infant was intubated, compensating for respiratory depression. Hypotension results in an increased heart rate initially in an attempt to bolster cardiac output. A vagal response results in bradycardia, which may then be followed by desaturation.

References: Camerota, A. J., and Arnold, J. H.: Anesthesia and analgesia. *In* Avery, G. B., Fletcher, M. A., and MacDonald, M. G. (Eds.): *Neonatology: Pathophysiology and Management of the Newborn,* 5th ed. Philadelphia, Lippincott, Williams & Wilkins, 1999, p. 1447.
Martin, R. G.: Pharmacology in neonatal care. *In* Deacon, J., and O'Neill, P. (Eds.): *Core Curriculum for Neonatal Intensive Care Nursing,* 2nd ed. Philadelphia, W. B. Saunders, p. 652.

10. (**B**) Sodium bicarbonate cannot be given with the maintenance fluid containing calcium. A precipitate of calcium carbonate will form. No medications should be administered through a peripheral arterial line, since arterial spasm and vascular compromise distally to the line may result. Penicillin is incompatible with dobutamine. Dopamine and dobutamine are compatible with vecuronium. Additionally, a line with inotropes should not be used for the bolus administration of any medication, as this could cause significant blood pressure fluctuations.

References: Taketomo, C. K., Hodding, J. H., and Kraus, D. M.: *Pediatric Dosage Handbook,* 6th ed. Cleveland, Lexi-Comp, 1999.

Tissel, L. A.: Handbook of injectable drugs, 10th ed. American Society of Health-System Pharmacists, 1995.

Section II
Pathophysiology

CHAPTER 12
CARDIOVASCULAR DISORDERS

1. (**D**) Zero referencing is done by opening the zeroing stopcock to atmosphere and aligning it with the patient's phlebostatic axis. Soft, compliant tubing and long tubing decrease the natural frequency of the monitoring system and can lead to an overestimation of systolic pressure.

Reference: Darovic, G. O., Vanriper, S., and Vanriper, J.: Fluid-filled monitoring systems. *In* Darovic, G. O.: *Hemodynamic Monitoring: Invasive and Noninvasive Clinical Application,* 2nd ed. Philadelphia, W. B. Saunders, 1995, p. 149.

2. (**A**) A ventricular septal defect (VSD) is associated with a left-to-right shunt, resulting in increased pulmonary blood flow. Infants with a VSD often present with congestive heart failure and pulmonary infections. Hepatomegaly results from the congestive heart failure (CHF). Polycythemia occurs primarily in infants with cyanotic heart lesions as a compensatory mechanism to increase oxygen delivery.

References: Crockett, M.: Cardiovascular disorders. *In* Deacon, J., and O'Neill, P. (Eds.): *Core Curriculum for Neonatal Intensive Care Nursing,* 2nd ed. Philadelphia, W. B. Saunders, 1999, p. 206.
Hazinski, M. F.: *Manual of Pediatric Critical Care.* St. Louis, Mosby, 1999, p. 84.

3. (**C**) The Blalock-Taussig shunt connects the subclavian artery to the pulmonary artery. The Blalock-Taussing shunt is a palliative procedure performed in infants with congenital heart lesions associated with decreased pulmonary blood flow.

Reference: Crockett, M.: Cardiovascular disorders. *In* Deacon, J., and O'Neill, P. (Eds.): *Core Curriculum for Neonatal Intensive Care Nursing,* 2nd ed. Philadelphia, W. B. Saunders, 1999, p. 206.

4. (**A**) Cyanosis that is caused by a congenital heart lesion results from unoxygenated systemic venous blood shunting into the systemic arterial system (right-to-left shunt), bypassing the lungs. In tricuspid atresia, there is a complete absence of a

tricuspid valve. Blood cannot flow from the right atrium to the right ventricle. There must be an intra-atrial communication for the blood in the right atrium to exit, resulting in a right-to-left shunt. Ventricular septal defect (VSD), patent ductus arteriosus (PDA), and atrial septal defect (ASD) are associated with a left-to-right shunt.

Reference: Hazinski, M. F.: *Manual of Pediatric Critical Care.* St. Louis, Mosby, 1999, p. 84.

5. **(A)** Preload is the amount of stretch in the myocardial fibers just prior to contraction. In the clinical setting, preload is evaluated by assessing the pressure in the ventricles at end diastole. In the absence of tricuspid valve disease, right ventricular end diastolic pressure is the same as right atrial pressure. In the absence of central venous obstruction, central venous pressure is the same as right atrial pressure.

Reference: Hazinski, M. F.: *Manual of Pediatric Critical Care.* St. Louis, Mosby, 1999, p. 84.

6. **(A)** All congenital heart defects, with the exception of the secundum type of atrial septal defect (ASD), predispose the infant to subacute bacterial endocarditis. Primary cardiomyopathy, an abnormality of the ventricular myocardium, is not caused by congenital heart defects (CHDs). Kawasaki disease is a microvascular inflammatory disease of unknown etiology. Rheumatic fever is an infectious inflammatory disorder that is most commonly precipitated by group A streptococcus-induced pharyngitis.

References: Ayoub, E. M.: Acute rheumatic fever. *In* Emmanoulides, G. C., Riemenschneider, T. A., Allen, D. H., and Gutgesell, H. P. (Eds.): *Moss and Adams' Heart Disease in Infants, Children, and Adolescents Including the Fetus and Young Adult,* 5th ed. Baltimore, Williams & Wilkins, 1995, p. 1400.
Hazinski, M. F.: *Manual of Pediatric Critical Care.* St. Louis, Mosby, 1999, p. 84.
Lott, J. W.: Assessment and management of cardiovascular dysfunction. *In* Kenner, C., Lott, J. W., and Flandermeyer, A. A. (Eds.): *Comprehensive Neonatal Nursing: A Physiologic Perspective,* 2nd ed. Philadelphia, W. B. Saunders, 1998, p. 306.

7. **(D)** Echocardiography is a noninvasive tool utilizing sound waves to visualize cardiac structures and measure cardiac function. Intracardiac pressures and oxygen saturation are evaluated by cardiac catheterization. The electrocardiogram

measures electrical activity of the heart. Myocardial perfusion is best assessed by radionuclide imaging.

References: Callow, L., Suddaby, E. C., and Slota, M. C.: Cardiovascular system. *In* Slota, M. C. (Ed.): *Core Curriculum for Pediatric Intensive Care Nursing.* Philadelphia, W. B. Saunders, 1998, p. 144.
Hazinski, M. F.: *Manual of Pediatric Critical Care.* St. Louis, Mosby, 1999, p. 84.

8. **(C)** Clinical features of a patent ductus arteriosus (PDA) include a murmur heard best at the left sternal border in the second and third intercostal spaces, an active precordium, and widened pulse pressure. Because of the lower pulmonary vascular resistance, blood shunts from left to right across the ductus. As the left-to-right shunt increases, the peripheral pulses become more prominent and there is an increase in pulmonary blood flow with a consequential "steal" of blood that would normally perfuse the body. The incidence of PDA is inversely proportional to gestational age, with the incidence close to 80% in infants less than 1200 g.

References: Brook, M. M., and Heymann, M. A.: Patent ductus arteriosus. *In* Emmanoulides, G. C., Riemenschneider, T. A., Allen, D. H., and Gutgesell, H. P. (Eds.): *Moss and Adams' Heart Disease in Infants, Children, and Adolescents Including the Fetus and Young Adult,* 5th ed. Baltimore, Williams & Wilkins, 1995, p. 746.
Lott, J. W.: Assessment and management of cardiovascular dysfunction. *In* Kenner, C., Lott, J. W., and Flandermeyer, A. A. (Eds.): *Comprehensive Neonatal Nursing: A Physiologic Perspective,* 2nd ed. Philadelphia, W. B. Saunders, 1998, p. 306.

9. **(B)** The goal of treatment for this infant is to close the ductus arteriosus. Endogenous and exogenous prostaglandins play a significant role in maintaining the patency of the ductus. Indomethacin is a prostaglandin synthetase inhibitor and is used to constrict the ductus.

References: Brook, M. M., and Heymann, M. A.: Patent ductus arteriosus. *In* Emmanoulides, G. C., Riemenschneider, T. A., Allen, D. H., and Gutgesell, H. P. (Eds.): *Moss and Adams' Heart Disease in Infants, Children, and Adolescents Including the Fetus and Young Adult,* 5th ed. Baltimore, Williams & Wilkins, 1995, p. 746.
Lott, J. W.: Assessment and management of cardiovascular dysfunction. *In* Kenner, C., Lott, J. W., and Flandermeyer, A. A. (Eds.): *Comprehensive Neonatal Nursing: A Physiologic Perspective,* 2nd ed. Philadelphia, W. B. Saunders, 1998, p. 306.

10. **(B)** During fetal life, alveoli are fluid-filled and hypoxic, leading to pulmonary artery constriction and increased pulmonary vascular resistance and pressure. Sys-

temic vascular pressure and resistance are low, because a majority of the fetal systemic circulation flows to the placenta, which is a low-resistance organ.

Reference: Hazinski, M. F.: *Manual of Pediatric Critical Care.* St. Louis, Mosby, 1999, p. 84.

11. **(B)** In normal anatomy, the pulmonary artery arises from the right ventricle and the aorta arises from the left ventricle. Transposition of the great vessels is a congenital heart defect in which the pulmonary artery arises from the left ventricle and the aorta arises from the right ventricle, so the arteries are transposed.

Reference: Crockett, M.: Cardiovascular disorders. *In* Deacon, J., and O'Neill, P. (Eds.): *Core Curriculum for Neonatal Intensive Care Nursing,* 2nd ed. Philadelphia, W. B. Saunders, 1999, p. 206.

12. **(D)** The rhythm strip demonstrates supraventricular tachycardia (SVT). The heart rate is 238 beats/minute, the R-R interval is regular. The characteristic ECG of SVT includes a fixed rate over 200 beats/min, fixed R-R interval, and a regular narrow-complex QRS with a 1:1 relationship between the P wave and QRS complex. P waves may come before or after the QRS, or be obscured. Infants with SVT often present with heart rates over 220 to 240 beats/minute.

References: Daberkow-Carson, E., and Washington, R. L.: Cardiovascular diseases and surgical interventions. *In* Merenstein, G. B., and Gardner, S. L. (Eds.): *Handbook of Neonatal Intensive Care Nursing,* 4th ed. St. Louis, Mosby, 1998, p. 500.
Page, J., and Hosking, M.: *An approach to the neonate with sudden dysrhythmia: Diagnosis, mechanisms, and management. Neonatal Network* 16(6):7, 1997.

13. **(B)** Adenosine is the drug of choice in the acute treatment of supraventricular tachycardia (SVT). Verapamil is not recommended in infants less than 1 year of age. Defibrillation is a form of counter-shock used for the treatment of pulseless ventricular tachycardia or ventricular fibrillation. Eyeball massage should never be done on infants.

References: Daberkow-Carson, E., and Washington, R. L.: Cardiovascular diseases and surgical interventions. *In* Merenstein, G. B., and Gardner, S. L. (Eds.): *Handbook of Neonatal Intensive Care Nursing,* 4th ed. St. Louis, Mosby, 1998, p. 500.
Hazinski, M. F.: *Manual of Pediatric Critical Care.* St. Louis, Mosby, 1999, p. 84.

14. **(A)** Frank and Starling demonstrated that, to a point, the greater the stretch of myo-

cardial fibers prior to contraction, the greater the tension generated by the myocardial fibers during contraction. Stretch of the myocardial fibers prior to contraction is synonymous with preload. Tension generated by the myocardial fibers during contraction is synonymous with cardiac output. Therefore, to a point, the greater the preload is, the greater the cardiac output, and interventions that increase preload will result in an increased cardiac output.

Reference: Hazinski, M. F.: *Manual of Pediatric Critical Care.* St. Louis, Mosby, 1999, p. 84.

15. **(A)** Myocarditis can be caused by almost any bacteria, virus, rickettsia, fungus, or parasite. However, coxsackievirus is the most common agent.

Reference: Lewis, A. B.: Myocarditis. *In* Emmanoulides, G. C., Riemenschneider, T. A., Allen, D. H., and Gutgesell, H. P. (Eds.): *Moss and Adams' Heart Disease in Infants, Children, and Adolescents Including the Fetus and Young Adult,* 5th ed. Baltimore, Williams & Wilkins, 1995, p. 1381.

16. **(D)** During diastole, the aortic and pulmonic valves are closed, and the tricuspid and mitral valves are open. Unless there is stenosis of the tricuspid valve, the pressure in the right ventricle at end diastole equals the pressure in the right atrium (central venous pressure) due to this common communication.

Reference: Hazinski, M. F.: *Manual of Pediatric Critical Care.* St. Louis, Mosby, 1999, p. 84.

17. **(D)** Transient ischemia due to vasospasm is a frequent complication of umbilical artery catheterization. The ischemia is characterized by blue toes. Warming the opposite foot causes a reflex vasodilation and improved blood flow to the extremity. Ischemia that is recurrent or does not go away should prompt removal of the catheter.

Reference: Short-Bartlett, S. C.: Arterial catheterization. *In* Taeusch, H. W., Christiansoen, R. O., and Buescher, E. S. (Eds.): *Pediatric and Neonatal Tests and Procedures.* Philadelphia, W. B. Saunders, 1996, p. 160.

18. **(A)** The optimal site of dopamine infusion is into a central vein, such as the umbilical venous catheter. To avoid liver damage, infusion of dopamine into the umbilical vein should be done only if the tip of the catheter is in the inferior vena cava. Medications should never be infused into

a peripheral artery. If central venous access is not available, dopamine may be administered into a peripheral IV line. In such cases, a peripheral site closest to the heart should be chosen. Vasopressors also should not be infused via the umbilical artery line.

References: Bell, S. G.: Neonatal cardiovascular pharmacology. *Neonatal Network* 17(2):7, 1998.
Green, C., and Yohannan, M. D.: Umbilical arterial and venous catheters: placement, use, and complications. *Neonatal Network* 17(6):23, 1998.

19. **(A)** Prostaglandin E_1 is indicated to maintain patency of the ductus arteriosus. Isolated patent ductus arteriosus, ventricular septal defect, and atrial septal defect are all characterized by increased pulmonary blood flow. Maintaining the ductus open in these defects would increase pulmonary blood flow further, increasing the risk of pulmonary edema, and compromising the infant. Tricuspid atresia is characterized by a complete obstruction of unoxygenated blood from the right atrium to the right ventricle. Venous blood is shunted across a patent foramen ovale to the left atrium, mixing with oxygenated blood. Maintaining patency of the ductus arteriosus is critical for pulmonary blood flow.

References: Bell, S. G.: Neonatal cardiovascular pharmacology. *Neonatal Network* 17(2):7, 1998.
Crockett, M.: Cardiovascular disorders. *In* Deacon, J., and O'Neill, P. (Eds.): *Core Curriculum for Neonatal Intensive Care Nursing,* 2nd ed. Philadelphia, W. B. Saunders, 1999, p. 206.

20. **(B)** This infant is having a hypercyanotic ("tet") spell. Hypercyanotic spells are characterized by hyperpnea (increased respiratory rate and depth), irritability, increasing cyanosis, and a decreased intensity of murmur. These spells occur in infants with tetralogy of Fallot (TOF) as well as other congenital heart defects (CHDs) having mixed arterial and venous blood. Decreased systemic vascular resistance or increased resistance to right ventricular outflow increases right-to-left shunting, which then leads to hyperpnea. Hyperpnea leads to increased systemic venous return, which increases the amount of right-to-left shunting. A vicious cycle ensues. Morphine is indicated because it suppresses the respiratory center and eradicates the hyperpnea.

References: Bell, S. G.: Neonatal cardiovascular pharmacology. *Neonatal Network* 17(2):7, 1998.
Park, M. K.: *The Pediatric Cardiology Handbook,* 2nd ed. St. Louis, Mosby, 1997.

21. **(D)** Goals of therapy for congestive heart failure (CHF) are aimed at improving cardiac function and decreasing demands on the heart. Reducing cardiac demands can be accomplished by maintaining a neutral thermal environment, providing a quiet environment, placing the infant in a semi-Fowler position (as can be accomplished with a cardiac chair), and restricting fluids.

References: Lott, J. W.: Assessment and management of cardiovascular dysfunction. *In* Kenner, C., Lott, J. W., and Flandermeyer, A. A. (Eds.): *Comprehensive Neonatal Nursing: A Physiologic Perspective,* 2nd ed. Philadelphia, W. B. Saunders, 1998, p. 306.
Park, M. K.: *The Pediatric Cardiology Handbook,* 2nd ed. St. Louis, Mosby, 1997.

22. **(D)** The second heart sound is produced by the closure of the aortic and pulmonic valves at the end of ventricular systole.

Reference: Crockett, M.: Cardiovascular disorders. *In* Deacon, J., and O'Neill, P. (Eds.): *Core Curriculum for Neonatal Intensive Care Nursing,* 2nd ed. Philadelphia, W. B. Saunders, 1999, p. 206.

23. **(A)** Pulsus paradoxus is found in pericardial effusion, cardiac tamponade, or severe asthma. Pulsus paradoxus is defined as a drop in systolic blood pressure of 10 mm Hg or more during inspiration.

Reference: Callow, L., Suddaby, E. C., and Slota, M. C.: Cardiovascular system. *In* Slota, M. C. (Ed.): *Core Curriculum for Pediatric Critical Care Nursing.* Philadelphia, W. B. Saunders, 1998, p. 144.

24. **(C)** In infants, a weight gain of over 50 g/day is significant and should be verified and reported to the physician. Significant weight gain may represent fluid retention as a compensatory mechanism in congestive heart failure.

Reference: Hazinski, M. F.: Cardiovascular disorders. *In* Hazinski, M. F. (Ed.): *Nursing Care of the Critically Ill Child,* 2nd ed. St. Louis, Mosby-Year Book, 1992, p. 117.

25. **(A)** During a balloon septostomy, a balloon-tipped catheter is threaded from the inferior vena cava into the right atrium. The tip is then passed across the foramen ovale to the left atrium, the tip is inflated and the catheter is quickly pulled back, tearing a hole in the atrial septum. This hole will allow mixing of blood at the

atrial level. The balloon atrial septostomy can be a life-saving procedure in infants with transposition of the great vessels (TOGV) and poor intercirculatory mixing.

References: Paul, M. H., and Wernovsky, G.: Transposition of the great arteries. *In* Emmanoulides, G. C., Riemenschneider, T. A., Allen, D. H., and Gutgesell, H. P. (Eds.): *Moss and Adams' Heart Disease in Infants, Children, and Adolescents Including the Fetus and Young Adults,* 5th ed. Baltimore, Williams & Wilkins, 1995, p. 1154.
Witt, C.: Cyanotic heart lesions with increased pulmonary blood flow. *Neonatal Network* 17(7):7, 1998.

26. **(C)** Cardiac output is determined by heart rate, preload, contractility, and afterload. The neonatal myocardium is relatively noncompliant and has fewer contractile fibers. As a result, response to preload is diminished. Calcium uptake by the sacroplasmic reticulum is limited in the neonatal myocardium, therefore, there is less calcium available for contractility. Additionally, sympathetic innervation to the myocardium is incomplete. Contractility in the neonate is limited because of these two factors. The neonate's myocardium is very sensitive to afterload because of the heart's limited compliance. Thus, increasing afterload (the resistance against which the heart has to pump) can lead to decreased cardiac output in the neonate. Cardiac output in neonates is primarily dependent on heart rate.

References: Furdon, S. A.: Recognizing congestive heart failure in the neonatal period. *Neonatal Network* 16(7):5, 1997.
Ruth-Sanchez, V.: Cardiac anomalies restricting blood flow to the left atrium. *Neonatal Network* 17(6):7, 1998.

27. **(C)** The atrial rate is 166, the ventricular rate is 71, and there is no association between the atrial and ventricular beats. The rhythm strip demonstrates complete heart block. Complete heart block is characterized by a ventricular rate slower than the atrial rate, and no association between the atrial and ventricular rates. Maternal systemic lupus erythematosus is frequently associated with complete heart block in newborns.

References: Daberkow-Carson, E., and Washington, R. L.: Cardiovascular diseases and surgical interventions. *In* Merenstein, G. B., and Gardner, S. L. (Eds.): *Handbook of Neonatal Intensive Care Nursing,* 4th ed. St. Louis, Mosby, 1998, p. 500.
Park, M. K.: *The Pediatric Cardiology Handbook,* 2nd ed. St. Louis, Mosby, 1997.

28. **(D)** Tall, peaked T waves are seen in hyperkalemia. Hypokalemia is associated with a prominent U wave. Hypocalcemia is associated with prolonged QT interval but no effect on the shape of the T wave. Hypercalcemia is associated with a shortened QT interval.

Reference: Vargo, L.: The basics of neonatal EKG interpretation. *Neonatal Network* 17(8):7, 1998.

29. **(C)** The electrolyte results reflect hypocalcemia. Hypocalcemia is associated with a prolonged ST segment, which will lengthen the QT interval.

References: Tsang, R. C., Demarini, S., and Rath, L.: Fluids, electrolytes, vitamins, and trace minerals: basis of ingestions, digestion, elimination, and metabolism. *In* Kenner, C., Lott, J. W., and Flandermeyer, A. A. (Eds.): *Comprehensive Neonatal Nursing: A Physiologic Perspective,* 2nd ed. Philadelphia, W. B. Saunders, 1998, p. 336.
Vargo, L.: The basics of neonatal EKG interpretation. *Neonatal Network* 17(8):7, 1998.

30. **(B)** As a compensatory mechanism to chronic hypoxemia, the kidneys increase erythropoietin production, leading to increased red blood cells, hemoglobin levels, and oxygen-carrying capacity. Increased red blood cell production leads to polycythemia. Pulmonary edema and pneumonia are consequences of heart defects associated with increased pulmonary blood flow. Pneumothorax is not associated with congenital heart defects.

Reference: Spilman, L. J., and Furdon, S. A.: Recognition, understanding, and current management of cardiac lesions with decreased pulmonary blood flow. *Neonatal Network* 17(4):7, 1998.

31. **(A)** Prerenal failure results from renal hypoperfusion. In congestive heart failure (CHF), renal arteries constrict in an effort to send blood flow to more important organs such as the brain and myocardium. Additionally, the renin-angiotensin-aldosterone system is activated, resulting in further vasoconstriction and decreased renal blood flow.

References: Bernhardt, J.: Renal and genitourinary disorders. *In* Deacon, J., and O'Neill, P. (Eds.): *Core Curriculum for Neonatal Intensive Care Nursing,* 2nd ed. Philadelphia, W. B. Saunders, 1999, p. 442.
Furdon, S. A.: Recognizing congestive heart failure in the neonatal period. *Neonatal Network* 16(7):5, 1997.

32. **(B)** Early stages of septic shock are distinguished by a hyperdynamic state. Characteristics include tachycardia, tachypnea,

increased cardiac output, and warm extremities. The patient may also appear flushed as a result of vasodilation.

Reference: McConnell, M. S., and Perkin, R. M.: Shock states. *In* Fuhrman, B. P., and Zimmerman, J. J. (Eds.): *Pediatric Critical Care,* 2nd ed. St. Louis, Mosby, 1998, p. 293.

33. (**A**) This infant is demonstrating clinical signs of adequate cardiac output and requires no treatment at this time. Most infants with complete heart block are asymptomatic and do not require immediate intervention. Defibrillation is indicated only for the treatment of pulseless ventricular tachycardia and ventricular fibrillation. Synchronized cardioversion and adenosine are both indicated for the treatment of fast supraventricular rhythms.

References: Flanagan, M. F., Yeager, S. B., and Weindling, S. N.: Cardiac disease. *In* Avery, G. B., Fletcher, M. A., and MacDonald, M. G. (Eds.): *Neonatology: Pathophysiology and Management of the Newborn,* 5th ed. Philadelphia, Lippincott, Williams & Wilkins, 1999, p. 577.
Klassen, L. R.: Complete congenital heart block: a review and case study. *Neonatal Network* 18(3):33, 1999.

34. (**D**) Effectiveness of adenosine is dependent on the dose, injection speed, site of injection, and circulation time from the vein to the heart. Adenosine should not be administered via the umbilical artery catheter because the drug is metabolized by the time it reaches the heart. Adenosine has a half-life of 10 to 15 seconds and must be administered rapidly and at the site most proximal to the heart. Adenosine administration should be followed immediately with a normal saline flush. Adenosine is never given via the endotracheal tube.

References: Chronister, C.: Clinical management of supraventricular tachycardia with adenosine. *Am J Crit Care* 2:41, 1993.
Taketomo, C. K., Hodding, J. H., and Kraus, D. M.: *Pediatric Dosage Handbook,* 6th ed. Hudson, OH, Lexi-Comp, Inc., 1999.
Young, T. E., and Magnum, O. B.: *Neofax: A Manual of Drugs Used in Neonatal Care,* 13th ed. Raleigh, NC, Acorn Publishing Co., 2000.

35. (**C**) In transposition of the great vessels (TOGV), the aorta arises from the right ventricle, and the pulmonary artery arises from the left ventricle. Unoxygenated blood returns from the body to the right atrium and exits back to the body via the aorta. Oxygenated blood returns from the lungs to the left atrium and exits back to the lungs via the pulmonary artery. The infant born with TOGV is dependent on either an intracardiac shunt or patent ductus arteriosus for survival. As pulmonary vascular resistance drops after birth, pulmonary blood flow increases through these shunts. Tricuspid atresia, tetralogy of Fallot, and pulmonary atresia with intact ventricular septum are all associated with an obstruction to blood flow from the right side of the heart and consequently decreased pulmonary blood flow.

Reference: Witt, C.: Cyanotic heart lesions with increased pulmonary blood flow. *Neonatal Network* 17(7):7, 1998.

36. (**D**) Tetralogy of Fallot is associated with decreased pulmonary blood flow. The degree of hypoxemia and cyanosis is dependent on the degree of right ventricular outflow tract obstruction and the amount of shunting across the ventricular septal defect (VSD). Supplemental oxygen has little effect on the degree of hypoxemia and cyanosis.

References: Spilman, L. J., and Furdon, S. A.: Recognition, understanding, and current management of cardiac lesions with decreased pulmonary blood flow. *Neonatal Network* 17(4):7, 1998.
Zuberbuhler, J. R.: Tetralogy of Fallot. *In* Emmanoulides, G. C., Riemenschneider, T. A., Allen, D. H., and Gutgesell, H. P. (Eds.): *Moss and Adams' Heart Disease in Infants, Children, and Adolescents Including the Fetus and Young Adult,* 5th ed. Baltimore, Williams & Wilkins, 1995, p. 998.

37. (**D**) Indomethacin is a nonsteroidal anti-inflammatory agent that inhibits the production of prostaglandin. Prostaglandins play a role in maintaining patency of the ductus arteriosus as well as the cerebral, mesenteric, and renal arteries. A slow infusion of indomethacin has been recommended to minimize the decreased blood flow velocities in the cerebral, gastrointestinal, and renal arterial systems.

Reference: Young, T. E., and Mangum, O. B.: *Neofax: A Manual of Drugs Used in Neonatal Care,* 13th ed. Raleigh, NC, Acorn Publishing, Inc., 2000.

38. (**D**) Transient renal dysfunction is the most significant recognizable side effect of indomethacin. Hyponatremia is also a side effect of indomethacin. Apnea and hypotension generally do not occur after indomethacin administration but are side effects of prostaglandin E_1.

Reference: Bell, S. G.: Neonatal cardiovascular pharmacology. *Neonatal Network* 17(2):7, 1998.

39. (**A**) Pneumatosis intestinalis is diagnostic of necrotizing enterocolitis (NEC). NEC is a contraindication to indomethacin administration.

References: McCollum, L. L., and Thigpen, J. L.: Assessment and management of gastrointestinal dysfunction. *In* Kenner, C., Lott, J. W., and Flandermeyer, A. A. (Eds.): *Comprehensive Neonatal Nursing: A Physiologic Perspective.* Philadelphia, W. B. Saunders, 1998, p. 371.
Young, T. E., and Mangum, O. B.: *Neofax: A Manual of Drugs Used in Neonatal Care,* 13th ed. Raleigh, NC, Acorn Publishing, Inc., 2000.

40. (**D**) Because apnea is a worrisome side effect of prostaglandin E$_1$ infusion, the nurse should be prepared to provide ventilatory support if needed.

Reference: Bell, S. G.: Neonatal cardiovascular pharmacology. *Neonatal Network* 17(2):7, 1998.

41. (**B**) Dopamine administered at low doses, generally 2 to 5 μg/kg/min, will dilate the renal arteries, resulting in increased urine output. Dopamine exerts its inotropic and chronotropic effects at moderate doses, generally 5 to 10 μg/kg/min. Increase in systemic vascular resistance and blood pressure is seen at high doses, generally greater than 10 μg/kg/min.

Reference: Bell, S. G.: Neonatal cardiovascular pharmacology. *Neonatal Network* 17(2):7, 1998.

42. (**C**) Dobutamine is a synthetic catecholamine with primarily B$_1$-adrenergic activity. Although it may decrease systemic and pulmonary vascular resistance in adults, it improves cardiac output mostly by improving cardiac contractility. Dopamine has little effect on heart rate and is not a venodilator.

Reference: Young, T. E., and Mangum, O. B.: *Neofax: A Manual of Drugs Used in Neonatal Care,* 13th ed. Raleigh, NC, Acorn Publishing, Inc., 2000.

43. (**C**) A positive inotrope, digoxin improves cardiac output. Digoxin is also a negative chronotrope, thereby decreasing heart rate. Dobutamine improves cardiac contractility, which will improve cardiac output and subsequently blood pressure. Epinephrine increases heart rate and cardiac contractility, both effects improving cardiac output. Digoxin is the only drug that is used as an antiarrhythmic; it has been used in the management of supraventricular tachycardia (SVT), atrial flutter, and atrial fibrillation.

Reference: Young, T. E., and Mangum, O. B.: *Neofax: A Manual of Drugs Used in Neonatal Care,* 13th ed. Raleigh, NC, Acorn Publishing, Inc., 2000.

44. (**C**) When the tip of an umbilical catheter is in the inferior vena cava, the catheter is an umbilical venous catheter. Central venous pressure can be monitored with a catheter in the inferior vena cava.

Reference: Morrison, S. C., and Fletcher, B. D.: Diagnostic imaging. *In* Fanaroff, A. A., and Martin, R. J.: *Neonatal-Perinatal Medicine: Diseases of the Fetus & Infant,* 6th ed. St. Louis, Mosby, 1997, p. 639.

45. (**D**) A dampened waveform indicates that the waveform is not being effectively transmitted to the transducer. Causes include blood clots in the monitoring system, loose connections, kinked tubing, compliant tubing, and a catheter tip that is against a vessel wall. The pulsatile energy that distends the tubing with each heart beat (systole) is diminished by increasing the length of the monitoring system.

Reference: Darovic, G. O., Vanriper, S., and Vanriper, J.: Fluid-filled monitoring systems. *In* Darovic, G. O. (Ed.): *Hemodynamic Monitoring: Invasive and Noninvasive Clinical Application,* 2nd ed. Philadelphia, W. B. Saunders, 1995, p. 149.

46. (**B**) An infant with congestive heart failure (CHF) has a cardiac output that is unable to meet the demands of the body. CHF results in systemic and venous congestion. The goals of therapy are to improve the functioning of the heart and minimize the work that it has to do. Therapy often includes the use of digoxin to improve cardiac contractility and a diuretic to eliminate excess intravascular fluid.

Reference: Lott, J. W.: Assessment and management of cardiovascular dysfunction. *In* Kenner, C., Lott, J. W., and Flandermeyer, A. A. (Eds.): *Comprehensive Neonatal Nursing: A Physiologic Perspective,* 2nd ed. Philadelphia, W. B. Saunders, 1998, p. 306.

47. (**D**) Normal PR interval varies with age and heart rate. The upper limit of normal for the PR interval in a 1- to 3-week-old newborn with a heart rate between 120 and 140 is 0.11 seconds. First-degree atrioventricular (AV) block is defined as a prolongation of the PR interval beyond the upper limit of normal for the patient's age and heart rate.

Reference: Park, M. K., and Guntheroth, W. G.: *How to Read Pediatric ECGs,* 3rd ed. St. Louis, Mosby, 1992.

48. (**C**) Causes of first-degree atrioventricular (AV) block include digitalis toxicity, myocarditis, certain congenital heart defects (CHDs, endocardial cushion defect, atrial septal defect [ASD], Ebstein's anomaly), and hyperkalemia.

Reference: Park, M. K.: *The Pediatric Cardiology Handbook,* 2nd ed. St. Louis, Mosby, 1997.

49. (**C**) Common signs of congestive heart failure (CHF) are tachycardia, tachypnea, hepatomegaly, and rales. Given the history of atrioventricular (AV) canal defect, congestive heart failure (CHF) is the most likely problem. It is common for an infant with AV canal defect to develop CHF at this age because of the decreasing pulmonary vascular resistance and increasing left-to-right shunting of blood. An infant with dehydration would not demonstrate the pulmonary and venous congestion symptoms of rales and hepatomegaly. A septic infant may be tachycardic and tachypneic but is unlikely to have hepatomegaly.

References: Crockett, M.: Cardiovascular disorders. *In* Deacon, J., and O'Neill, P. (Eds.): *Core Curriculum for Neonatal Intensive Care Nursing,* 2nd ed. Philadelphia, W. B. Saunders, 1999, p. 206.
Park, M. K.: *The Pediatric Cardiology Handbook,* 2nd ed. St. Louis, Mosby, 1997.

50. (**D**) The mainstay of therapy for congestive heart failure (CHF) is diuretics and inotropes. Hydralazine is used in the treatment of hypertension due to its ability to cause relaxation of the smooth muscle of the arteriolar resistance vessels.

References: Crockett, M.: Cardiovascular disorders. *In* Deacon, J., and O'Neill, P. (Eds.): *Core Curriculum for Neonatal Intensive Care Nursing,* 2nd ed. Philadelphia, W. B. Saunders, 1999, p. 206.
Young, T. E., and Mangum, O. B.: *Neofax: A Manual of Drugs Used in Neonatal Care,* 13th ed. Raleigh, NC, Acorn Publishing, Inc., 2000.

51. (**D**) Coarctation of the aorta is associated with an obstruction to blood flow in the aortic arch segment. The obstruction is most commonly distal to the left subclavian artery. A pressure difference is created between the upper extremities, which receive their blood supply proximal to the obstruction, and the lower extremities, which receive their blood supply distal to obstruction. The pressure difference results in upper extremity pulses and blood pressure that are greater than lower extremity pulses and blood pressure. When the obstruction is preductal, unoxygenated blood enters the descending aorta from the ductus, leading to cyanosis visible over only the lower body.

Reference: Lott, J. W.: Assessment and management of cardiovascular dysfunction. *In* Kenner, C., Lott, J. W., and Flandermeyer, A. A. (Eds.): *Comprehensive Neonatal Nursing: A Physiologic Perspective,* 2nd ed. Philadelphia, W. B. Saunders, 1998, p. 306.

52. (**C**) Oxygenated blood enters the fetus via the umbilical vein. The ductus venosus is a low-resistance channel that connects the portal sinus to the inferior vena cava. The ductus venosus allows a significant portion of the oxygenated blood to bypass the liver and proceed directly to the inferior vena cava, where it can enter the heart quickly.

Reference: Zabloudil, C.: Adaptation to extrauterine life. *In* Deacon, J., and O'Neill, P. (Eds.): *Core Curriculum for Neonatal Intensive Care Nursing,* 2nd ed. Philadelphia, W. B. Saunders, 1999, p. 40.

53. (**B**) The ductus arteriosus is a channel connecting the pulmonary artery and the aorta. The direction of blood flow across the ductus is determined by resistance in the pulmonary and systemic circuits. In the fetus, the pulmonary circuit is a higher resistance circuit. Consequently, in the fetus, blood flows from the pulmonary artery to the aorta across the ductus arteriosus.

Reference: Lott, J. W.: Assessment and management of cardiovascular dysfunction. *In* Kenner, C., Lott, J. W., and Flandermeyer, A. A. (Eds.): *Comprehensive Neonatal Nursing: A Physiologic Perspective,* 2nd ed. Philadelphia, W. B. Saunders, 1998, p. 306.

54. (**D**) Cyanosis is difficult to evaluate in the newborn. Cyanosis occurs when there is at least 5 g/100 mL of deoxygenated hemoglobin. The appearance of cyanosis is dependent on the degree of hemoglobin. Infants with high hemoglobin levels may appear cyanotic despite having sufficient amounts of oxygen saturated hemoglobin. Acrocyanosis is common in the first 24 to 48 hours of life; central cyanosis is not.

Reference: Crockett, M.: Cardiovascular disorders. *In* Deacon, J., and O'Neill, P. (Eds.): *Core Curriculum for Neonatal Intensive Care Nursing,* 2nd ed. Philadelphia, W. B. Saunders, 1999, p. 206.

55. (**C**) Renal vein thrombosis from umbilical artery catheter placement is the most

common cause of hypertension in neonates.

Reference: Crockett, M.: Cardiovascular disorders. *In* Deacon, J., and O'Neill, P. (Eds.): *Core Curriculum for Neonatal Intensive Care Nursing,* 2nd ed. Philadelphia, W. B. Saunders, 1999, p. 206.

56. **(C)** Oxygen is a potent pulmonary artery vasodilator. Dilation of the pulmonary arteries in hypoplastic left heart syndrome (HLHS) results in increased pulmonary blood flow and decreased systemic blood flow. A PaO_2 greater than 60 mm Hg in infants with HLHS often results in metabolic acidosis. Hyperoxic ventilation should be avoided in these infants.

Reference: Freedom, R. M., and Benson, L. N.: Hypoplastic left heart syndrome. *In* Emmanoulides, G. C., Riemenschneider, T. A., Allen, D. H., and Gutgesell, H. P. (Eds.): *Moss and Adams' Heart Disease in Infants, Children, and Adolescents Including the Fetus and Young Adult,* 5th ed. Baltimore, Williams & Wilkins, 1995, p. 1133.

57. **(A)** The infant is demonstrating clinical signs of shock, most likely due to hypovolemia. During volume therapy, systemic perfusion and end-organ function should improve. As vascular volume is restored, perfusion should improve, resulting in increased extremity warmth, improved capillary refill, improved extremity warmth, and normalization of heart rate.

Reference: Hazinski, M. F.: *Manual of Pediatric Critical Care.* St. Louis, Mosby, 1999, p. 84.

58. **(C)** Zeroing a fluid-filled monitoring system eliminates the effect of atmospheric pressure on the patient's physiologic pressures. To eliminate the effect of hydrostatic pressure within the monitoring system, the air-fluid interface of the zeroing stopcock must be at the same level as the catheter tip when zeroing. If the air-fluid interface of the zeroing stopcock is below the catheter tip, the positive pressure in the fluid column will be transmitted from the monitored site to the transducer, resulting in a pressure reading higher than the patient's actual pressure.

Reference: Darovic, G. O., Vanriper, S., and Vanriper, J.: Fluid-filled monitoring systems. *In* Darovic, G. O. (Eds.): *Hemodynamic Monitoring: Invasive and Noninvasive Clinical Application,* 2nd ed. Philadelphia, W. B. Saunders, 1995, p. 149.

CHAPTER 13
PULMONARY DISORDERS

1. **(A)** The canalicular stage of fetal lung development I (16–25 weeks' gestation) is characterized by the transformation of the pre-viable lung to a potentially viable organ capable of gas exchange. Three major events occur during this stage of fetal lung development: (1) formation of the acinus; (2) beginning development of pulmonary capillaries; and (3) initiation of surfactant synthesis in type II pneumocytes. The formation of respiratory bronchioles represents the first gas-exchanging units (acini) within the tracheobronchial tree and delineates the gas exchange portion of the lung from the conducting airways. Continued development of the gas exchanging units leads to the creation of new respiratory alveolar ducts and alveoli during the terminal sac stage (25–37 weeks' gestation).

References: Elliot, S. J., and Leuthner, S. R.: Anatomy and development of the lung. *In* Hansen, T. N., Cooper, T. R., and Weisman, L. E. (Eds.): *Contemporary Diagnosis and Management of Neonatal Respiratory Diseases,* 2nd ed. Newtown, Handbooks in Health Care, 1998, p. 1.
Hagedorn, M. E., Gardner, S. L., and Abman, S. H.: Respiratory diseases. *In* Merenstein, G. B., and Gardner, S. L. (Eds.): *Handbook of Neonatal Intensive Care,* 4th ed. St. Louis, Mosby-Year Book, 1998, p. 437.

2. **(C)** The terminal sac phase of fetal lung development (25–37 weeks' gestation) is the period of lung differentiation: (1) proliferation of pulmonary vascular bed; (2) decrease in amount of interstitial mesenchyme allows for the fusion of gas exchange epithelium to the pulmonary capillaries, requisite for the development of the air-blood barrier necessary for pulmonary gas exchange; and (3) progressive increase in the numbers of alveoli, lung volumes, and respiratory surface area. The differentiation of the fetal lung during the terminal sac stage indicates the first anatomic potential for supporting gas exchange in an extrauterine environment.

References: Casey, P.: Respiratory distress. *In* Deacon, J., and O'Neill, P. (Eds.): *Core Curriculum for Neonatal Intensive Care Nursing,* 2nd ed. Philadelphia, W. B. Saunders, 1999, p. 118.
Jobe, A. L.: The respiratory system, part I: Lung development. *In* Fanaroff, A. A., and Martin, R. J. (Eds.): *Neonatal-Perinatal Medicine,* 6th ed. St. Louis, Mosby, 1997, p. 991.

3. **(C)** Prior to 24 weeks' gestation, the fetal lungs are incapable of maintaining ade-

quate gaseous exchange necessary for extrauterine life due to insufficient alveolar surface area and insufficient pulmonary vascular development.

References: Hagedorn, M. E., Gardner, S. L., and Abman, S. H.: Respiratory diseases. *In* Merenstein, G. B., and Gardner, S. L. (Eds.): *Handbook of Neonatal Intensive Care*, 4th ed. St. Louis, Mosby-Year Book, 1998, p. 437.
Jobe, A. L.: The respiratory system, part I: Lung development. *In* Fanaroff, A. A., and Martin, R. J. (Eds.): *Neonatal-Perinatal Medicine*, 6th ed. St. Louis, Mosby, 1997, p. 991.

4. **(D)** The alveolar phase of lung development extends from 37 weeks' gestation until 8 to 10 years of life. During this period, there is further alveolar proliferation and differentiation, which maximizes the amount of exposed surface area for gaseous exchange.

References: Casey, P.: Respiratory distress. *In* Deacon, J., and O'Neill, P. (Eds.): *Core Curriculum for Neonatal Intensive Care Nursing*, 2nd ed. Philadelphia, W. B. Saunders, 1999, p. 118.
Hagedorn, M. E., Gardner, S. L., and Abman, S. H.: Respiratory diseases. *In* Merenstein, G. B., and Gardner, S. L. (Eds.): *Handbook of Neonatal Intensive Care*, 4th ed. St. Louis, Mosby-Year Book, 1998, p. 437.

5. **(A)** Surfactant is a surface-active material that lines alveoli and works against surface tension forces to prevent alveolar collapse at the end of expiration. The presence of adequate quantities of surfactant in the alveoli improves lung function by reducing surface tension, which enables the alveoli to remain open during expiration (alveolar stability), thereby facilitating gaseous exchange and the improvement of lung function.

References: Casey, P.: Respiratory distress. *In* Deacon, J., and O'Neill, P. (Eds.): *Core Curriculum for Neonatal Intensive Care Nursing*, 2nd ed. Philadelphia, W. B. Saunders, 1999, p. 118.
Hagedorn, M. E., Gardner, S. L., and Abman, S. H.: Respiratory diseases. *In* Merenstein, G. B., and Gardner, S. L. (Eds.) *Handbook of Neonatal Intensive Care*, 4th ed. St. Louis, Mosby-Year Book, 1998, p. 437.

6. **(D)** Infants born to class A, B, and C diabetic mothers prior to 38 weeks' gestation may develop respiratory distress syndrome due to the inhibitory effects of excess insulin on surfactant production. Antenatal factors associated with acceleration in fetal lung maturity include the following: exposure to prenatal heroin addiction, maternal hypertension, and intrauterine growth retardation.

References: Casey, P.: Respiratory distress. *In* Deacon, J., and O'Neill, P. (Eds.): *Core Curriculum for Neonatal Intensive Care Nursing*, 2nd ed. Philadelphia, W. B. Saunders, 1999, p. 118.
Hagedorn, M. E., Gardner, S. L., and Abman, S. H.: Respiratory diseases. *In* Merenstein, G. B., and Gardner, S. L. (Eds.): *Handbook of Neonatal Intensive Care*, 4th ed. St. Louis, Mosby-Year Book, 1998, p. 437.

7. **(B)** The type II pneumocyte is responsible for the synthesis, storage, secretion, and recycling of surfactant in the lung. Surfactant protein-A is one of four surfactant-specific proteins within the surfactant lipoprotein complex. The acinus is the gas-exchanging respiratory unit within the lung.

References: Casey, P.: Respiratory distress. *In* Deacon, J., and O'Neill, P. (Eds.): *Core Curriculum for Neonatal Intensive Care Nursing*, 2nd ed. Philadelphia, W. B. Saunders, 1999, p. 118.
Jobe, A. L.: The respiratory system, part I: Lung development. *In* Fanaroff, A. A., and Martin, R. J. (Eds.): *Neonatal-Perinatal Medicine*, 6th ed. St. Louis, Mosby, 1997, p. 991.

8. **(D)** Peripheral cyanosis of the hands and feet (acrocyanosis) is a normal finding in the first 24 hours of life. Respiratory rates of 30 to 60 breaths per minute is normal in the early neonatal period, with rates above 60 (tachypnea) generally the earliest sign of respiratory distress in the neonate. Hypotension may be associated with respiratory diseases but is often a late sign of respiratory distress. Expiratory grunting, nasal flaring, and chest wall retractions are indicative of a marked increase in the work of breathing, and therefore indicators of respiratory distress.

References: Casey, P.: Respiratory distress. *In* Deacon, J., and O'Neill, P. (Eds.): *Core Curriculum for Neonatal Intensive Care Nursing*, 2nd ed. Philadelphia, W. B. Saunders, 1999, p. 118.
Hagedorn, M. E., Gardner, S. L., and Abman, S. H.: Respiratory diseases. *In* Merenstein, G. B., and Gardner, S. L. (Eds.): *Handbook of Neonatal Intensive Care*, 4th ed. St. Louis, Mosby-Year Book, 1998, p. 437.

9. **(A)** Respiratory distress syndrome (RDS) is predominantly a disease of immature lung anatomy and physiology. Anatomically, the ability of the preterm lung to support adequate ventilation and perfusion depends greatly on the degree of development of the pulmonary vasculature and alveolar surface areas. Physiologically, the absence of sufficient quantities of surfactant leads to alveolar

collapse, ventilation-perfusion mismatch, and, ultimately, respiratory failure. The more immature the lung, the greater the incidence of RDS, with 60 to 80% of infants born at less than 28 weeks' gestation affected. RDS is more common in males and second-born twins.

References: Hagedorn, M. E., Gardner, S. L., and Abman, S. H.: Respiratory diseases. *In* Merenstein, G. B., and Gardner, S. L. (Eds.): *Handbook of Neonatal Intensive Care*, 4th ed. St. Louis, Mosby-Year Book, 1998, p. 437.
Martin, R. J., and Fanaroff, A. A.: The respiratory system, Part III: Respiratory distress syndrome and its management. *In* Fanaroff, A. A., and Martin, R. J. (Eds.): *Neonatal-Perinatal Medicine*, 6th ed. St. Louis, Mosby, 1997, p. 1018.

10. **(C)** A history of prematurity and tachypnea, grunting, flaring, and retractions within the first minutes to hours of life is characteristic with respiratory distress syndrome.

Reference: Hagedorn, M. E., Gardner, S. L., and Abman, S. H.: Respiratory diseases. *In* Merenstein, G. B., and Gardner, S. L. (Eds.): *Handbook of Neonatal Intensive Care*, 4th ed. St. Louis, Mosby-Year Book, 1998, p. 437.

11. **(A)** Grunting is defined as a forced exhalation against a partially closed glottis and represents the infant's attempt to keep the alveoli open at the end of expiration. Grunting prevents alveolar collapse by producing a positive end-expiratory pressure (PEEP) that serves to splint the airways open and thereby improves gaseous exchange by maintaining functional residual capacity (FRC). FRC is defined as the volume of air that remains in the lung after a normal expiration. It has been shown that grunting can sustain an FRC and a PaO_2 equivalent to that which is produced through the application of 2 to 3 cm of H_2O of continuous distending pressure (CPAP).

References: Carlo, W. A.: The respiratory system, Part II: Assessment of pulmonary function. *In* Fanaroff, A. A., and Martin, R. J. (Eds.): *Neonatal-Perinatal Medicine*, 6th ed. St. Louis, Mosby, 1997, p. 1009.
Casey, P.: Respiratory distress. *In* Deacon, J., and O'Neill, P. (Eds.): *Core Curriculum for Neonatal Intensive Care Nursing*, 2nd ed. Philadelphia, W. B. Saunders, 1999, p. 118.
Hagedorn, M. E., Gardner, S. L., and Abman, S. H.: Respiratory diseases. *In* Merenstein, G. B., and Gardner, S. L. (Eds.): *Handbook of Neonatal Intensive Care*, 4th ed. St. Louis, Mosby-Year Book, 1998, p. 437.

12. **(B)** The definitive diagnosis of neonatal sepsis is based on the presence of a positive blood culture. The isolation of bacte-

ria from blood, cerebrospinal fluid (CSF), and urine specimens are considered to be valid indicators of bacterial sepsis and should be obtained when neonatal sepsis is suspected. It is important to note that in many neonatal centers, lumbar puncture (i.e., spinal tap) is not a routine component of the diagnostic work-up for suspected neonatal sepsis. However, in the presence of a positive blood culture, cerebral spinal fluid should be obtained prior to the administration of antibiotics. Surface cultures (i.e., skin, nares, rectum) are not indicative of systemic infection but are indicative of bacterial colonization.

References: Merenstein, G. B., Adams, K., and Weisman, L. E.: Infection in the neonate. *In* Merenstein, G. B., and Gardner, S. L. (Eds.): *Handbook of Neonatal Intensive Care*, 4th ed. St. Louis, Mosby-Year Book, 1998, p. 413.
Hickey, S. M., and McCracken, G.: The immune system, Part II: Postnatal bacterial infections. *In* Fanaroff, A. A., and Martin, R. J. (Eds.): *Neonatal-Perinatal Medicine*, 6th ed. St. Louis, Mosby, 1997, p. 1018.

13. **(C)** The granular or ground-glass appearance is primarily caused by alveolar atelectasis or nonaerated alveoli. The air bronchograms represent aerated bronchioles superimposed on a background of nonaerated alveoli/atelectatic alveoli.

Reference: Martin, R. J., and Fanaroff, A. A.: The respiratory system, Part III: Respiratory distress syndrome and its management. *In* Fanaroff, A. A., and Martin, R. J. (Eds.): *Neonatal-Perinatal Medicine*, 6th ed. St. Louis, Mosby, 1997, p. 1018.

14. **(C)** The pH of 7.25 is indicative of acidosis. The $PaCO_2$ of 70 indicates a respiratory component of the acidosis. The HCO_3 of 21 is within normal range.

References: Kirby, E.: Assisted ventilation. *In* Deacon, J., and O'Neill, P. (Eds.): *Core Curriculum for Neonatal Intensive Care Nursing*, 2nd ed. Philadelphia, W. B. Saunders, 1999, p. 164.
Parry, W. H., and Zimmer, J.: Acid-base homeostasis and oxygenation. *In* Merenstein, G. B., and Gardner, S. L. (Eds.): *Handbook of Neonatal Intensive Care*, 4th ed. St. Louis, Mosby-Year Book, 1998, p. 160.

15. **(B)** Increasing agitation, "see-saw" respirations, and secretions "bubbling" up the endotracheal tube may be indications that the infant requires suctioning. The first action should be to assess the patient, to determine whether the infant is still intubated and to assess the need for suctioning.

References: Garcia-Pratts, J. A., and Adams, J. M.: Respiratory therapy—general considerations: Management of the airway. *In* Hansen, T. N., Cooper, T. R., and Weisman, L. E. (Eds.): *Contemporary Diagnosis and Management of Neonatal Respiratory Diseases,* 2nd ed. Newtown, Handbooks in Healthcare, 1998, p. 235.

Hagedorn, M. E., Gardner, S. L., and Abman, S. H.: Respiratory diseases. *In* Merenstein, G. B., and Gardner, S. L. (Eds.): *Handbook of Neonatal Intensive Care,* 4th ed. St. Louis, Mosby-Year Book, 1998, p. 437.

16. **(C)** Patent ductus arteriosus (PDA) associated with respiratory distress syndrome results from failure of the ductus to close after birth or from its reopening after functional closure. There is an increased incidence of PDA in infants younger than 30 weeks' gestation and weighing less than 1500 g. PDA should be considered when there is a delay in clinical improvement from respiratory distress syndrome (RDS) or when there is a prolonged or increased requirement for ventilator and/or oxygen support. The key pathophysiologic abnormalities associated with PDA are increased blood flow to pulmonary circulation and volume overload to the left ventricle. This leads to rales, tachypnea, machinery-like murmur, hyperdynamic precordium, bounding peripheral pulses, diminished capillary refill, tissue mottling, and oliguria.

Reference: Daberkow-Carson, E., and Washington, R. L.: Cardiovascular diseases and surgical interventions. *In* Merenstein, G. B., and Gardner, S. L. (Eds.): *Handbook of Neonatal Intensive Care,* 4th ed. St. Louis, Mosby-Year Book, 1998, p. 500.

17. **(A)** Indomethacin, fluid restriction, and diuretic therapy are possible components of medical management for infants with symptomatic PDA. Prostaglandin E_1 is used to maintain ductal patency in newborns with specific types of congenital heart defects (e.g., ductal-dependent lesions, coarctation of aorta, transposition of great vessels, tricuspid atresia, pulmonary atresia, hypoplastic left heart).

References: Drummon, W. H.: Ductus arteriosus. *In* Spitzer, A. R. (Ed.): *Intensive Care of the Fetus & Neonate.* St. Louis, Mosby, 1996, p. 760.
Merenstein, G. B., and Gardner, S. L. (Eds.): *Handbook of Neonatal Intensive Care,* 4th ed. St. Louis, Mosby-Year Book, 1998, p. 500.

18. **(B)** The left-to-right shunting of blood from the aorta to the pulmonary artery via the ductus arteriosus results in increased blood flow to the lungs and decreased blood flow to the lower aorta, with resultant signs of systemic hyper-

fusion (i.e., tissue mottling, diminished capillary refill, oliguria) and pulmonary congestion (i.e., tachypnea, hypercarbia).

References: Daberkow-Carson, E., and Washington, R. L.: Cardiovascular diseases and surgical interventions. *In* Merenstein, G. B., and Gardner, S. L. (Eds.): *Handbook of Neonatal Intensive Care,* 4th ed. St. Louis, Mosby-Year Book, 1998, p. 500.
Drummon, W. H.: Ductus arteriosus. *In* Spitzer, A. R. (Ed.): *Intensive Care of the Fetus & Neonate.* St. Louis, Mosby, 1996, p. 760.

19. **(D)** The pulmonary consequences of a patent ductus arteriosus (PDA) in a preterm infant with underlying respiratory distress syndrome are directly dependent on the following factors: (1) the amount of blood that is shunting left to right from the aorta to the lungs; (2) gestational age; (3) underlying pulmonary disease; and (4) the presence of other medical conditions. In infants with prior lung disease, the increase in pulmonary interstitial fluid as a result of left-to-right shunting across the PDA leads to a further reduction in pulmonary compliance, and frequently necessitates the use of increased ventilatory pressures to optimize pulmonary status. Pulmonary interstitial emphysema, pulmonary hemorrhage, and long-term ventilatory dependency are pulmonary complications of PDA associated with the excessive use of ventilatory pressures. Pulmonary hypoplasia is an anatomic malformation. It is either an isolated entity or secondary to lesions that restrict lung growth.

References: Drummon, W. H.: Ductus arteriosus. *In* Spitzer, A. R. (Ed.): *Intensive Care of the Fetus & Neonate.* St. Louis, Mosby, 1996, p. 760.
Miller, M. J., Fanaroff, A. A., and Martin, R. J.: Respiratory disorders in preterm and term infants. *In* Fanaroff, A. A., and Martin, R. J. (Eds.): *Neonatal Perinatal Medicine: Diseases of the Fetus and Infant,* 6th ed. St. Louis, Mosby, 1997, p. 1040.

20. **(A)** An optimal thermal environment based on the neonate's gestational age and birth weight is necessary to minimize oxygen consumption and oxygen requirements. Hypothermia (cold stress) leads to peripheral vasoconstriction, anaerobic metabolism, and metabolic acidosis. This, in turn, causes pulmonary vessel constriction, leading to further hypoxia, anaerobic metabolism, acidosis, and decreased surfactant production. It is a vicious cycle that may further complicate the infant's respiratory status.

References: Blake, W. W., and Murray, A. A.: Heat balance. *In* Merenstein, G. B., and Gardner, S. L. (Eds.): *Handbook of Neonatal Intensive Care,* 4th ed. St. Louis, Mosby-Year Book, 1998, p. 100.

Hagedorn, M. E., Gardner, S. L., and Abman, S. H.: Respiratory diseases. *In* Merenstein, G. B., and Gardner, S. L. (Eds.): *Handbook of Neonatal Intensive Care,* 4th ed. St. Louis, Mosby-Year Book, 1998, p. 437.

21. **(B)** Fluid retention and edema are characteristic findings during the early phase of respiratory distress syndrome. A spontaneous diuresis that occurs between 48 and 72 hours of life precedes the onset of the recovery phase of respiratory distress syndrome and subsequent improvement in lung function.

Reference: Martin, R. J., and Fanaroff, A. A.: The respiratory system, Part III: Respiratory distress syndrome and its management. *In* Fanaroff, A. A., and Martin, R. J. (Eds.): *Neonatal-Perinatal Medicine,* 6th ed. St. Louis, Mosby, 1997, p. 1018.

22. **(D)** Bacteria responsible for early onset pneumonia or sepsis are acquired from the birth canal before or during delivery. Predisposing risk factors include chorioamnionitis with maternal fever, premature rupture of membranes, prolonged labor, or excessive obstetric manipulations (internal monitors, fetal scalp monitors, etc.).

References: Merenstein, G. B., Adams, K., and Weisman, L. E.: Infection in the neonate. *In* Merenstein, G. B., and Gardner, S. L. (Eds.): *Handbook of Neonatal Intensive Care,* 4th ed. St. Louis, Mosby-Year Book, 1998, p. 500.

Orlando, S.: Pathophysiology of acute respiratory diseases. *In* Askin, D. F. (Ed.): *Acute Respiratory Care of the Neonate.* Petaluma, NICU Ink Books, 1997, p. 37.

23. **(A)** The following criteria are indications for starting oxygen supplementation: (1) PaO_2 less than 60 mm Hg, (2) respiratory distress, (3) central cyanosis, (4) hypotonia, and (5) apnea. Although tachypneic, there are no indications of apnea, and the neonate is able to maintain PaO_2 levels within normal range with oxygen supplementation. On the basis of the clinical data, neither intubation nor nitric oxide is required at this time.

References: Casey, P.: Respiratory distress. *In* Deacon, J., and O'Neill, P. (Eds.): *Core Curriculum for Neonatal Intensive Care Nursing,* 2nd ed. Philadelphia, W. B. Saunders, 1999, p. 118.

Hagedorn, M. E., Gardner, S. L., and Abman, S. H.: Respiratory diseases. *In* Merenstein, G. B., and Gardner, S. L. (Eds.): *Handbook of Neonatal Intensive Care,* 4th ed. St. Louis, Mosby-Year Book, 1998, p. 437.

Miller, M. J., Fanaroff, A. A., and Martin, R. J.: The respiratory system, Part V: Respiratory disorders in preterm and term infants. *In* Fanaroff, A. A., and Martin, R. J. (Eds.): *Neonatal-Perinatal Medicine,* 6th ed. St. Louis, Mosby, 1997, p. 1040.

24. **(C)** In transient tachypnea of the newborn (TTN), chest radiographic findings typically reveal prominent perihilar streaking, hyperaeration, and a mildly to moderately enlarged heart. The perihilar streaking is thought to represent engorgement of the periarterial lymphatics that participate in the clearance of alveolar fluid. Hyperaeration (hyperexpansion) of the lungs is thought to be due to retained lung fluid that obstructs the lower airways, resulting in overdistention from a ball-valve phenomenon.

References: Casey, P.: Respiratory distress. *In* Deacon, J., and O'Neill, P. (Eds.): *Core Curriculum for Neonatal Intensive Care Nursing,* 2nd ed. Philadelphia, W. B. Saunders, 1999, p. 118.

Hagedorn, M. E., Gardner, S. L., and Abman, S. H.: Respiratory diseases. *In* Merenstein, G. B., and Gardner, S. L. (Eds.): *Handbook of Neonatal Intensive Care,* 4th ed. St. Louis, Mosby-Year Book, 1998, p. 437.

Miller, M. J., Fanaroff, A. A., and Martin, R. J.: The respiratory system, Part V: Respiratory disorders in preterm and term infants. *In* Fanaroff, A. A., and Martin, R. J. (Eds.): *Neonatal-Perinatal Medicine,* 6th ed. St. Louis, Mosby, 1997, p. 1040.

25. **(A)** Transient tachypnea of the newborn (TTN) is thought to be due to delayed resorption of fetal alveolar fluid from the pulmonary lymphatic system. The increased fluid leads to airway obstruction and air-trapping, which in turn is responsible for the clinical signs of respiratory distress in the neonate.

References: Hagedorn, M. E., Gardner, S. L., and Abman, S. H.: Respiratory diseases. *In* Merenstein, G. B., and Gardner, S. L. (Eds.): *Handbook of Neonatal Intensive Care,* 4th ed. St. Louis, Mosby-Year Book, 1998, p. 437.

Miller, M. J., Fanaroff, A. A., and Martin, R. J.: The respiratory system, Part V: Respiratory disorders in preterm and term infants. *In* Fanaroff, A. A., and Martin, R. J. (Eds.): *Neonatal-Perinatal Medicine,* 6th ed. St. Louis, Mosby, 1997, p. 1040.

26. **(D)** Several conditions may have a clinical presentation that mimics transient tachypnea of the newborn (TTN) or have radiographic findings similar to those characteristic of TTN. Bacterial pneumonia, respiratory distress syndrome (RDS), and TTN all clinically present with tachypnea, oxygen requirements, and increased work of breathing during the early neonatal period. However, infants with TTN are sickest at birth, and then begin a gradual

improvement with complete resolution within 48 to 72 hours, whereas infants with RDS or pneumonia will progressively worsen over time. Chest radiographs are helpful in distinguishing TTN from RDS. On a radiograph, TTN is characterized as a "high-volume," or hyperinflated, lung, whereas RDS is characterized as a "low-volume" lung. Pulmonary edema associated with cardiac defects can also mimic TTN but is distinguished from TTN based on other signs of cardiac disease and by failure to show improvement over time. A pneumothorax, on the other hand, is not considered in the differential diagnosis of TTN.

Reference: Speer, M. E., and Hansen, T. N.: Transient tachypnea of the newborn. *In* Hansen, T. N., Cooper, R., and Weisman, L. E. (Eds.): *Contemporary Diagnosis and Management of Neonatal Respiratory Diseases*, 2nd ed. Newtown, Handbooks in Healthcare, 1998, p. 95.

27. **(C)** Asphyxia is defined as increased inadequate tissue perfusion, which fails to meet the metabolic demands of the tissue for oxygen and waste removal. Asphyxia is characterized by progressive hypoxia ($\downarrow$ Po_2), hypercarbia ($\uparrow$ Pco_2) and acidosis ($\downarrow$ pH).

Reference: Niermeyer, S., and Clarke, S.: Delivery room care. *In* Merenstein, G. B., and Gardner, S. L. (Eds.): *Handbook of Neonatal Intensive Care*, 4th ed. St. Louis, Mosby-Year Book, 1998, p. 46.

28. **(B)** From a clinical perspective, it is difficult to discriminate between primary and secondary apnea at birth. Both are characterized by hypotonia, apnea, and heart rate less than 100 bpm. Whereas blow-by-oxygen and tactile stimulation may be all that are required to initiate spontaneous respiration in primary apnea, infants born with secondary apnea require resuscitation with assisted ventilation and oxygen to induce spontaneous respiration.

References: Goodwin, M.: Apnea of the newborn infant. *In* Deacon, J., and O'Neill, P. (Eds.): *Core Curriculum for Neonatal Intensive Care Nursing*, 2nd ed. Philadelphia, W. B. Saunders, 1999, p. 151.
Niermeyer, S., and Clarke, S.: Delivery room care. *In* Merenstein, G. B., and Gardner, S. L. (Eds.): *Handbook of Neonatal Intensive Care Nursing*, 4th ed. St. Louis, Mosby, 1998, p. 46.

29. **(D)** Fetal and/or neonatal asphyxia may significantly impair the physiologic transition from intrauterine to extrauterine life. In the presence of severe hypoxemia and acidosis, the pulmonary vasculature

remains constricted, which in turn leads to hypoperfusion of the lungs, and a return to a persistent fetal type of circulation.

Reference: Niermeyer, S., and Clarke, S.: Delivery room care. *In* Merenstein, G. B., and Gardner, S. L. (Eds.): *Handbook of Neonatal Intensive Care*, 4th ed. St. Louis, Mosby-Year Book, 1998, p. 46.

30. **(B)** Central apnea is defined as the absence of airflow and respiratory effort.

Reference: Goodwin, M.: Apnea of the newborn infant. *In* Deacon, J., and O'Neill, P. (Eds.): *Core Curriculum for Neonatal Intensive Care Nursing*, 2nd ed. Philadelphia, W. B. Saunders, 1999, p. 151.

31. **(A)** There are significant differences between the adult and neonatal response to hypoxemia and changes in Pco_2. Adults respond with a sustained increase in ventilation, whereas neonates demonstrate a brief period of increased ventilation followed by respiratory depression.

References: Goodwin, M.: Apnea of the newborn infant. *In* Deacon, J., and O'Neill, P. (Eds.): *Core Curriculum for Neonatal Intensive Care Nursing*, 2nd ed. Philadelphia, W. B. Saunders, 1999, p. 151.
Hagedorn, M. E., Gardner, S. L., and Abman, S. H.: Respiratory diseases. *In* Merenstein, G. B., and Gardner, S. L. (Eds.): *Handbook of Neonatal Intensive Care*, 4th ed. St. Louis, Mosby-Year Book, 1998, p. 437.
Miller, M. J., Fanaroff, A. A., and Martin, R. J.: The respiratory system, Part V: Respiratory disorders in preterm and term infants. *In* Fanaroff, A. A., and Martin, R. J. (Eds.): *Neonatal-Perinatal Medicine*, 6th ed. St. Louis, Mosby, 1997, p. 1040.

32. **(D)** A number of pathophysiologic disorders may predispose the infant to apnea. Hypotension has been identified as a possible cause of apnea. Hypertension has not been identified as an underlying cause of apnea.

References: Goodwin, M.: Apnea of the newborn infant. *In* Deacon, J., and O'Neill, P. (Eds.): *Core Curriculum for Neonatal Intensive Care Nursing*, 2nd ed. Philadelphia, W. B. Saunders, 1999, p. 151.
Miller, M. J., Fanaroff, A. A., and Martin, R. J.: The respiratory system, Part V: Respiratory disorders in preterm and term infants. *In* Fanaroff, A. A., and Martin, R. J. (Eds.): *Neonatal-Perinatal Medicine*, 6th ed. St. Louis, Mosby, 1997, p. 1040.

33. **(C)** Observations of chest wall movements during rapid eye movement (REM) versus quiet sleep have noted that chest wall movements are predominantly "out of phase" (paradoxical) during REM sleep in comparison to the synchronous expansion of rib cage and abdomen during quiet sleep. It is suggested that the para-

doxical chest wall movements in REM sleep are caused by decreased intercostal muscle activity. Other mechanisms have also been proposed to explain the high incidence of apnea during REM sleep: (1) a fall in functional residual capacity (FRC) and a drop of 6 to 10 mm Hg in PaO_2 during REM sleep; (2) increased depression of ventilation in response to hypoxia during active or REM sleep; (3) "blunted" response to rising levels of carbon dioxide during REM or active sleep; and (4) decreased skeletal muscle tone of tongue and pharynx during sleep, which may lead to airway obstruction.

References: Goodwin, M.: Apnea of the newborn infant. *In* Deacon, J., and O'Neill, P. (Eds.): *Core Curriculum for Neonatal Intensive Care Nursing,* 2nd ed. Philadelphia, W. B. Saunders, 1999, p. 151.
Hagedorn, M. E., Gardner, S. L., and Abman, S. H.: Respiratory diseases. *In* Merenstein, G. B., and Gardner, S. L. (Eds.): *Handbook of Neonatal Intensive Care,* 4th ed. St. Louis, Mosby-Year Book, 1998, p. 437.
Miller, M. J., Fanaroff, A. A., and Martin, R. J.: The respiratory system, Part V: Respiratory disorders in preterm and term infants. *In* Fanaroff, A. A., and Martin, R. J. (Eds.): *Neonatal-Perinatal Medicine,* 6th ed. St. Louis, Mosby, 1997, p. 1040.

34. **(D)** Although apnea may be caused by a multitude of physiologic factors, apnea can also be induced iatrogenically. Iatrogenic causes of apnea include the following: (1) increased and/or sudden changes in environmental temperature; (2) vagal response to suctioning, insertion of nasogastric tubes, gastroesophageal reflux, and obstruction of airway; (3) noxious stimuli, including loud noises, tapping on isolette, and excessive handling; and (4) obstructive apnea due to improper neck positioning or aspiration. Weighing an infant on a cold scale exposes an infant to a sudden environmental change, which in turn may cause an apneic episode in an "at-risk" preterm infant.

References: Goodwin, M.: Apnea of the newborn infant. *In* Deacon, J., and O'Neill, P. (Eds.): *Core Curriculum for Neonatal Intensive Care Nursing,* 2nd ed. Philadelphia, W. B. Saunders, 1999, p. 151.
Hagedorn, M. E., Gardner, S. L., and Abman, S. H.: Respiratory diseases. *In* Merenstein, G. B., and Gardner, S. L. (Eds.): *Handbook of Neonatal Intensive Care,* 4th ed. St. Louis, Mosby-Year Book, 1998, p. 437.

35. **(A)** The most common side effects associated with prostaglandin E_1 include bradycardia, cutaneous flushing, hyperthermia, hypotension, and apnea.

References: Bell, S. G.: Neonatal cardiovascular pharmacology. *Neonatal Network* 17(2):7, 1998.
Pettet, G., Sewell, S., and Merenstein, G. B.: Delivery room care. *In* Merenstein, G. B., and Gardner, S. L. (Eds.): *Handbook of Neonatal Intensive Care,* 4th ed. St. Louis, Mosby-Year Book, 1998, p. 30.

36. **(B)** Doxapram is a potent respiratory stimulant for apnea that is refractory to methylxanthine therapy. Aminophylline, theophylline, and caffeine are methylxanthines.

References: Goodwin, M.: Apnea of the newborn infant. *In* Deacon, J., and O'Neill, P. (Eds.): *Core Curriculum for Neonatal Intensive Care Nursing,* 2nd ed. Philadelphia, W. B. Saunders, 1999, p. 151.
Miller, M., and Martin, R. J.: Pathophysiology of apnea of prematurity. *In* Polin, R., and Fox, W. (Eds.): *Fetal and Neonatal Physiology,* 2nd ed. Philadelphia, W. B. Saunders, 1998, p. 1129.

37. **(B)** Tachycardia is a side effect of theophylline and may be one of the signs of theophylline toxicity. The physician should be notified when tachycardia is present prior to administration of the drug. Serum concentration must be monitored to avoid toxic levels with potentially adverse effects.

References: Calhoun, L. K.: Pharmacologic management of apnea of prematurity. *J Perinatal Neonatal Nursing* 9:56, 1996.
Miller, M. J., Fanaroff, A. A., and Martin, R. J.: The respiratory system, Part V: Respiratory disorders in preterm and term infants. *In* Fanaroff, A. A., and Martin, R. J. (Eds.): *Neonatal-Perinatal Medicine,* 6th ed. St. Louis, Mosby, 1997, p. 1040.

38. **(A)** The recommended dose of theophylline is 5 mg/kg loading dose followed by 1 to 2 mg/kg every 8 to 12 hours to achieve an adequate therapeutic level of 5 to 15 µg/mL.

References: Calhoun, L. K.: Pharmacologic management of apnea of prematurity. *J Perinatal Neonatal Nursing* 9:56, 1996.
Goodwin, M.: Apnea of the newborn infant. *In* Deacon, J., and O'Neill, P. (Eds.): *Core Curriculum for Neonatal Intensive Care Nursing,* 2nd ed. Philadelphia, W. B. Saunders, 1999, p. 151.

39. **(B)** The therapeutic advantages to caffeine are as follows:

1. Oral and intravenous preparations are available.
2. Caffeine is administered only once a day.
3. Caffeine has a longer half-life, resulting in smaller changes in its plasma concentration, which decreases the risk of toxicity.

4. Caffeine has a wider therapeutic index.

References: Calhoun, L. K.: Pharmacologic management of apnea of prematurity. *J Perinatal Neonatal Nursing* 9:56, 1996.
Goodwin, M.: Apnea of the newborn infant. *In* Deacon, J., and O'Neill, P. (Eds.): *Core Curriculum for Neonatal Intensive Care Nursing*, 2nd ed. Philadelphia, W. B. Saunders, 1999, p. 151.
Miller, M. J., Fanaroff, A. A., and Martin, R. J.: The respiratory system, Part V: Respiratory disorders in preterm and term infants. *In* Fanaroff, A. A., and Martin, R. J. (Eds.): *Neonatal-Perinatal Medicine*, 6th ed. St. Louis, Mosby, 1997, p. 1040.

40. **(B)** The most appropriate immediate response is to confirm the absence of respiration and then to apply "gentle" tactile stimulation as the first intervention employed to reestablish breathing. For most infants, gentle tactile stimulation may be all that is required to reestablish respiration. Noxious stimuli, such as loud noises, can induce apneic episodes in infants. If gentle tactile stimuli is ineffective in reversing the apnea episode, then it may be necessary to provide assisted ventilation.

Reference: Hagedorn, M. E., Gardner, S. L., and Abman, S. H.: Respiratory diseases. *In* Merenstein, G. B., and Gardner, S. L. (Eds.): *Handbook of Neonatal Intensive Care*, 4th ed. St. Louis, Mosby-Year Book, 1998, p. 437.

41. **(A)** When evaluating teaching effectiveness regarding home apnea monitoring, the nurse should assess the parent's ability to:

1. State reason for apnea.
2. Demonstrate electrode application.
3. Demonstrate ability to differentiate between "real" alarms versus "technical" alarms.
4. Demonstrate appropriate response to apnea monitor alarms.
5. State safety measures for the use of apnea monitors in the home environment.

Reference: Hagedorn, M. E., Gardner, S. L., and Abman, S. H.: Respiratory diseases. *In* Merenstein, G. B., and Gardner, S. L. (Eds.): *Handbook of Neonatal Intensive Care*, 4th ed. St. Louis, Mosby-Year Book, 1998, p. 437.

42. **(D)** Side effects of methylxanthine therapy include the following:

1. cardiovascular (e.g., tachycardia, hypotension, cardiac dysrhythmias)
2. central nervous system (e.g., jitteriness, increased wakefulness, seizures, increased REM sleep)
3. gastrointestinal (e.g., feeding intoler-

ance, gastroesophageal reflux, gastrointestinal bleeding)
4. genitourinary (e.g., increased diuresis with sodium loss)

References: Goetzman, B. W., and Milstein, J. M.: Pharmacologic adjuncts I. *In* Goldsmith, J. P., and Karotkin, E. H. (Eds.): *Assisted Ventilation of the Neonate*, 3rd ed. Philadelphia, W. B. Saunders, 1999, p. 291.
Goodwin, M.: Apnea of the newborn infant. *In* Deacon, J., and O'Neill, P. (Eds.): *Core Curriculum for Neonatal Intensive Care Nursing*, 2nd ed. Philadelphia, W. B. Saunders, 1999, p. 151.

43. **(C)** Abdominal distention is a potential complication associated with nasal continuous positive airway pressure (CPAP). Orogastric tubes should be used for gastric decompression. Because neonates are obligate nasal breathers, nasogastric tubes should be avoided to minimize problems associated with nasal occlusion.

Reference: Ahumada, C. A., and Goldsmith, J. P.: Continuous distending pressure. *In* Goldsmith, J. P., and Karotkin, E. H. (Eds.): *Assisted Ventilation of the Neonate*, 3rd ed. Philadelphia, W. B. Saunders, 1996, p. 151.

44. **(C)** A major contraindication to the use of extracorporeal membrane oxygenation (ECMO) therapy is prematurity. Research indicates a greater risk of spontaneous intraventricular hemorrhage when preterm infants of less than 35 weeks' gestation participated in ECMO trials.

Reference: Stork, E. K.: The respiratory system, Part VIII: Rescue therapy for cardiorespiratory failure. *In* Fanaroff, A. A., and Martin, R. J. (Eds.): *Neonatal-Perinatal Medicine*, 6th ed. St. Louis, Mosby, 1997, p. 1089.

45. **(D)** Extracorporeal membrane oxygenation (ECMO) is contraindicated in cases of irreversible respiratory disease (i.e., pulmonary hypoplasia incompatible with life). ECMO does not reverse serious preexisting lung damage, as is seen in infants with chronic lung disease (e.g., bronchopulmonary dysplasia). ECMO would not be indicated for infants with transient tachypnea of the newborn (TTN) due to the transient nature of respiratory distress that is observed in these patients. However, a medical indication for ECMO is respiratory failure that is associated with persistent pulmonary hypertension of the newborn.

References: Lund, C. H.: Extracorporeal membrane oxygenation in the neonate. *In* Deacon, J., and O'Neill, P. (Eds.): *Core Curriculum for Neonatal Intensive Care*

Nursing, 2nd ed. Philadelphia, W. B. Saunders, 1999, p. 192.

Stork, E. K.: The respiratory system, Part VIII: Rescue therapy for cardiorespiratory failure. *In* Fanaroff, A. A., and Martin, R. J. (Eds.): *Neonatal-Perinatal Medicine,* 6th ed. St. Louis, Mosby, 1997, p. 1089.

46. **(A)** Extracorporeal membrane oxygenation (ECMO) has generally been considered as a treatment of last resort for neonates with life-threatening cardiorespiratory disease unresponsive to conventional or high-frequency ventilation. Unfortunately, ECMO is extremely invasive, expensive, and associated with serious outcomes. Alternative therapies, such as inhaled nitric oxide (NO) have increasingly proven useful in the reduction of pulmonary hypertension and, as such, have reduced the need for ECMO intervention for term infants with hypoxemia unresponsive to conventional ventilation.

References: Hagedorn, M. E., Gardner, S. L., and Abman, S. H.: Respiratory diseases. *In* Merenstein, G. B., and Gardner, S. L. (Eds.): *Handbook of Neonatal Intensive Care,* 4th ed. St. Louis, Mosby-Year Book, 1998, p. 437.

Stork, E. K.: The respiratory system, Part VIII: Rescue therapy for cardiorespiratory failure. *In* Fanaroff, A. A., and Martin, R. J. (Eds.): *Neonatal-Perinatal Medicine,* 6th ed. St. Louis, Mosby, 1997, p. 1089.

47. **(D)** The most frequent cause of death during extracorporeal membrane oxygenation (ECMO) is thrombocytopenia and low platelet function. During ECMO, approximately 80% of cardiac output is exposed to a large artificial surface (membrane oxygenator) each minute. Platelets show the most adverse effects when exposed to the artificial surface, as demonstrated by thrombocytopenia and impaired platelet function, which may lead to hemorrhage and, ultimately, death.

References: Lund, C. H.: Extracorporeal membrane oxygenation in the neonate. *In* Deacon, J., and O'Neill, P. (Eds.): *Core Curriculum for Neonatal Intensive Care Nursing,* 2nd ed. Philadelphia, W. B. Saunders, 1999, p. 192.

Stork, E. K.: The respiratory system, Part VIII: Rescue therapy for cardiorespiratory failure. *In* Fanaroff, A. A., and Martin, R. J. (Eds.): *Neonatal-Perinatal Medicine,* 6th ed. St. Louis, Mosby, 1997, p. 1089.

48. **(A)** Final eligibility criteria for extracorporeal membrane oxygenation (ECMO) therapy is based on objective data derived from one of two numeric scoring systems (i.e., alveolar/arterial oxygen gradient and oxygenation index) used to estimate the mortality risk. Assuming that other

exclusion criteria have been ruled out, ECMO is considered when it is estimated that the mortality risk is greater than 80%.

References: Torosian, M. B., Statter, M. B., and Arensman, R. M.: Extracorporeal membrane oxygenation. *In* Goldsmith, J. P., and Karotkin, E. H. (Eds.): *Assisted Ventilation of the Neonate,* 3rd ed. Philadelphia, W. B. Saunders, 1996, p. 241.

Stork, E. K.: The respiratory system, Part VIII: Rescue therapy for cardiorespiratory failure. *In* Fanaroff, A. A., and Martin, R. J. (Eds.): *Neonatal-Perinatal Medicine,* 6th ed. St. Louis, Mosby, 1997, p. 1089.

49. **(C)** After extracorporeal membrane oxygenation (ECMO), patients frequently experience morbidity related to poor somatic growth, oral feeding dysfunction, chronic lung disease and subsequent ventilator dependency, neurologic dysfunction, and long-term neurodevelopmental delays. Necrotizing enterocolitis has not been identified as a complication of ECMO.

Reference: Lund, C. H.: Extracorporeal membrane oxygenation in the neonate. *In* Deacon, J., and O'Neill, P. (Eds.): *Core Curriculum for Neonatal Intensive Care Nursing,* 2nd ed. Philadelphia, W. B. Saunders, 1999, p. 192.

50. **(C)** Surfactant replacement therapy directly addresses the underlying etiology of respiratory distress syndrome, which is surfactant deficiency.

Reference: Moise, A. A., and Hansen, T. N.: Acute, acquired parenchymal lung disease: Hyaline membrane disease. *In* Hansen, T. N., Cooper, T. R., and Weisman, L. E. (Eds.): *Contemporary Diagnosis and Management of Neonatal Respiratory Diseases,* 2nd ed. Newtown, Handbooks in Health Care, 1998, p. 79.

51. **(B)** Surfactant replacement increases pulmonary compliance and reduces pulmonary vascular resistance, thereby reducing the distending pressures needed to inflate the lung and the work of breathing, which ultimately improves oxygenation.

Reference: Moise, A. A., and Hansen, T. N.: Hyaline membrane disease. *In* Hansen, T. N., Cooper, T. R., and Weisman, L. E. (Eds.): *Contemporary Diagnosis and Management of Neonatal Respiratory Diseases,* 2nd ed. Newtown, Handbooks in Health Care, 1998, p. 79.

52. **(B)** Surfactant may be given as a preventive treatment (prophylactic) prior to the establishment of respiratory distress syndrome (RDS) as a diagnosis, or can be given as a rescue therapy once the diagnosis of RDS has been established. As a prophylaxis, surfactant is administered into the infant's trachea as soon as possi-

ble following delivery. For rescue therapy, surfactant is administered following the diagnosis of RDS.

References: Martin, R. J., and Fanaroff, A. A.: The respiratory system, Part III: Respiratory distress syndrome and its management. *In* Fanaroff, A. A., and Martin, R. J. (Eds.): *Neonatal-Perinatal Medicine,* 6th ed. St. Louis, Mosby, 1997, p. 1018.
Moise, A. A., and Gest, A. L.: Surfactant administration. *In* Hansen, T. N., Cooper, T. R., and Weisman, L. E. (Eds.): *Contemporary Diagnosis and Management of Neonatal Respiratory Diseases,* 2nd ed. Newtown, Handbooks in Health Care, 1998, p. 241.

53. **(A)** Transient bradycardia and oxygen desaturation are the most common adverse effects related to surfactant administration. If when dosing, the infant becomes bradycardic and/or decreases oxygen saturation by pulse oximetry, the appropriate action is to stop surfactant dosing and allow the infant time for recovery.

Reference: Donovan, E. F., Schwartz, J. E., and Moles, L. M.: New technologies applied to the management of respiratory dysfunction. *In* Kenner, C., Lott, J. W., and Flandemeyer, A. (Eds.): *Comprehensive Neonatal Nursing,* 2nd ed. Philadelphia, W. B. Saunders, 1998, p. 268.

54. **(C)** Unless clinically necessary, the endotracheal tube should not be suctioned for at least 1 to 2 hours following dosing to prevent the removal of surfactant from the tracheobronchial tree.

References: Hagedorn, M. E., Gardner, S. L., and Abman, S. H.: Respiratory diseases. *In* Merenstein, G. B., and Gardner, S. L. (Eds.): *Handbook of Neonatal Intensive Care,* 4th ed. St. Louis, Mosby-Year Book, 1998, p. 437.
Moise, A. A., and Gest, A. L.: Surfactant administration. *In* Hansen, T. N., Cooper, T. R., and Weisman, L. E. (Eds.): *Contemporary Diagnosis and Management of Neonatal Respiratory Diseases,* 2nd ed. Newtown, Handbooks in Health Care, 1998, p. 241.

55. **(B)** The risk for meconium aspiration may initially occur in utero if repeated incidences of asphyxia have induced gasping respirations and the inhalation of meconium-stained fluid into the trachea. At the time of delivery, the risk for meconium aspiration may occur if the infant takes a breath or is stimulated to breathe prior to clearing the mouth and trachea of residual meconium. Meconium staining of amniotic fluid is present in approximately 12% of all deliveries and is predominantly present in those infants who are postmature and small for gestational age.

References: Casey, P.: Respiratory distress. *In* Deacon, J., and O'Neill, P. (Eds.): *Core Curriculum for Neonatal Intensive Care Nursing,* 2nd ed. Philadelphia, W. B. Saunders, 1999, p. 118.
Miller, M. J., Fanaroff, A. A., and Martin, R. J.: The respiratory system, Part V: Respiratory disorders in preterm and term infants. *In* Fanaroff, A. A., and Martin, R. J. (Eds.): *Neonatal-Perinatal Medicine,* 6th ed. St. Louis, Mosby, 1997, p. 1040.

56. **(D)** The pH of 7.28 indicates acidosis. There is both a respiratory and metabolic component to this acidosis. The PCO_2 value of 56 is outside the normal range of 7.35 to 7.45, reflecting the respiratory component, whereas the bicarbonate value of 11 mEq/L and negative base excess reflect the metabolic component to the acidosis. The normal range of bicarbonate is 22 to 24 mEq/L.

References: Kirby, E.: Assisted ventilation. *In* Deacon, J., and O'Neill, P. (Eds.): *Core Curriculum for Neonatal Intensive Care Nursing,* 2nd ed. Philadelphia, W. B. Saunders, 1999, p. 164.
Parry, W. H., and Zimmer, J.: Acid-base homeostasis and oxygenation. *In* Merenstein, G. B., and Gardner, S. L. (Eds.): *Handbook of Neonatal Intensive Care,* 4th ed. St. Louis, Mosby, 1998, p. 160.

57. **(C)** Signs and symptoms of a tension pneumothorax include sudden, acute deterioration in cardiopulmonary status; profound cyanosis, bradycardia, and severe hypotension; diminished peripheral pulses; asymmetry in chest rise; diminished and/or shifted breath sounds; and diminished and/or muffled heart tones.

References: Casey, P.: Respiratory distress. *In* Deacon, J., and O'Neill, P. (Eds.): *Core Curriculum for Neonatal Intensive Care Nursing,* 2nd ed. Philadelphia, W. B. Saunders, 1999, p. 118.
Hagedorn, M. E., Gardner, S. L., and Abman, S. H.: Respiratory diseases. *In* Merenstein, G. B., and Gardner, S. L. (Eds.): *Handbook of Neonatal Intensive Care,* 4th ed. St. Louis, Mosby-Year Book, 1998, p. 437.

58. **(B)** The diagnosis of persistent fetal circulation (PFC) (i.e., persistent pulmonary hypertension of the newborn [PPHN]) should be suspected in infants with severe hypoxemia despite maximal oxygen therapy. These infants present with respiratory distress and are labile with "wide-swings" in oxygen saturations. The diagnosis of PFC or PPHN is confirmed by documenting extrapulmonary right-to-left shunting of blood in the absence of congenital heart disease. This can be demonstrated by pre- and post-ductal readings of oxygen saturation by pulse oximetry or by simultaneous drawing of right

radial and umbilical artery blood gases. A difference of 10 to 15 mm between pre- and postductal readings is indicative of right-to-left-shunting at the level of ductus arteriosus and foramen ovale.

References: Casey, P.: Respiratory distress. *In* Deacon, J., and O'Neill, P. (Eds.): *Core Curriculum for Neonatal Intensive Care Nursing*, 2nd ed. Philadelphia, W. B. Saunders, 1999, p. 118.
Hagedorn, M. E., Gardner, S. L., and Abman, S. H.: Respiratory diseases. *In* Merenstein, G. B., and Gardner, S. L. (Eds.): *Handbook of Neonatal Intensive Care*, 4th ed. St. Louis, Mosby-Year Book, 1998, p. 437.
Morin, F. C., and Davis, J. M.: Persistent pulmonary hypertension. *In* Spitzer, A. R. (Ed.): *Intensive Care of the Fetus and Neonate*. St. Louis, Mosby, 1996, p. 506.

59. **(A)** For infants with persistent pulmonary hypertension of the newborn (PPHN), the major goals are as follows: (1) correct hypoxia and acidosis; (2) reverse pulmonary vascular resistance; (3) support extrapulmonary systems; and (4) treat underlying cause, if indicated. Oxygen is a potent pulmonary vasodilator, and is administered in amounts necessary to maintain PaO_2 greater than 90 mm Hg. Hyperventilation is provided in an effort to lower $PaCO_2$ (hypocarbia) and raise pH levels (alkalosis), which has a direct vasodilatory effect on the pulmonary vasculature. Pharmacologic agents (i.e., tolazoline, isoproterenol, prostaglandin E_1, nifedipine) may be used to help promote pulmonary vasodilation. Muscle-paralyzing agents (e.g., pancuronium, vecuronium) are frequently administered when the infant's spontaneous respirations interfere with mechanical ventilation or when the infant is "fighting" assisted ventilation. Sedatives (e.g., fentanyl citrate, morphine sulfate) are provided, particularly when the infant requires muscle paralysis. Finally, vasopressors (e.g., dopamine, dobutamine) are used to keep systemic blood pressure above pulmonary vascular pressure in an attempt to reverse the right-to-left shunting.

References: Casey, P.: Respiratory distress. *In* Deacon, J., and O'Neill, P. (Eds.): *Core Curriculum for Neonatal Intensive Care Nursing*, 2nd ed. Philadelphia, W. B. Saunders, 1999, p. 118.
Hagedorn, M. E., Gardner, S. L., and Abman, S. H.: Respiratory diseases. *In* Merenstein, G. B., and Gardner, S. L. (Eds.): *Handbook of Neonatal Intensive Care*, 4th ed. St. Louis, Mosby-Year Book, 1998, p. 437.
Morin, F. C., and Davis, J. M.: Persistent pulmonary hypertension. *In* Spitzer, A. R. (Ed.): *Intensive Care of the Fetus and Neonate*. St. Louis, Mosby, 1996, p. 506.

60. **(B)** Research studies suggest that low-dose nitric oxide therapy (1 to 10 parts per million) is a selective and potent pulmonary vasodilator when inhaled directly into the lungs. Inhaled nitric oxide exerts its effects on pulmonary vasculature and does not affect systemic arterial pressure.

References: Casey, P.: Respiratory distress. *In* Deacon, J., and O'Neill, P. (Eds.): *Core Curriculum for Neonatal Intensive Care Nursing*, 2nd ed. Philadelphia, W. B. Saunders, 1999, p. 118.
Morin, F. C., and Davis, J. M.: Persistent pulmonary hypertension. *In* Spitzer, A. R. (Ed.): *Intensive Care of the Fetus and Neonate*. St. Louis, Mosby, 1996, p. 506.
Stork, E. K.: The respiratory system, Part VIII: Rescue therapy for cardiorespiratory failure. *In* Fanaroff, A. A., and Martin, R. J. (Eds.): *Neonatal-Perinatal Medicine*, 6th ed. St. Louis, Mosby, 1997, p. 1089.

61. **(D)** Methemoglobinemia, pulmonary edema, and platelet dysfunction are potential complications to nitric oxide administration. Apnea has not been documented as a side effect.

References: Morin, F. C., and Davis, J. M.: Persistent pulmonary hypertension. *In* Spitzer, A. R. (Ed.): *Intensive Care of the Fetus and Neonate*. St. Louis, Mosby, 1996, p. 506.
Stork, E. K.: The respiratory system, Part VIII: Rescue therapy for cardiorespiratory failure. *In* Fanaroff, A. A., and Martin, R. J. (Eds.): *Neonatal-Perinatal Medicine*, 6th ed. St. Louis, Mosby, 1997, p. 1089.

62. **(A)** Infants with persistent pulmonary hypertension of the newborn may be at risk for renal dysfunction and/or failure associated with decreased blood flow to the kidneys related to asphyxia and hypotension.

Reference: Casey, P.: Respiratory distress. *In* Deacon, J., and O'Neill, P. (Eds.): *Core Curriculum for Neonatal Intensive Care Nursing*, 2nd ed. Philadelphia, W. B. Saunders, 1999, p. 118.

63. **(A)** Milking and stripping a chest tube is generally not necessary if only air is being evacuated. Gentle kneading of the tube may be necessary if clots or debris are visible and are not free-flowing within the tube. Research has shown that damage to lung tissue may occur as a result of high pressures generated by milking and stripping chest tubes. Frequent repositioning of the patient promotes maximum drainage and lung expansion. Continuous bubbling in the water seal chamber may be a sign of a leak within the system and, as such, is not an indication of effective functioning of the chest tube and drainage apparatus. However, an important aspect

of care is the frequent monitoring and documentation of tube patency and oscillation of fluid within the drainage system.

Reference: Hagedorn, M. E., Gardner, S. L., and Abman, S. H.: Respiratory diseases. *In* Merenstein, G. B., and Gardner, S. L. (Eds.): *Handbook of Neonatal Intensive Care,* 4th ed. St. Louis, Mosby-Year Book, 1998, p. 437.

64. **(C)** Pulmonary air leaks are caused by overdistention of alveoli and subsequent rupture. As air leaks from the alveoli, it travels along the tracheobronchial tree and may accumulate in the mediastinum (pneumomediastinum), in the pleural space (pneumothorax), in the space surrounding the heart (pneumopericardium), or in the peritoneum (pneumoperitoneum). The clinical presentation of pneumopericardium is often one of rapid deterioration and cardiac tamponade as characterized by initial tachycardia, then profound bradycardia accompanied by hypotension, narrowed pulse pressure, and muffled heart tones. Chest radiograph reveals air surrounding the heart, producing a halo effect.

References: Casey, P.: Respiratory distress. *In* Deacon, J., and O'Neill, P. (Eds.): *Core Curriculum for Neonatal Intensive Care Nursing,* 2nd ed. Philadelphia, W. B. Saunders, 1999, p. 118.
Goldberg, R. N., and Abdenour, G. E.: Air leak syndrome. *In* Spitzer, A. (Ed.): *Intensive Care of the Fetus and Neonate.* St. Louis, Mosby, 1996, p. 629.
Hagedorn, M. E., Gardner, S. L., and Abman, S. H.: Respiratory diseases. *In* Merenstein, G. B., and Gardner, S. L. (Eds.): *Handbook of Neonatal Intensive Care,* 4th ed. St. Louis, Mosby-Year Book, 1998, p. 437.

65. **(A)** Respiratory distress immediately following delivery accompanied by diminished breath sounds, scaphoid abdomen, and mediastinal shift are key indicators of congenital diaphragmatic hernia (CDH). The severity of respiratory distress is directly related to the degree of pulmonary hypoplasia. In the early newborn period, the diagnosis of CDH is confirmed by the presence of dilated loops of bowel in the thoracic cavity, the absence of gas within the abdomen, and a mediastinal shift towards the contralateral side by radiographic examination.

References: Guillory, C., and Cooper, T. R.: Diseases affecting the diaphragm and chest wall. *In* Hansen, T. N., Cooper, T. R., and Weisman, L. E. (Eds.): *Contemporary Diagnosis and Management of Neonatal Respiratory Diseases,* 2nd ed. Newtown, Handbooks in Health Care, 1998, p. 188.
Holland, R. M., Price, F. N., and Bensard, D. D.: Neonatal surgery. *In* Merenstein, G. B., and Gardner, S. L.

(Eds.): *Handbook of Neonatal Intensive Care,* 4th ed. St. Louis, Mosby-Year Book, 1998, p. 625.

66. **(D)** The underlying lung pathology in congenital diaphragmatic hernia is pulmonary hypoplasia. The presence of abdominal contents in the thoracic cavity compresses the developing lung, leading to inhibited and/or defective growth of the affected lung. Pulmonary hypoplasia is characterized by decreased numbers and size of alveoli, bronchioles, and pulmonary vasculature. These anatomic changes lead to a decrease in pulmonary blood flow and resultant persistent pulmonary hypertension of the newborn.

References: Casey, P.: Respiratory distress. *In* Deacon, J., and O'Neill, P. (Eds.): *Core Curriculum for Neonatal Intensive Care Nursing,* 2nd ed. Philadelphia, W. B. Saunders, 1999, p. 118.
Miller, M. J., Fanaroff, A. A., and Martin, R. J.: The respiratory system, Part V: Respiratory disorders in preterm and term infants. *In* Fanaroff, A. A., and Martin, R. J. (Eds.): *Neonatal-Perinatal Medicine,* 6th ed. St. Louis, Mosby, 1997, p. 1040.

67. **(D)** As soon as the diagnosis of congenital diaphragmatic hernia is confirmed, a double lumen orogastric tube should be inserted and connected to low, intermittent suction. This minimizes the amount of air in the stomach and helps relieve compression on the hypoplastic lung.

Reference: Guillory, C., and Cooper, T. R.: Diseases affecting the diaphragm and chest wall. *In* Hansen, T. N., Cooper, T. R., and Weisman, L. E. (Eds.): *Contemporary Diagnosis and Management of Neonatal Respiratory Diseases,* 2nd ed. Newtown, Handbooks in Health Care, 1998, p. 188.

68. **(C)** The timing of the surgical repair should be delayed until the infant has been "stabilized" from a pulmonary perspective. Early repair is contraindicated when there is evidence of severe pulmonary insufficiency. Early management of pulmonary status includes mechanical ventilation with low peak inspiratory pressure (PIP), rapid rates, and minimal positive end-expiratory pressure (PEEP), sedation and paralysis, frequent monitoring of arterial blood gases from indwelling arterial catheters, inotropic support for systemic hypotension, and correction of metabolic acidosis. Extracorporeal membrane oxygenation (ECMO), nitric oxide, and partial liquid ventilation may be indicated in cases in which maximal conventional support has failed to

achieve adequate stabilization prior to surgery.

References: Guillory, C., and Cooper, T. R.: Diseases affecting the diaphragm and chest wall. *In* Hansen, T. N., Cooper, T. R., and Weisman, L. E. (Eds.): *Contemporary Diagnosis and Management of Neonatal Respiratory Diseases,* 2nd ed. Newtown, Handbooks in Health Care, 1998, p. 188.
Miller, M. J., Fanaroff, A. A., and Martin, R. J.: The respiratory system, Part V: Respiratory disorders in preterm and term infants. *In* Fanaroff, A. A., and Martin, R. J. (Eds.): *Neonatal-Perinatal Medicine,* 6th ed. St. Louis, Mosby, 1997, p. 1040.

69. **(D)** Congenital lobar emphysema, eventration of the diaphragm, and cystic adenomatoid malformation are three pulmonary disorders with clinical presentations similar to that of congenital diaphragmatic hernia (CDH). Because these conditions "mimic" CDH, they must be ruled out as the cause of the neonate's respiratory distress. On the other hand, pulmonary interstitial emphysema is not included in the differential diagnosis of CDH.

Reference: Guillory, C., and Cooper, T. R.: Diseases affecting the diaphragm and chest wall. *In* Hansen, T. N., Cooper, T. R., and Weisman, L. E. (Eds.): *Contemporary Diagnosis and Management of Neonatal Respiratory Diseases,* 2nd ed. Newtown, Handbooks in Health Care, 1998, p. 188.

70. **(A)** Gastroesophageal reflux (GER) is a potentially serious long-term complication following diaphragmatic hernia repair. The incidence of GER is highest for infants who require large prosthetic patches for repair of the diaphragm. Other long-term postoperative complications include recurrence of hernia, small bowel obstruction, thoracolumbar scoliosis, and chronic pulmonary insufficiency.

References: Guillory, C., and Cooper, T. R.: Diseases affecting the diaphragm and chest wall. *In* Hansen, T. N., Cooper, T. R., and Weisman, L. E. (Eds.): *Contemporary Diagnosis and Management of Neonatal Respiratory Diseases,* 2nd ed. Newtown, Handbooks in Health Care, 1998, p. 188.
Miller, M. J., Fanaroff, A. A., and Martin, R. J.: The respiratory system, Part V: Respiratory disorders in preterm and term infants. *In* Fanaroff, A. A., and Martin, R. J. (Eds.): *Neonatal-Perinatal Medicine,* 6th ed. St. Louis, Mosby, 1997, p. 1040.

71. **(B)** Infants with pulmonary hemorrhage frequently present with a sudden cyanosis and deterioration of cardiopulmonary status accompanied by the presence of pink or bloody secretions in the trachea or endotracheal tube.

References: Casey, P.: Respiratory distress. *In* Deacon, J., and O'Neill, P. (Eds.): *Core Curriculum for Neonatal Intensive Care Nursing,* 2nd ed. Philadelphia, W. B. Saunders, 1999, p. 118.
Miller, M. J., Fanaroff, A. A., and Martin, R. J.: The respiratory system, Part V: Respiratory disorders in preterm and term infants. *In* Fanaroff, A. A., and Martin, R. J. (Eds.): *Neonatal-Perinatal Medicine,* 6th ed. St. Louis, Mosby, 1997, p. 1040.
Weltry, S. E., and Hansen, T. N.: Pulmonary hemorrhage. *In* Hansen, T. N., Cooper, T. R., and Weisman, L. E. (Eds.): *Contemporary Diagnosis and Management of Neonatal Respiratory Diseases,* 2nd ed. Newtown, Handbooks in Health Care, 1998, p. 117.

72. **(B)** Positive pressure ventilation with positive end-expiratory pressure is provided to improve oxygenation and ventilation until edema lung fluid clears. Suction only as needed to maintain patent airway, as pulmonary hemorrhage may be due to trauma or injury to the trachea caused by suctioning. Pulmonary hemorrhage may be a complication associated with surfactant administration. Blood transfusions may be required to replace acute blood loss.

References: Casey, P.: Respiratory distress. *In* Deacon, J., and O'Neill, P. (Eds.): *Core Curriculum for Neonatal Intensive Care Nursing,* 2nd ed. Philadelphia, W. B. Saunders, 1999, p. 118.
Weltry, S. E., and Hansen, T. N.: Pulmonary hemorrhage. *In* Hansen, T. N., Cooper, T. R., and Weisman, L. E. (Eds.): *Contemporary Diagnosis and Management of Neonatal Respiratory Diseases,* 2nd ed. Newtown, Handbooks in Health Care, 1998, p. 117.

73. **(B)** Choanal atresia is a rare disorder that is characterized by a bony or membranous protrusion into the nasal passages, which causes airway obstruction or blockage. Choanal atresia can be unilateral or bilateral. Infants with bilateral choanal atresia present with cyanosis and difficulty in breathing in the early neonatal period, with improvement in cyanosis observed when the infant cries or mouth-breathes. The diagnosis of choanal atresia is confirmed by the inability to pass a catheter through the nasal passages into the posterior oropharynx.

References: Casey, P.: Respiratory distress. *In* Deacon, J., and O'Neill, P. (Eds.): *Core Curriculum for Neonatal Intensive Care Nursing,* 2nd ed. Philadelphia, W. B. Saunders, 1999, p. 118.
Miller, M. J., Fanaroff, A. A., and Martin, R. J.: The respiratory system, Part V: Respiratory disorders in preterm and term infants. *In* Fanaroff, A. A., and Martin, R. J. (Eds.): *Neonatal-Perinatal Medicine,* 6th ed. St. Louis, Mosby, 1997, p. 1040.

74. **(A)** Choanal atresia frequently occurs in association with other congenital anoma-

lies, such as CHARGE association, Treacher-Collins syndrome, tracheo-esophageal fistula, palatal abnormalities, and Crouzon syndrome. Choanal atresia is one of the anomalies of the CHARGE association, which also includes coloboma, heart defects, retarded growth and development, genital hypoplasia, and ear anomalies. Because there is a 50 to 60% occurrence of heart defects in patients with choanal atresia, a cardiac evaluation is highly recommended.

References: Cabrera-Meza, G., and Cooper, T. R.: Diseases of the upper airway: Disorders of the nose, mouth and pharynx. *In* Hansen, T. N., Cooper, T. R., and Weisman, L. E. (Eds.): *Contemporary Diagnosis and Management of Neonatal Respiratory Diseases,* 2nd ed. Newtown, Handbooks in Health Care, 1998, p. 198.
Casey, P.: Respiratory distress. *In* Deacon, J., and O'Neill, P. (Eds.): *Core Curriculum for Neonatal Intensive Care Nursing,* 2nd ed. Philadelphia, W. B. Saunders, 1999, p. 118.
Miller, M. J., Fanaroff, A. A., and Martin, R. J.: The respiratory system, Part V: Respiratory disorders in preterm and term infants. *In* Fanaroff, A. A., and Martin, R. J. (Eds.): *Neonatal-Perinatal Medicine,* 6th ed. St. Louis, Mosby, 1997, p. 1040.

75. (**A**) Pierre Robin sequence is characterized by the following triad of congenital defects: micrognathia (small jaw), glossoptosis (downward drooping of the tongue), and cleft palate. Micrognathia is the primary defect that causes a cascade of secondary effects (i.e., glossoptosis and cleft palate).

References: Casey, P.: Respiratory distress. *In* Deacon, J., and O'Neill, P. (Eds.): *Core Curriculum for Neonatal Intensive Care Nursing,* 2nd ed. Philadelphia, W. B. Saunders, 1999, p. 118.
Cabrera-Meza, G., and Cooper, T. R.: Diseases of the upper airway: Disorders of the nose, mouth and pharynx. *In* Hansen, T. N., Cooper, T. R., and Weisman, L. E. (Eds.): *Contemporary Diagnosis and Management of Neonatal Respiratory Diseases,* 2nd ed. Newtown, Handbooks in Health Care, 1998, p. 198.
Prows, C. A., and Bender, P. L.: Beyond Pierre Robin sequence. *Neonatal Network* 18(5):13, 1999.

76. (**D**) Obstructive apnea occurs when the tongue falls backward into the hypopharynx, thereby blocking the airways. Chronic airway obstruction with carbon dioxide retention and hypoxia may ultimately lead to the development of cor pulmonale. These infants are also at risk for feeding difficulties and failure to thrive. Extra calories are needed to compensate for the calories expended as a result of the increased work of breathing and cardiac effort to overcome chronic

airway obstruction. Subglottic stenosis is not a complication associated with micrognathia or glossoptosis.

References: Cabrera-Meza, G., and Cooper, T. R.: Diseases of the upper airway: Disorders of the nose, mouth and pharynx. *In* Hansen, T. N., Cooper, T. R., and Weisman, L. E. (Eds.): *Contemporary Diagnosis and Management of Neonatal Respiratory Diseases,* 2nd ed. Newtown, Handbooks in Health Care, 1998, p. 198.
Prows, C. A., and Bender, P. L.: Beyond Pierre Robin sequence. *Neonatal Network* 18(5):13, 1999.

77. (**C**) There is an inverse relationship between the incidence of bronchopulmonary dysplasia (BPD) and the birth weight and gestational age of the infant. BPD is primarily a disease of small and extremely immature infants, with an incidence rate of 85% for infants with birth weights less than 700 g.

References: Adams, J. M., and Wearden, M. E.: Sub-acute and chronic acquired parenchymal lung diseases: Bronchopulmonary dysplasia. *In* Hansen, T. N., Cooper, T. R., and Weisman, L. E. (Eds.): *Contemporary Diagnosis and Management of Neonatal Respiratory Diseases,* 2nd ed. Newtown, Handbooks in Health Care, 1998, p. 150.
Casey, P.: Respiratory distress. *In* Deacon, J., and O'Neill, P. (Eds.): *Core Curriculum for Neonatal Intensive Care Nursing,* 2nd ed. Philadelphia, W. B. Saunders, 1999, p. 118.

78. (**A**) Bronchopulmonary dysplasia (BPD) is an iatrogenic disorder caused by the effects of oxygen toxicity and barotrauma from mechanical ventilation on an immature lung. The incidence of BPD is extremely low in infants born close to term. Transient tachypnea of the newborn and hypovolemia have not been identified as risk factors for the development of BPD.

References: Bancalari, E.: Part VII: Neonatal chronic lung disease. *In* Fanaroff, A. A., and Martin, R. J. (Eds.): *Neonatal-Perinatal Medicine,* 6th ed. St. Louis, Mosby, 1997, p. 1074.
Cabrera-Meza, G., and Cooper, T. R.: Diseases of the upper airway: disorders of the nose, mouth and pharynx. *In* Hansen, T. N., Cooper, T. R., and Weisman, L. E. (Eds.): *Contemporary Diagnosis and Management of Neonatal Respiratory Diseases,* 2nd ed. Newtown, Handbooks in Health Care, 1998, p. 198.

79. (**C**) The clinical presentation of bronchopulmonary dysplasia (BPD) is characterized by hypoxia, hypercapnia, and respiratory acidosis, not alkalosis. Rales, rhonchi, wheezing, and retractions are also clinical characteristics of BPD.

References: Bancalari, E.: Part VII: Neonatal chronic lung disease. *In* Fanaroff, A. A., and Martin, R. J. (Eds.):

Neonatal-Perinatal Medicine, 6th ed. St. Louis, Mosby, 1997, p. 1074.

Casey, P.: Respiratory distress. *In* Deacon, J., and O'Neill, P. (Eds.): *Core Curriculum for Neonatal Intensive Care Nursing,* 2nd ed. Philadelphia, W. B. Saunders, 1999, p. 118.

80. **(A)** The pathogenesis of bronchopulmonary dysplasia is characterized by a constant cycle of recurring lung injury accompanied by healing and repair that affects all areas of the tracheobronchial tree. Postmortem examination of the surface of the lung reveals emphysematous areas alternating with areas of collapse (atelectasis). The chest radiograph of severe bronchopulmonary dysplasia (BPD) has often been described as "cystic," with areas of emphysematous alveoli (hyperinflated) that have often coalesced into larger cysts surrounded by dense fibrotic or collapsed alveoli.

References: Bancalari, E.: Part VII: Neonatal chronic lung disease. *In* Fanaroff, A. A., and Martin, R. J. (Eds.): *Neonatal-Perinatal Medicine,* 6th ed. St. Louis, Mosby, 1997, p. 1074.

Adams, J. M., and Wearden, M. E.: Sub-acute and chronic acquired parenchymal lung diseases: Bronchopulmonary dysplasia. *In* Hansen, T. N., Cooper, T. R., and Weisman, L. E. (Eds.): *Contemporary Diagnosis and Management of Neonatal Respiratory Diseases,* 2nd ed. Newtown, Handbooks in Health Care, 1998, p. 150.

81. **(B)** Infants with bronchopulmonary dysplasia (BPD) are at risk for bronchoconstriction and bronchospasm due to bronchiole smooth muscle hypertrophy and increased airway hyperreactivity. Infants with BPD are extremely sensitive to hypoxia, which can cause severe bronchoconstriction with resultant bronchospasm. These spells are thought to be caused by either pulmonary bronchospasm or pulmonary hypertension and are characterized by irritability, agitation, cyanosis, increased respiratory effort, hypoxia, and hypercapnia.

References: Bancalari, E.: Part VII: Neonatal chronic lung disease. *In* Fanaroff, A. A., and Martin, R. J. (Eds.): *Neonatal-Perinatal Medicine,* 6th ed. St. Louis, Mosby, 1997, p. 1074.

Casey, P.: Respiratory distress. *In* Deacon, J., and O'Neill, P. (Eds.): *Core Curriculum for Neonatal Intensive Care Nursing,* 2nd ed. Philadelphia, W. B. Saunders, 1999, p. 118.

82. **(B)** Albuterol is a bronchodilator that when given via inhalation has been shown to reduce airway constriction in patients with bronchopulmonary dyspla-

sia. Albuterol is the recommended drug of choice for severe episodes of airway hyperreactivity.

References: Adams, J. M., and Wearden, M. E.: Bronchopulmonary dysplasia. *In* Hansen, T. N., Cooper, T. R., and Weisman, L. E. (Eds.): *Contemporary Diagnosis and Management of Neonatal Respiratory Diseases,* 2nd ed. Newtown, Handbooks in Health Care, 1998, p. 150.

Bancalari, E.: Part VII: Neonatal chronic lung disease. *In* Fanaroff, A. A., and Martin, R. J. (Eds.): *Neonatal-Perinatal Medicine,* 6th ed. St. Louis, Mosby, 1997, p. 1074.

83. **(A)** Right-sided heart failure (i.e., cor pulmonale) is characterized by increasing respiratory distress, full pulses, poor peripheral circulation, hepatomegaly, and a loud pansystolic murmur.

Reference: Verklan, M. T.: Bronchopulmonary dysplasia: Its effects upon the heart and lungs. *Neonatal Network* 16(8):5, 1999.

84. **(A)** Nephrocalcinosis, a form of renal calculi, is associated with long-term diuretic therapy with Lasix.

Reference: Bancalari, E.: Part VII: Neonatal chronic lung disease. *In* Fanaroff, A. A., and Martin, R. J. (Eds.): *Neonatal-Perinatal Medicine,* 6th ed. St. Louis, Mosby, 1997, p. 1074.

85. **(D)** When assessing compensation status, it is important to examine the pH, and the two acid-base determinants. For this infant, the arterial blood gases (ABGs) reflect a beginning of partial compensation, in which both acid-base components remain abnormal in opposite directions with the pH beginning to move toward a more normal range. Full compensation is characterized by the return of the pH to a normal range (7.35–7.45). A PaO_2 of 49 mm Hg is indicative of hypoxemia, as it falls outside the normally accepted range of 60 to 80 mm Hg.

References: Askin, D. F.: Interpretation of neonatal blood gases, part II: Disorders of acid-base balance. *Neonatal Network* 16(6):23, 1997.

Parry, W. H., and Zimmer, J.: Acid-base homeostasis and oxygenation. *In* Merenstein, G. B., and Gardner, S. L. (Eds.): *Handbook of Neonatal Intensive Care,* 4th ed. St. Louis, Mosby-Year Book, 1998, p. 160.

86. **(A)** Multiple side effects have been identified with steroid use, including hypertension, hyperglycemia, hypocalcemia and other electrolyte disturbances, increased risk for infection, immunosuppression, and nephrocalcinosis. Pulmonary edema has not been identified as a complication

of steroid therapy; indeed, the decrease in pulmonary edema can be viewed as a beneficial effect of steroid therapy.

References: Bancalari, E.: Part VII: Neonatal chronic lung disease. *In* Fanaroff, A. A., and Martin, R. J. (Eds.): *Neonatal-Perinatal Medicine,* 6th ed. St. Louis, Mosby, 1997, p. 1074.
Casey, P.: Respiratory distress. *In* Deacon, J., and O'Neill, P. (Eds.): *Core Curriculum for Neonatal Intensive Care Nursing,* 2nd ed. Philadelphia, W. B. Saunders, 1999, p. 118.

87. **(D)** Adequate nutrition is critical for the healing and growth of lung tissue as well as for overall growth and development for infants with bronchopulmonary dysplasia (BPD). Unfortunately, many infants with BPD suffer from growth failure owing to the increased energy expenditure associated with increased work of breathing and cardiac effort. What would be considered adequate for normal infant growth and development is very inadequate for the infant with BPD. Often, these infants will require 150 to 200 kcal/kg/day to support adequate growth.

Reference: Hagedorn, M. I., Gardner, S. L., and Abman, S. H.: Respiratory diseases. *In* Merenstein, G. B., and Gardner, S. L. (Eds.): *Handbook of Neonatal Intensive Care,* 4th ed. St. Louis, Mosby, 1998, p. 437.

88. **(A)** Oxygen is a powerful pulmonary vasodilator and serves to reduce the pulmonary vascular resistance that is associated with hypoxia and acidosis. Increased pulmonary vascular resistance leads to pulmonary hypertension and right-sided heart failure (cor pulmonale). For infants with bronchopulmonary dysplasia (BPD), supplemental oxygen is frequently required well past the time of extubation to decrease pulmonary vascular resistance and to support optimal growth.

References: Adams, J. M., and Wearden, M. E.: Bronchopulmonary dysplasia. *In* Hansen, T. N., Cooper, T. R., and Weisman, L. E. (Eds.): *Contemporary Diagnosis and Management of Neonatal Respiratory Diseases,* 2nd ed. Newtown, Handbooks in Health Care Company, 1998, p. 150.
Casey, P.: Respiratory distress. *In* Deacon, J., and O'Neill, P. (Eds.): *Core Curriculum for Neonatal Intensive Care Nursing,* 2nd ed. Philadelphia, W. B. Saunders, 1999, p. 118.

89. **(A)** Functional residual capacity (FRC) is defined as the volume of gas that remains in the lungs after a normal expiration. Tidal volume (TV) is defined as the amount of air that moves into or out of the lungs with each single breath at rest. Vital capacity (VC) is defined as the volume of air maximally inspired and maximally expired. Physiologic dead space is composed of anatomic and alveolar dead space.

Reference: Kirby, E.: Assisted ventilation. *In* Deacon, J., and O'Neill, P. (Eds.): *Core Curriculum for Neonatal Intensive Care Nursing,* 2nd ed. Philadelphia, W. B. Saunders, 1999, p. 164.

90. **(B)** Pulmonary interstitial emphysema (PIE), a potentially life-threatening complication of assisted ventilation, occurs when air leaks from ruptured alveoli into the pulmonary interstitium, thereby forming cystic and linear radiolucencies throughout affected areas. PIE is a "radiographic" diagnosis characterized by unilateral and/or bilateral microcystic areas. The lungs may also appear hyperinflated with a flattened diaphragm. Radiographic findings of grainy or ground-glass appearance are consistent with hyaline membrane disease.

References: Casey, P.: Respiratory distress. *In* Deacon, J., and O'Neill, P. (Eds.): *Core Curriculum for Neonatal Intensive Care Nursing,* 2nd ed. Philadelphia, W. B. Saunders, 1999, p. 118.
Korones, S. B.: Complications: Bronchopulmonary dysplasia, air leak syndromes, and retinopathy of prematurity. *In* Goldsmith, J. P., and Karotkin, E. H. (Eds.): *Assisted Ventilation of the Neonate,* 3rd ed. Philadelphia, W. B. Saunders, 1996, p. 327.

91. **(C)** Fetal hemoglobin is one of several factors that directly influence the ease with which hemoglobin releases oxygen to the tissues. In the presence of fetal hemoglobin, there is an increased affinity for oxygen (i.e., shift of oxygen dissociation curve to the left). Subsequently, hemoglobin holds onto oxygen, which in turn decreases the amount of oxygen released to the tissues (i.e., tissue hypoxia). Because fetal hemoglobin shifts the oxygen dissociation curve toward the left, a neonate may have a higher oxygen saturation value at a lower PaO_2. Clinically, this means that a neonate may be pink in color until the PaO_2 drops to a very low and dangerous level (i.e., less than 40 mm Hg). Therefore, the absence of cyanosis does not ensure that the neonate is well oxygenated; indeed, the presence of central cyanosis is often a late and very serious sign of respiratory insufficiency.

References: Hagedorn, M. E., Gardner, S. L., and Abman, S. H.: Respiratory diseases. *In* Merenstein, G. B., and

Gardner, S. L. (Eds.): *Handbook of Neonatal Intensive Care*, 4th ed. St. Louis, Mosby, 1998, p. 437.

Kirby, E.: Assisted ventilation. *In* Deacon, J., and O'Neill, P. (Eds.): *Core Curriculum for Neonatal Intensive Care Nursing*, 2nd ed. Philadelphia, W. B. Saunders, 1999, p. 164.

Parry, W. H., and Zimmer, J.: Acid-base homeostasis and oxygenation. *In* Merenstein, G. B., and Gardner, S. L. (Eds.): *Handbook of Neonatal Intensive Care*, 4th ed. St. Louis, Mosby, 1998, p. 160.

92. (**A**) Many factors are known to influence the accuracy in pulse oximetry monitoring. Of primary importance is the adequacy of perfusion to the limbs in which the probes are attached. If perfusion is diminished to the limb in which a probe is attached (i.e., shock, vasoconstriction due to dopamine infusion, inflated blood pressure cuff), the oximeter probe will be unable to detect the arterial pulsations necessary for the determination of oxygen saturation. Inaccurate readings may also occur in the following situations: (1) exposure of the probe to infrared or phototherapy lights; (2) increased limb movement; (3) dyes or inks as are used in obtaining foot-prints; and (4) in the presence of meconium-stained skin.

References: Kirby, E.: Assisted ventilation. *In* Deacon, J., and O'Neill, P. (Eds.): *Core Curriculum for Neonatal Intensive Care Nursing*, 2nd ed. Philadelphia, W. B. Saunders, 1999, p. 164.

Pierce, J. R., and Turner, B. S.: Physiologic monitoring. *In* Merenstein, G. B., and Gardner, S. L. (Eds.): *Handbook of Neonatal Intensive Care*, 4th ed. St. Louis, Mosby, 1998, p. 116.

93. (**C**) It is recommended that the liter flow be maintained between 5 and 7 L/min to prevent the buildup of carbon dioxide within the hood.

Reference: Kirby, E.: Assisted ventilation. *In* Deacon, J., and O'Neill, P. (Eds.): *Core Curriculum for Neonatal Intensive Care*, 2nd ed. Philadelphia, W. B. Saunders, 1999, p. 164.

94. (**A**) Indications of extubation include decreased chest wall movement, lack of fogging or condensation in endotracheal tube, cyanosis, bradycardia, sudden deterioration in clinical condition, audible crying, increasing abdominal distention, and breath sounds audible in the stomach. In the event that an endotracheal tube is accidentally "displaced" into the esophagus, it may be possible to hear mechanical or hand ventilated breaths within the stomach region.

Reference: Kirby, E.: Assisted ventilation. *In* Deacon, J., and O'Neill, P. (Eds.): *Core Curriculum for Neonatal Intensive Care*, 2nd ed. Philadelphia, W. B. Saunders, 1999, p. 164.

95. (**C**) Carbon dioxide elimination is controlled by both oscillatory amplitude (i.e., size of pressure wave generated by oscillator) and by breathing rate (i.e., Hertz).

Reference: Kirby, E.: Assisted ventilation. *In* Deacon, J., and O'Neill, P. (Eds.): *Core Curriculum for Neonatal Intensive Care*, 2nd ed. Philadelphia, W. B. Saunders, 1999, p. 164.

96. (**A**) For patients receiving high-frequency ventilation (HFV), the degree of chest wall vibrations is an indicator of lung compliance, airway patency, tidal volume, and effectiveness in ventilator parameters. A sudden decrease in chest wall vibration may indicate an obstructed airway and/or pneumothorax.

Reference: Kirby, E.: Assisted ventilation. *In* Deacon, J., and O'Neill, P. (Eds.): *Core Curriculum for Neonatal Intensive Care*, 2nd ed. Philadelphia, W. B. Saunders, 1999, p. 164.

97. (**C**) Positional therapy with affected side downward, selective intubation of contralateral mainstem bronchus, and high-frequency ventilation are a few of the treatment options for localized pulmonary interstitial emphysema (PIE). On the other hand, PIE is not an indication for extracorporeal membrane oxygenation (ECMO), as it is predominantly seen in preterm infants on prolonged mechanical ventilation. ECMO is contraindicated for preterm infants with respiratory failure.

References: Goldberg, R. N., and Abdenour, G. E.: Air leak syndrome. *In* Spitzer, A. R. (Ed.): *Intensive Care of the Fetus and Neonate*. St. Louis, Mosby, 1997, p. 629.

Miller, M. J., Fanaroff, A. A., and Martin, R. J.: The respiratory system, Part V: Respiratory disorders in preterm and term infants. *In* Fanaroff, A. A., and Martin, R. J. (Eds.): *Neonatal-Perinatal Medicine*, 6th ed. St. Louis, Mosby, 1997, p. 1040.

98. (**D**) The pH of 7.50 is indicative of alkalosis. The $PaCO_2$ of 30 indicates a respiratory component of the alkalosis. The HCO_3 of 22 is within normal range.

Reference: Kirby, E.: Assisted ventilation. *In* Deacon, J., and O'Neill, P. (Eds.): *Core Curriculum for Neonatal Intensive Care Nursing*, 2nd ed. Philadelphia, W. B. Saunders, 1999, p. 164.

99. (**B**) The ventilator rate (i.e., IMV, SIMV) affects the lung's ability to "blow off"

carbon dioxide. Hyperventilation may lead to respiratory alkalosis, as evidenced by a pH greater than 7.45 and a $Paco_2$ less than 35. Decreasing the ventilator rate may normalize the pH and CO_2 values.

Reference: Kirby, E.: Assisted ventilation. *In* Deacon, J., and O'Neill, P. (Eds.): *Core Curriculum for Neonatal Intensive Care Nursing,* 2nd ed. Philadelphia, W. B. Saunders, 1999, p. 164.

CHAPTER 14
METABOLIC/ENDOCRINE DISORDERS

1. **(B)** Hypoglycemia in an IDM should be anticipated. Providing early feeds can help avert hypoglycemia if the infant is medically stable. Serum glucose levels should be monitored frequently.

Reference: Stokowski, L. C.: Metabolic disorders. *In* Deacon, J., and O'Neill, P. (Eds.): *Core Curriculum for Neonatal Intensive Care Nursing,* 2nd ed. Philadelphia, W. B. Saunders, 1999, p. 326.

2. **(A)** Patient care management of the infant with hypercalcemia includes promoting the excretion of calcium. Furosemide has calciuretic action.

Reference: Stokowski, L. C.: Metabolic disorders. *In* Deacon, J., and O'Neill, P. (Eds.): *Core Curriculum for Neonatal Intensive Care Nursing,* 2nd ed. Philadelphia, W. B. Saunders, 1999, p. 326.

3. **(C)** Rapid infusion of calcium can cause bradycardia or cardiac arrest.

Reference: Stokowski, L. C.: Metabolic disorders. *In* Deacon, J., and O'Neill, P. (Eds.): *Core Curriculum for Neonatal Intensive Care Nursing,* 2nd ed. Philadelphia, W. B. Saunders, 1999, p. 326.

4. **(A)** There is no uniform policy on newborn screening; however, every state and the District of Columbia test for PKU and congenital hypothyroidism.

Reference: Kenner, C., and Amlung, S.: Newborn genetic screening: Blessing or curse. *Neonatal Network* 18(7):11, 1999.

5. **(B)** Maternal Graves disease is the most common cause of neonatal hyperthyroidism.

Reference: Stokowski, L. C.: Endocrine disorders. *In* Deacon, J., and O'Neill, P. (Eds.): *Core Curriculum for Neonatal Intensive Care Nursing,* 2nd ed. Philadelphia, W. B. Saunders, 1999, p. 357.

6. **(C)** In the syndrome of inappropriate antidiuretic hormone (SIADH), osmolalities and sodium levels of urine and serum are diagnostic. Urine output is low with high specific gravity and high sodium levels.

Reference: Stokowski, L. C.: Metabolic disorders. *In* Deacon, J., and O'Neill, P. (Eds.): *Core Curriculum for Neonatal Intensive Care Nursing,* 2nd ed. Philadelphia, W. B. Saunders, 1999, p. 326.

7. **(B)** The primary cause of metabolic bone disease is inadequate intake of calcium and phosphorus rather than vitamin D deficiency.

Reference: Stokowski, L. C.: Metabolic disorders. *In* Deacon, J., and O'Neill, P. (Eds.): *Core Curriculum for Neonatal Intensive Care Nursing,* 2nd ed. Philadelphia, W. B. Saunders, 1999, p. 326.

8. **(C)** Hypocalcemia and hypomagnesemia are major metabolic problems exhibited by infants of diabetic mothers. Hypocalcemia develops within 3 days of life and is seen primarily in the infant of an insulin-dependent mother. It is thought to be secondary to decreased hypoparathyroid functioning.

Reference: Kenner, C., Amlung, S. R., and Flandermyer, A. A.: Assessment and management of endocrine dysfunction. *In Protocols in Neonatal Nursing.* Philadelphia, W. B. Saunders, 1998, p. 295.

9. **(D)** Glucose reaches the fetus by facilitated diffusion across the placenta at a concentration of about 80% of the mother's.

Reference: Stokowski, L. C.: Metabolic disorders. *In* Deacon, J., and O'Neill, P. (Eds.): *Core Curriculum for Neonatal Intensive Care Nursing,* 2nd ed. Philadelphia, W. B. Saunders, 1999, p. 326.

10. **(B)** Galactosemia is the most common disorder of carbohydrate metabolism with the onset in the neonatal period. Vomiting and diarrhea occur with the introduction of lactose feedings.

Reference: Stokowski, L. C.: Metabolic disorders. *In* Deacon, J., and O'Neill, P. (Eds.): *Core Curriculum for Neonatal Intensive Care Nursing,* 2nd ed. Philadelphia, W. B. Saunders, 1999, p. 326.

11. **(C)** Hypophosphatemia is a common feature in preterm infants with rickets. Rickets is caused by an insufficient intake of calcium and phosphorus.

Reference: Tsang, R. C., Demarini, S., and Rath, L. L.: Fluids, electrolytes, vitamins, and trace minerals: Basis of ingestion, digestion, elimination, and metabolism. *In* Kenner, C., Lott, J. W., and Flandermyer, A. A. (Eds.): *Comprehensive Neonatal Nursing: A Physiologic Perspective,* 2nd ed. Philadelphia, W. B. Saunders, 1998, p. 336.

12. (**D**) Rickets is a disorder caused by inadequate calcium and phosphorus intake and not vitamin D deficiency.

Reference: Stokowski, L. C.: Metabolic disorders. *In* Deacon, J., and O'Neill, P. (Eds.): *Core Curriculum for Neonatal Intensive Care Nursing*, 2nd ed. Philadelphia, W. B. Saunders, 1999, p. 326.

13. (**A**) The fetus is usually not affected by inborn errors of metabolism because the placenta has effectively removed the toxins. Neonates with metabolic disease can appear normal at birth.

Reference: Stokowski, L. C.: Metabolic disorders. *In* Deacon, J., and O'Neill, P. (Eds.): *Core Curriculum for Neonatal Intensive Care Nursing*, 2nd ed. Philadelphia, W. B. Saunders, 1999, p. 326.

14. (**A**) Most newborn genetic screening tests are for diseases that are autosomal recessive. This type of inheritance pattern is particularly characteristic of inborn metabolic errors. The Y-recessive mode is impossible. The X-linked dominant is not very common.

Reference: Kenner, C., and Amlung, S.: Newborn genetic screening: Blessing or curse. *Neonatal Network* 18(7):11, 1999.

15. (**B**) The most common cause of ambiguous genitalia in the newborn is congenital adrenal hyperplasia (CAH), but not all patients with the disorder show sexual ambiguity.

Reference: Gamblian, V., Bivens, K., Burton, K. S., Hoell Kitler, C., Kleeman, T. A., and Prows, C.: Assessment and management of endocrine dysfunction. *In* Kenner, C., Lott, J. W., and Flandermeyer, A. A. (Eds.): *Comprehensive Neonatal Nursing: A Physiologic Perspective*, 2nd ed. Philadelphia, W. B. Saunders, 1998, p. 336.

16. (**D**) The level of blood glucose concentration considered to be safe in the newborn is controversial. There is general agreement that a level less than 40 mg/dL in preterm or full-term infants requires treatment.

Reference: Stokowski, L. C.: Metabolic disorders. *In* Deacon, J., and O'Neill, P. (Eds.): *Core Curriculum for Neonatal Intensive Care Nursing*, 2nd ed. Philadelphia, W. B. Saunders, 1999, p. 326.

17. (**C**) Mental development of infants with congenital hypothyroidism is correlated with the onset of treatment. Delay in treating congenital hypothyroidism leads to mental retardation. Thyrotoxicosis and cortisol insufficiency are complications of hyperthyroidism and congenital adrenal hyperplasia, respectively. Untreated galactosemia can lead to severe sepsis.

Reference: Stokowski, L. C.: Endocrine disorders. *In* Deacon, J., and O'Neill, P. (Eds.): *Core Curriculum for Neonatal Intensive Care Nursing*, 2nd ed. Philadelphia, W. B. Saunders, 1999, p. 357.

CHAPTER 15
GASTROINTESTINAL DISORDERS

1. (**C**) In duodenal atresia, air fills the stomach and blind ending duodenum, forming the "double bubble."

Reference: Muise, K., Judge, N. E., and Morrison, S. C.: Perinatal ultrasound. *In* Fanaroff, A. A., and Martin, R. J. (Eds.): *Neonatal-Perinatal Medicine: Diseases of the Infant*, 6th ed. St. Louis, Mosby, 1997, p. 84.

2. (**C**) Thirty percent of all babies with duodenal atresia have Down syndrome.

Reference: Muise, K., Judge, N. E., and Morrison, S. C.: Perinatal ultrasound. *In* Fanaroff, A. A., and Martin, R. J. (Eds.): *Neonatal-Perinatal Medicine: Diseases of the Infant*, 6th ed. St. Louis, Mosby-Year Book, 1997, p. 84.

3. (**D**) Hyperviscous secretions from the glands of the small intestine result in meconium with low water content. This meconium is abnormally sticky and adheres to the intestinal mucosal lining.

Reference: Flake, A. W., and Ryckman, F. C.: Selected anomalies and intestinal disorders. *In* Fanaroff, A. A., and Martin, R. J. (Eds.): *Neonatal-Perinatal Medicine: Diseases of the Infant*, 6th ed. St. Louis, Mosby-Year Book, 1997, p. 1307.

4. (**B**) There is delayed gastric emptying time in preterm infants. The amplitude of the gastric contractions increases with gestational age with a fourfold increase noted between 28 and 38 weeks' gestation.

Reference: Premji, S. S.: Ontogeny of the gastrointestinal system and its impact on feeding the preterm infant. *Neonatal Network* 17(2):17, 1998.

5. (**C**) Risk factors that have been shown to be strongly associated with the pathogenesis of necrotizing enterocolitis (NEC) include prematurity, bacterial colonization of the gastrointestinal tract, and rapid advancement of enteral feedings. Other fac-

tors that contribute to NEC include components of the premature gastrointestinal tract such as decreased gastric acidity and poor intestinal barrier function. Many studies have shown that early minimal feedings can be protective to the premature gastrointestinal tract and are not associated with an increased incidence of NEC or other morbidity. Additionally, the use of breast milk has shown to be protective against NEC.

References: Schanler, R. J., Schulman, R. J., Lau, C., et al.: Feeding strategies for premature infants: Randomized trial of gastrointestinal priming and tube feeding method. *Pediatrics* 103:434, 1999.
Neu, J.: Necrotizing enterocolitis: The search for a uniform pathogenic theory leading to prevention. *Pediatr Clin North Am* 43:409, 1996.

6. **(D)** The most common form of tracheoesophageal fistula (TEF), esophageal atresia with lower segment TEF, occurs in 85% of patients with esophageal malformations.

Reference: Ryckman, F. C., Flake, A. W., and Balistreri, W. F.: Upper gastrointestinal disorders. *In* Fanaroff, A. A., and Martin, R. J. (Eds.): *Neonatal-Perinatal Medicine: Diseases of the Infant*, 6th ed. St. Louis, Mosby, 1997, p. 1295.

7. **(A)** Certain anomalies are associated with malrotation, those being congenital diaphragmatic hernias, abdominal wall defects, and intestinal atresias. Any episode of vomiting or obstructive symptoms should be vigorously pursued.

Reference: Flake, A. W., and Ryckman, F. C.: Selected anomalies and intestinal obstruction. *In* Fanaroff, A. A., and Martin, R. J. (Eds.): *Neonatal-Perinatal Medicine: Diseases of the Infant*, 6th ed. St. Louis, Mosby, 1997, p. 1307.

8. **(C)** Tracheoesophageal fistula (TEF) is associated with multiple coexisting anomalies comprising the VATER syndrome, which includes vertebral abnormalities, anal anomalies, renal malformations, and dysplasias of the radius.

Reference: Ryckman, F. C., Flake, A. W., and Balistreri, W. F.: Upper gastrointestinal disorders. *In* Fanaroff, A. A., and Martin, R. J. (Eds.): *Neonatal-Perinatal Medicine: Diseases of the Infant*, 6th ed. St. Louis, Mosby, 1997, p. 1295.

9. **(C)** Omphalocele is associated with chromosomal anomalies such as trisomy 13, 18, and 21. It is also associated with Beckwith-Wiedeman syndrome, prune belly syndrome, and other cardiac and genitourinary anomalies.

Reference: Howell, K.: Understanding gastroschisis: An abdominal wall defect. *Neonatal Network* 17(8):17, 1998.

10. **(A)** A postoperative complication of returning a large amount of bowel to a small abdominal cavity may be pressure on the inferior vena cava (IVC). Decreased blood return from the IVC can result in respiratory and cardiovascular complications. The surgical team should be called immediately for evaluation.

Reference: Flake, A. W., and Ryckman, F. C.: Selected anomalies and intestinal obstruction. *In* Fanaroff, A. A., and Martin, R. J. (Eds.): *Neonatal-Perinatal Medicine: Diseases of the Infant*, 6th ed. St. Louis, Mosby, 1997, p. 1307.

11. **(A)** Aggressive treatment must be initiated as soon as necrotizing enterocolitis (NEC) is suspected. The infant should be placed on NPO status immediately to provide bowel rest. Antibiotics are administered after blood cultures are obtained. A urinary drainage catheter may be utilized to monitor urine output.

Reference: McCollum, L. L., and Thigpen, J. L.: Assessment and management of gastrointestinal dysfunction. *In* Kenner, C., Lott, J. W., and Flandermeyer, A. A. (Eds.): *Comprehensive Neonatal Nursing: A Physiologic Perspective*, 2nd ed. Philadelphia, W. B. Saunders, 1998, p. 371.

12. **(B)** With volvulus about the superior mesenteric vascular pedicle, the ischemic intestine can extend from mid-duodenum to the transverse colon. Volvulus will result in midintestinal ischemia and bilious vomiting, occasional rectal bleeding, and shock.

Reference: Flake, A. W., and Ryckman, F. C.: Selected anomalies and intestinal obstruction. *In* Fanaroff, A. A., and Martin, R. J. (Eds.): *Neonatal-Perinatal Medicine: Diseases of the Infant*, 6th ed. St. Louis, Mosby, 1997, p. 1307.

13. **(C)** Respiratory status should be monitored during daily reduction by the surgical team. Insertion of more bowel into the abdominal cavity during reduction causes increased pressure on the diaphragm, which can increase respiratory difficulty. If respiratory distress develops, the bowel may need to be unreduced and the reduction performed more gradually.

Reference: Molenaar, J., and Tibbuel, D.: Gastroschisis and omphalocele. *World J Surg* 17(3):337, 1993.
Howell, K.: Understanding gastroschisis: An abdominal wall defect. *Neonatal Network* 17(8):17, 1998.

14. **(D)** Infants status post repair of gastroschisis are at great risk for infection (wound dehiscence, infection, and systemic infection); antibiotics should be given as scheduled. Nasogastric aspirates may total as much as 100 ml/day during the first 24 hours after surgery; replacement will most likely be needed. The baby should be kept in a neutral thermal environment. Most infants are maintained on NPO status for 1 to 4 weeks. Kangaroo care would not be an immediate priority.

References: Molenaar, J., and Tibbuel, D.: Gastroschisis and omphalocele. *World J Surg* 17(3):337, 1993.
Howell, K.: Understanding gastroschisis: An abdominal wall defect. *Neonatal Network* 17(8):17, 1998.

15. **(C)** The ileocecal valve acts as a barrier to colonic bacteria. Loss of the ileocecal valve, as may occur during intestinal resection for necrotizing colitis, can lead to an overgrowth of colonic bacteria in the small intestine.

Reference: Cohen, M. B., and Balistreri, W. F.: Disorders of digestion. *In* Fanaroff, A. A., and Martin, R. J. (Eds.): *Neonatal-Perinatal Medicine: Diseases of the Fetus and Infant*, 6th ed. St. Louis, Mosby, 1997, p. 1299.

16. **(B)** Although usually apparent, an omphalocele may present only as an unusually thickened umbilical cord. Patent urachus is characterized by clear fluid draining from the umbilical cord. Prune belly syndrome presents with a flat flabby abdomen. A granuloma presents as a red mass deep in the umbilicus.

Reference: McCollum, L. L., and Thigpen, J. L.: Assessment and management of gastrointestinal dysfunction. *In* Kenner, C., Lott, J. W., and Flandermeyer, A. A. (Eds.): *Comprehensive Neonatal Nursing: A Physiologic Perspective*, 2nd ed. Philadelphia, W. B. Saunders, 1998, p. 371.

17. **(C)** The exact cause of necrotizing enterocolitis (NEC) remains unknown. Although polycythemia and formula feeding may play a role in the pathogenesis of NEC, this disorder is primarily a disease of prematurity. Clinical reports indicate that 62% to 94% of infants with NEC are premature. The incidence of NEC decreases with increasing gestational age. No consistent associations between NEC and gender have been identified.

References: McCollum, L. L., and Thigpen, J. L.: Assessment and management of gastrointestinal dysfunc-

tion. *In* Kenner, C., Lott, J. W., and Flandermeyer, A. A. (Eds.): *Comprehensive Neonatal Nursing: A Physiologic Perspective*, 2nd ed. Philadelphia, W. B. Saunders, 1998, p. 371.
Stoll, B. J.: Epidemiology of NEC. *Clin Perinatol* 21:205, 1994.

18. **(B)** Gastroschisis is characterized by herniation of abdominal contents lateral to the umbilical cord. Omphalocele is a midline defect in which abdominal contents extrude through the umbilical cord. The omphalocele is usually covered by a translucent membrane, whereas gastroschisis is never covered with a membrane.

Reference: Hartman, G. E., Boyajian, M. J., Choi, S. S., Eichelberger, M. R., Newman, K. D., and Powel, D. M.: General surgery. *In* Avery, G. B., Fletcher, M. A., and MacDonald, M. G. (Eds.): *Neonatology: Pathophysiology and Management of the Newborn*, 5th ed. Philadelphia, Lippincott Williams & Wilkins, 1999, p. 1005.

19. **(B)** Cardinal signs of intestinal obstruction in the neonate are (1) maternal history of polyhydramnios, (2) vomiting, especially bilious, (3) abdominal distension, and (4) failure to pass meconium within the first 48 hours of life. Esophageal atresia is not associated with bilious gastric contents. Prune belly syndrome is characterized by the absence of abdominal musculature. Abdominal distension and the presence of bilious gastric contents may be present in necrotizing enterocolitis (NEC); however, NEC is rarely seen in full-term infants and is not associated with a maternal history of polyhydramnios.

Reference: McCollum, L. L., and Thigpen, J. L.: Assessment and management of gastrointestinal dysfunction. *In* Kenner, C., Lott, J. W., and Flandermeyer, A. A. (Eds.): *Comprehensive Neonatal Nursing: A Physiologic Perspective*, 2nd ed. Philadelphia, W. B. Saunders, 1998, p. 371.

20. **(A)** The history and assessment findings suggest the presence of a tracheoesophageal fistula (TEF). The most common type of TEF includes atresia of the esophagus and a fistula between the lower pouch and the trachea. Preventing gastric contents from being aspirated is a critical goal in the preoperative management of infants with TEF.

Reference: McCollum, L. L., and Thigpen, J. L.: Assessment and management of gastrointestinal dysfunction. *In* Kenner, C., Lott, J. W., and Flandermeyer, A. A. (Eds.): *Comprehensive Neonatal Nursing: A Physiologic Perspective*, 2nd ed. Philadelphia, W. B. Saunders, 1998, p. 371.

21. (**A**) The assessment findings should alert the nurse to the possibility of necrotizing enterocolitis (NEC). Pneumoperitoneum, free air in the abdominal cavity, indicates intestinal perforation. Pneumoperitoneum is an absolute indication for surgery. An orogastric tube to gravity drainage is not sufficient to decompress the stomach.

Reference: McCollum, L. L., and Thigpen, J. L.: Assessment and management of gastrointestinal dysfunction. *In* Kenner, C., Lott, J. W., and Flandermeyer, A. A. (Eds.): *Comprehensive Neonatal Nursing: A Physiologic Perspective*, 2nd ed. Philadelphia, W. B. Saunders, 1998, p. 371.

22. (**A**) Intestinal strictures occur in approximately 5% to 25% of infants with necrotizing enterocolitis (NEC) and are characterized by recurrent distention, residuals, vomiting, intractable constipation, and bloody stools. Strictures commonly occur 2 to 8 weeks following an acute episode of NEC. Bilious emesis is not usually associated with milk protein allergy or gastroesophageal reflux. The incidence of recurring NEC is relatively low. Infants with recurring NEC present with the typical features of NEC. This infant did not demonstrate symptoms of recurring NEC.

References: McCollum, L. L., and Thigpen, J. L.: Assessment and management of gastrointestinal dysfunction. *In* Kenner, C., Lott, J. W., and Flandermeyer, A. A. (Eds.): *Comprehensive Neonatal Nursing: A Physiologic Perspective*, 2nd ed. Philadelphia, W. B. Saunders, 1998, p. 371.
Crissinger, K. D.: Necrotizing enterocolitis. *In* Fanaroff, A. A., and Martin, R. J. (Eds.): *Neonatal-Perinatal Medicine: Diseases of the Fetus and Infant*, 6th ed. St. Louis, Mosby, 1997, p. 1333.

23. (**D**) Bilious vomiting in a neonate should be considered malrotation with volvulus until proven otherwise. Malrotation with volvulus is a potentially lethal condition if not surgically corrected immediately. The main risk to the infant is widespread intestinal ischemia and necrosis due to obstruction of the intestinal blood supply.

Reference: McCollum, L. L., and Thigpen, J. L.: Assessment and management of gastrointestinal dysfunction. *In* Kenner, C., Lott, J. W., and Flandermeyer, A. A. (Eds.): *Comprehensive Neonatal Nursing: A Physiologic Perspective*, 2nd ed. Philadelphia, W. B. Saunders, 1998, p. 371.

24. (**C**) Metochlopramide has several actions that are beneficial in the treatment of gastroesophageal reflux (GER). These actions include increase in the tone and ampli-

tude of gastric contractions, increase in the resting tone of the lower esophageal sphincter, increase in duodenal and jejunal peristalsis. H_2 antagonists and antacids increase gastric pH.

Reference: McCollum, L. L., and Thigpen, J. L.: Assessment and management of gastrointestinal dysfunction. *In* Kenner, C., Lott, J. W., and Flandermeyer, A. A. (Eds.): *Comprehensive Neonatal Nursing: A Physiologic Perspective*, 2nd ed. Philadelphia, W. B. Saunders, 1998, p. 371.

25. (**C**) Premature infants are at risk for gastroesophageal reflux (GER) due to immaturity of the esophagogastric junction. Infants with congenital diaphragmatic hernia are at risk for GER due to a number of factors, including esophageal deviation to affected side and increased gastric intraabdominal pressure. Infants with neurologic damage are at risk for GER likely due to reduced frequency of swallowing and a weaker esophageal sphincter.

References: McCollum, L. L., and Thigpen, J. L.: Assessment and management of gastrointestinal dysfunction. *In* Kenner, C., Lott, J. W., and Flandermeyer, A. A. (Eds.): *Comprehensive Neonatal Nursing: A Physiologic Perspective*, 2nd ed. Philadelphia, W. B. Saunders, 1998, p. 371.
Rychman, F., Flake, A. W., and Balistreri, W. F.: Upper gastrointestinal disorders. *In* Fanaroff, A. A., and Martin, R. J. (Eds.): *Neonatal-Perinatal Medicine: Diseases of the Fetus and Infant*, 6th ed. St. Louis, Mosby, 1997, p. 1294.

26. (**D**) Defects in which the rectal pouch ends above the puborectal muscle (high lesion) are associated with a higher mortality rate and higher rate of fecal incontinence than defects in which the rectal pouch ends at or below the puborectal muscle.

Reference: McCollum, L. L., and Thigpen, J. L.: Assessment and management of gastrointestinal dysfunction. *In* Kenner, C., Lott, J. W., and Flandermeyer, A. A. (Eds.): *Comprehensive Neonatal Nursing: A Physiologic Perspective*, 2nd ed. Philadelphia, W. B. Saunders, 1998, p. 371.

CHAPTER 16
HEMATOLOGIC DISORDERS

1. (**C**) Erythropoietin (EPO) production is increased in response to anemia and low oxygen availability to tissues.

References: Glass, S.: Hematologic disorders. *In* Deacon, J., and O'Neill, P. (Eds.): *Core Curriculum for Neonatal Intensive Care Nursing*, 2nd ed. Philadelphia, W. B. Saunders, 1999.

Mentzer, W., and Glader, B.: Erythrocyte disorders in infancy. *In* Taeusch, H. W., and Ballard, R. A. (Eds.): *Avery's Diseases of the Newborn*, 7th ed. Philadelphia, W. B. Saunders, 1998, p. 1080.

2. (**A**) Decreased CO_2, decreased temperature, decreased 2,3-DPG, and an increased pH cause the hemoglobin-oxygen dissociation curve to be shifted to the right or a decrease in oxygen affinity to occur.

Reference: Mentzer, W., and Glader, B.: Erythrocyte disorders in infancy. *In* Taeusch, H. W., and Ballard, R. A. (Eds.): *Avery's Diseases of the Newborn*, 7th ed. Philadelphia, W. B. Saunders, 1998, p. 1080.

3. (**D**) Preterm infants have a decreased level of albumin available in the blood for bilirubin transport.

References: Glass, S.: Hematologic disorders. *In* Deacon, J., and O'Neill, P. (Eds.): *Core Curriculum for Neonatal Intensive Care Nursing*, 2nd ed. Philadelphia, W. B. Saunders, 1999.
Watson, R.: Gastrointestinal disorders. *In* Deacon, J., and O'Neill, P. (Eds.): *Core Curriculum for Neonatal Intensive Care Nursing*, 2nd ed. Philadelphia, W. B. Saunders, 1999, p. 254.

4. (**C**) Positioning the unclamped cord below the level of the placenta, chronic hypoxia, and prematurity are all factors that increase the blood volume. Cord compression immediately prior to the delivery compresses the umbilical veins, resulting in a shunting of blood away from the fetus toward the mother.

Reference: Glass, S.: Hematologic disorders. *In* Deacon, J., and O'Neill, P. (Eds.): *Core Curriculum for Neonatal Intensive Care Nursing*, 2nd ed. Philadelphia, W. B. Saunders, 1999, p. 383.

5. (**B**) The two primary factors that put an infant at risk for bilirubin toxicity are decreased albumin binding and altered blood-brain barrier. Sepsis alters this barrier, allowing unbound indirect bilirubin to enter the central nervous system (CNS) and cause damage to the basal ganglia.

References: MacMahon, J., Stevenson, D., and Oski, F.: Management of neonatal hyperbilirubinemia. *In* Taeusch, H. W., and Ballard, R. A. (Eds.): *Avery's Diseases of the Newborn*, 7th ed. Philadelphia, W. B. Saunders, 1998, p. 1033.
Watson, R.: Gastrointestinal disorders. *In* Deacon, J., and O'Neill, P. (Eds.): *Core Curriculum for Neonatal Intensive Care Nursing*, 2nd ed. Philadelphia, W. B. Saunders, 1999, p. 254.

6. (**C**) Although ensuring the presence of emergency equipment is important, the metabolic acidosis must be corrected prior to the exchange. Acidosis increases the risk of bilirubin toxicity and causes the infant to be more susceptible to complications related to the exchange.

Reference: Watson, R.: Gastrointestinal disorders. *In* Deacon, J., and O'Neill, P. (Eds.): *Core Curriculum for Neonatal Intensive Care Nursing*, 2nd ed. Philadelphia, W. B. Saunders, 1999, p. 254.

7. (**B**) ABO incompatibility, blood accumulation, and constipation will all cause an increase in the indirect or unconjugated bilirubin. Liver cell injury (such as in cholestatic jaundice), hepatitis, or hepatic obstruction will cause the direct or conjugated bilirubin to rise.

Reference: Watson, R.: Gastrointestinal disorders. *In* Deacon, J., and O'Neill, P. (Eds.): *Core Curriculum for Neonatal Intensive Care Nursing*, 2nd ed. Philadelphia, W. B. Saunders, 1999, p. 254.

8. (**B**) Vitamin K is required for the conversion of precursor proteins produced by the liver into active factors having coagulant capability. It is especially necessary for the conversion of the prothrombin (or extrinsic) complex clotting factors and thus affects the PT time.

References: Glass, S.: Hematologic disorders. *In* Deacon, J., and O'Neill, P. (Eds.): *Core Curriculum for Neonatal Intensive Care Nursing*, 2nd ed. Philadelphia, W. B. Saunders, 1999, p. 383.
Shaw, H.: Assessment and management of hematologic dysfunction. *In* Kenner, C., Lott, J. W., and Flandermeyer, A. A. (Eds.): *Comprehensive Neonatal Nursing: A Physiologic Perspective*, 2nd ed. Philadelphia, W. B. Saunders, 1998, p. 520.

9. (**C**) ABO incompatibility is seen most often in mothers with O blood type carrying a fetus with A or B blood type. Signs of ABO incompatibility can be demonstrated during the first pregnancy because of naturally occurring A and B antigens. The bilirubin level would probably be higher than 7 mg/dl on day 4 and signs of mild hemolysis and anemia would be present. Petechiae, a prolonged PT, and oozing are signs of a probable coagulopathy. The presence of ascites, pleural effusion, and hepatosplenomegaly would suggest erythroblastosis fetalis.

Reference: Glass, S.: Hematologic disorders. *In* Deacon, J., and O'Neill, P. (Eds.): *Core Curriculum for Neonatal Intensive Care Nursing*, 2nd ed. Philadelphia, W. B. Saunders, 1999, p. 383.

10. (**B**) Acute loss of large amounts of blood (in this case 26% of infant's blood vol-

ume) will result in acute distress of the infant. A shock-type picture will appear immediately following the incident. The hematocrit will not drop until 4 to 12 hours later because of the vascular constriction that occurs.

Reference: Mentzer, W., and Glader, B.: Erythrocyte disorders in infancy. *In* Taeusch, H. W., and Ballard, R. A. (Eds.): *Avery's Diseases of the Newborn*, 7th ed. Philadelphia, W. B. Saunders, 1998, p. 1080.

11. (**D**) Infants with hypovolemia related to acute external blood loss show marked clinical improvement following rapid expansion of the vascular space. This can be accomplished with a colloid or noncolloid isotonic solution infusion immediately after the incident. Type-specific blood can be given afterwards.

Reference: Mentzer, W., and Glader, B.: Erythrocyte disorders in infancy. *In* Taeusch, H. W., and Ballard, R. A. (Eds.): *Avery's Diseases of the Newborn*, 7th ed. Philadelphia, W. B. Saunders, 1998, p. 1080.

12. (**A**) Based on the clinical signs exhibited by the infant and the coagulation panel results, it can be presumed that the infant is experiencing disseminated intravascular coagulation (DIC). As the probable underlying disease process (sepsis) has already been addressed, the next step would be the administration of plasma products to provide factors, some fibrinogen, and volume.

Reference: Edstrom, C., Christensen, R., and Andrew, M.: Developmental aspects of blood hemostasis and disorders of coagulation and fibrinolysis in the neonatal period. *In* Christensen, R. (Ed.): *Hematologic Problems of the Neonate*. Philadelphia, W. B. Saunders, 2000, p. 239.

13. (**B**) Although the actual mechanism by which phototherapy reduces unconjugated bilirubin is not clearly understood, photooxidation and photoisomerization are theorized to be the mechanisms responsible. Uptake, albumin binding, and conjugation through glucuronyl transferase all refer to other steps in bilirubin metabolism.

Reference: Shaw, H.: Assessment and management of hematologic dysfunction. *In* Kenner, C., Lott, J. W., and Flandermeyer, A. A. (Eds.): *Comprehensive Neonatal Nursing: A Physiologic Perspective*, 2nd ed. Philadelphia, W. B. Saunders, 1998, p. 520.

14. (**C**) In idiopathic thrombocytopenic purpura, maternal autoantibodies bind themselves to maternal platelets and cause them to prematurely destruct. The IgG antibodies then cross the placenta and destroy fetal platelets. As a result, both the mother's and the neonate's platelet count are low. If the neonatal thrombocytopenia is related to neonatal conditions, the mother's platelet count will remain normal.

Reference: Glass, S.: Hematologic disorders. *In* Deacon, J., and O'Neill, P. (Eds.): *Core Curriculum for Neonatal Intensive Care Nursing*, 2nd ed. Philadelphia, W. B. Saunders, 1999, p. 383.

15. (**D**) The 41-week-gestation woman with gestational diabetes has two factors that cause polycythemia in the neonate: postmaturity and maternal diabetes. While PIH is a factor for polycythemia, its effect would probably be neutralized by the decreased hematocrit related to prematurity.

References: Glass, S.: Hematologic disorders. *In* Deacon, J., and O'Neill, P. (Eds.): *Core Curriculum for Neonatal Intensive Care Nursing*, 2nd ed. Philadelphia, W. B. Saunders, 1999, p. 383.
Mentzer, W., Glader, B.: Erythrocyte disorders in infancy. *In* Taeusch, H. W., and Ballard, R. A. (Eds.): *Avery's Diseases of the Newborn*, 7th ed. Philadelphia, W. B. Saunders, 1998, p. 1080.

16. (**B**) Although the newborn in the case study does not strictly meet the criteria for polycythemia (venous hematocrit of 65%), the fact that she has some jitteriness and difficulty feeding may show that she is beginning to experience the effects of hyperviscosity. Immediately moving to a partial exchange transfusion, however, also increases the risk of gastrointestinal complications. Because coexisting hypoglycemia is an important determinant of adverse neurologic outcomes and the baby is stable at this point, the exchange could be delayed, provided close observation is maintained.

References: Glass, S.: Hematologic disorders. *In* Deacon, J., and O'Neill, P. (Eds.): *Core Curriculum for Neonatal Intensive Care Nursing*, 2nd ed. Philadelphia, W. B. Saunders, 1999, p. 383.
Mentzer, W. C., and Glader, B. E.: Erythrocyte disorders in infancy. *In* Taeusch, H. W., and Ballard, R. A. (Eds.): *Avery's Diseases of the Newborn*, 7th ed. Philadelphia, W. B. Saunders, 1998, p. 1080.

17. (**C**) While oxygen-carrying capacity may be adequate to maintain cardiopulmonary function with a hemoglobin level of 7 g/dl, this infant is showing signs of symp-

tomatic chronic anemia and possible hypoxia. In addition, he is on supplemental oxygen and has a low reticulocyte count. As a result, a transfusion at this point would be beneficial.

References: Glass, S.: Hematologic disorders. *In* Deacon, J., and O'Neill, P. (Eds.): *Core Curriculum for Neonatal Intensive Care Nursing*, 2nd ed. Philadelphia, W. B. Saunders, 1999, p. 383.
Mentzer, W. C., and Glader, B. E.: Erythrocyte disorders in infancy. *In* Tausch, H. W., and Ballard, R. A. (Eds.): *Avery's Diseases of the Newborn*, 7th ed. Philadelphia, W. B. Saunders, 1998, p. 1080.

CHAPTER 17
NEUROLOGIC DISORDERS

1. **(B)** The head usually grows a maximum of 0.5 to 1.0 cm/week in preterm infants during the first weeks of life. Serial measurements are important to identify alterations in rate of growth. Head circumference is essential to track brain growth and helpful in detecting and monitoring for hydrocephalus and other cranial abnormalities.

Reference: Blackburn, S.: Assessment and management of neurologic dysfunction. *In* Kenner, C., Lott, J., and Flandermeyer, A. A. (Eds.): *Comprehensive Neonatal Nursing: A Physiologic Perspective*, 2nd ed. Philadelphia, W. B. Saunders, 1998, p. 572.

2. **(B)** Noting of cafe-au-lait spots may lead to early diagnosis and treatment of neurofibromatosis, a condition in which tumors form on cutaneous nerves. Early recognition may promote genetic counseling for the family who may not have been aware of the disease.

Reference: McCulloch, M.: Neurologic disorders. *In* Deacon, J., and O'Neill, P. (Eds.): *Core Curriculum for Neonatal Intensive Care Nursing*, 2nd ed. Philadelphia, W. B. Saunders, 1999, p. 479.

3. **(D)** Autoregulation would keep cerebral blood flow fairly constant despite changes in systemic blood pressure. Preterm infants are subject to sudden changes in blood pressure from fluid boluses, sepsis, pneumothorax, in response to hypoxia or hypercarbia, seizures, birth process, and so on. Fragile vessels in the choroid plexus rupture and leak without protection from hypotension or hypertension.

Reference: McCulloch, M.: Neurologic disorders. *In* Deacon, J., and O'Neill, P. (Eds.): *Core Curriculum for Neonatal Intensive Care Nursing*, 2nd ed. Philadelphia, W. B. Saunders, 1999, p. 478.

4. **(D)** The history of perinatal asphyxia should promote assessment for HIE. Risk factors and signs include Apgar score less than 5 at 10 minutes, base deficit greater than 15, lethargy, hypotonia, hyperalertness, seizures, and poor feeding. Some babies have concurrent multiorgan involvement such as acute tubular necrosis, persistent pulmonary hypertension of the newborn, and stunned myocardium but frequently they are fairly stable and may go undetected until neurologic deficits occur.

Reference: Blackburn, S.: Assessment and management of neurologic dysfunction. *In* Kenner, C., Lott, J., and Flandermeyer, A. A. (Eds.): *Comprehensive Neonatal Nursing: A Physiologic Perspective*, 2nd ed. Philadelphia, W. B. Saunders, 1998, p. 591.

5. **(A)** Seizures are common with moderate encephalopathy and occur in first 6 to 12 hours. Most of these are subtle. Symptoms of newborn seizures include lip-smacking, staring, and vital sign changes.

References: Blackburn, S.: Assessment and management of neurologic dysfunction. *In* Kenner, C., Lott, J., and Flandermeyer, A. A. (Eds.): *Comprehensive Neonatal Nursing: A Physiologic Perspective*, 2nd ed. Philadelphia, W. B. Saunders, 1998, p. 580.
McCulloch, M.: Neurologic disorders. *In* Deacon, J., and O'Neill, P. (Eds.): *Core Curriculum for Neonatal Intensive Care Nursing*, 2nd ed. Philadelphia, W. B. Saunders, 1999, p. 500.

6. **(D)** Stopping the seizure activity quickly would be the goal. Phenobarbital is the drug of choice for neonatal seizures. An electroencephalogram would take time to obtain. The baby's history suggests predisposition and high index of suspicion for seizures. Although it is important to identify and treat hypoglycemia (either as the cause of or secondary to a seizure), treating the seizure should be started before the time it would take for a laboratory determination (approximately 1/2 hr).

Reference: McCulloch, M.: Neurologic disorders. *In* Deacon, J., and O'Neill, P. (Eds.): *Core Curriculum for Neonatal Intensive Care Nursing*, 2nd ed. Philadelphia, W. B. Saunders, 1999, p. 499.

7. **(C)** Most often the presentation of a neonatal seizure is subtle, followed by the tonic/clonic type.

Reference: McCulloch, M.: Neurologic disorders. *In* Deacon, J., and O'Neill, P. (Eds.): *Core Curriculum for Neonatal Intensive Care Nursing*, 2nd ed. Philadelphia, W. B. Saunders, 1999, p. 497.

8. **(B)** Phenobarbital is the drug of choice for neonatal seizures. A therapeutic level is 15 to 30 µg/mL. A therapeutic level should be achieved before adding other agents. Phenytoin may have cardiovascular side effects in an infant with shock.

Reference: McCulloch, M.: Neurologic disorders. *In* Deacon, J., and O'Neill, P. (Eds.): *Core Curriculum for Neonatal Intensive Care Nursing,* 2nd ed. Philadelphia, W. B. Saunders, 1999, p. 498.

9. **(D)** Long-term Diamox therapy will cause metabolic acidosis and increase renal excretion of bicarbonate. Replacement therapy may be required.

Reference: Siberry, G. K., and Ianrone, R. (Eds.): *The Harriet Lane Handbook,* 15th ed. Philadelphia, Mosby, 2000, p. 475.

10. **(C)** The repair of myelomeningocele is to cover exposed meninges to prevent infection and death. The neurologic deficits that are already present will not be reversed. Babies should be assessed and treated for pain postoperatively due to large amount of tissue manipulation especially with muscle flaps and other discomforts of surgery.

Reference: McCulloch, M.: Neurologic disorders. *In* Deacon, J., and O'Neill, P. (Eds.): *Core Curriculum for Neonatal Intensive Care Nursing,* 2nd ed. Philadelphia, W. B. Saunders, 1999, p. 485.

11. **(B)** More than 90% of babies with myelomeningocele whose head circumference is increased will develop hydrocephalus. If not already apparent, signs and symptoms will appear postoperatively once the defect is closed. Unless the babies are preterm, they are at no increased risk for IVH. Craniosynostosis is not typically associated with neural tube defects.

Reference: McCulloch, M.: Neurologic disorders. *In* Deacon, J., and O'Neill, P. (Eds.): *Core Curriculum for Neonatal Intensive Care Nursing,* 2nd ed. Philadelphia, W. B. Saunders, 1999, p. 485.

12. **(A)** Arnold-Chiari II malformation is almost always present with myelomeningocele, which occurs in up to 1 per 1000 live births (more frequently than the other above causes of neonatal hydrocephalus). It is important to recognize that Arnold-Chiari malformation can be associated with laryngeal stridor, feeding difficulties, and apnea in the newborn.

Reference: Halamek, L. P., and Stevenson, D. K.: Malformations of the central nervous system. *In* Spitzer,

A. R. (Ed.): Intensive Care of the Fetus and Neonate, Philadelphia, Mosby, 1996, p. 746.

13. **(B)** These are signs and symptoms of increasing intracranial pressure, which would indicate that the shunt was not removing cerebrospinal fluid (CSF) adequately. The nurse would need more information to assess if the infant was septic. If normal decompression of the ventricles occurs, the intracranial pressure (ICP) would be decreased. New intraventricular hemorrhage would be unlikely in a 2-month-old infant.

Reference: Blackburn, S.: Assessment and management of neurologic dysfunction. *In* Kenner, C., Lott, J., and Flandermeyer, A. A. (Eds.): *Comprehensive Neonatal Nursing: A Physiologic Perspective,* 2nd ed. Philadelphia, W. B. Saunders, 1998, p. 604.

14. **(D)** Infants with subgaleal bleed may exsanguinate from the amount of blood that can accumulate under the scalp and in the subcutaneous tissue of the neck. The blood is not intracranial, so head ultrasonography would not quantify the extent of the bleed. Tapping of cerebrospinal fluid (CSF) would not help this type of bleed. The infant may have seizures, but treatment of the seizure and shock would take priority over this diagnostic electroencephalogram (EEG).

Reference: McCulloch, M.: Neurologic disorders. *In* Deacon, J., and O'Neill, P. (Eds.): *Core Curriculum for Neonatal Intensive Care Nursing,* 2nd ed. Philadelphia, W. B. Saunders, 1999, p. 489.

15. **(D)** Positioning the infant with the head slightly elevated and in a midline, neutral position (avoiding neck flexion) helps decrease intracranial pressure.

Reference: Blackburn, S.: Assessment and management of neurologic dysfunction. *In* Kenner, C., Lott, J., and Flandermeyer, A. A. (Eds.): *Comprehensive Neonatal Nursing: A Physiologic Perspective,* 2nd ed. Philadelphia, W. B. Saunders, 1998, p. 588 (Table 29–11).

16. **(A)** Periventricular leukomalacia appears sonographically as an increase in the echogenicity of the parenchyma bordering the frontal horn and trigone region of the lateral ventricles. Periventricular echogenicity may resolve without any neurologic sequelae but often signal ischemia/infarcts and may be a precursor to periventricular leukomalacia. All the other above disorders have very different and distinguishing echogenic characteristics.

References: Alexander, A. A., and Sagerman, J. E.: Neonatal neurosonography. *In* Spitzer, A. R. (Ed.): *Intensive Care of the Fetus and Neonate*. Philadelphia, Mosby, 1996, p. 675.
Blackburn, S.: Assessment and management of neurologic dysfunction. *In* Kenner, C., Lott, J., and Flandermeyer, A. A. (Eds.): *Comprehensive Neonatal Nursing: A Physiologic Perspective*, 2nd ed. Philadelphia, W. B. Saunders, 1998, p. 594.

17. (**A**) A suppressed, low-voltage electroencephalogram (EEG) is a sign of moderate to severe hypoxic-ischemic encephalopathy. Poor differentiation of states may be due to sedation and immature sleep-awake pattern. A 60-cycle interference is noise in a signal that results from interference from the AC wall outlet power (e.g., bed, pumps, and other equipment plugged in) but should not be mistaken for seizure activity. Epileptiform activity may mean a low threshold to seizures, but they may be successfully treated.

Reference: Blackburn, S.: Assessment and management of neurologic dysfunction. *In* Kenner, C., Lott, J., and Flandermeyer, A. A. (Eds.): *Comprehensive Neonatal Nursing: A Physiologic Perspective*, 2nd ed. Philadelphia, W. B. Saunders, 1998, p. 722.

18. (**A**) Sedation should not necessarily be avoided if it can reduce response to noxious stimuli, swings in blood pressure with agitation, and crying and promote a nonstressful postnatal course.

Reference: McCulloch, M.: Neurologic disorders. *In* Deacon, J., and O'Neill, P. (Eds.): *Core Curriculum for Neonatal Intensive Care Nursing*, 2nd ed. Philadelphia, W. B. Saunders, 1999, p. 497.

19. (**B**) Fifty percent of infants have neurologic sequelae after meningitis. Hearing loss is the most frequent and it is easily screened in the newborn period. Meningitis does not usually cause structural damage or encephalopathies. Nerve palsies are typically from birth trauma.

Reference: McCulloch, M.: Neurologic disorders. *In* Deacon, J., and O'Neill, P. (Eds.): *Core Curriculum for Neonatal Intensive Care Nursing*, 2nd ed. Philadelphia, W. B. Saunders, 1999, p. 506.

20. (**C**) Fosphenytoin is beginning to replace phenytoin in neonates. It is a precursor to phenytoin and requires a different dose to achieve the same effects as phenytoin. Fosphenytoin has the same therapeutic levels. Slow administration and monitoring are needed for administration, as it also has cardiovascular side effects.

References: McCulloch, M.: Neurologic disorders. *In* Deacon, J., and O'Neill, P. (Eds.): *Core Curriculum for Neonatal Intensive Care Nursing*, 2nd ed. Philadelphia, W. B. Saunders, 1999, p. 499.
Young, T. E., and Mangum B.: *Neofax: A Manual of Drugs Used in Neonatal Care*, 13th ed. Raleigh, NC, Acorn Publishing, Inc., 2000.

CHAPTER 18
RENAL AND GENITOURINARY DISORDERS

1. (**C**) Posterior urethral valves obstruct the flow of urine from the kidney and bladder. Abnormalities of the bladder wall may develop along with vesicoureteral reflux (VUR), leading to parenchymal renal damage.

Reference: Bernhardt, J.: Renal and genitourinary disorders. *In* Deacon, J., and O'Neill, P. (Eds.): *Core Curriculum for Neonatal Intensive Care Nursing*, 2nd ed. Philadelphia, W. B. Saunders, 1999, p. 442.

2. (**A**) Ureteropelvic junction obstruction prevents flow of urine from the kidney into the bladder. This results in a back-up of urine and subsequent dilation of the structures of the kidney.

Reference: Bernhardt, J.: Renal and genitourinary disorders. *In* Deacon, J., and O'Neill, P. (Eds.): *Core Curriculum for Neonatal Intensive Care Nursing*, 2nd ed. Philadelphia, W. B. Saunders, 1999, p. 442.

3. (**D**) Furosemide is filtered by the glomerulus but primarily secreted in the proximal tubule. Potassium loss is well documented with its use.

Reference: Bonilla-Felix, M., Brannan, P., and Portman, R. J.: Neonatal nephrology. *In* Merenstein, G. B., and Gardner, S. L. (Eds.): *Handbook of Neonatal Intensive Care*, 4th ed. St. Louis, Mosby, 1998, p. 541.

4. (**D**) A blood pressure cuff that is too small for the extremity will cause the measurement to be higher than actual and a cuff that is too large will cause the measurement to be artificially low. Measuring with an appropriate-size cuff is critical to an accurate measurement, which will guide treatment.

Reference: Bernhardt, J.: Renal and genitourinary disorders. *In* Deacon, J., and O'Neill, P. (Eds.): *Core Curriculum for Neonatal Intensive Care Nursing*, 2nd ed. Philadelphia: W. B. Saunders, 1999, p. 442.

5. (**B**) Vomiting can be an early sign of incarceration of the hernia.

Reference: Kenner, C.: Assessment and management of genitourinary dysfunction. *In* Kenner, C., Lott, J. W., and Flandermeyer, A. A. (Eds.): *Comprehensive Neonatal Nursing: A Physiologic Perspective*, 2nd ed. Philadelphia, W. B. Saunders, 1998, p. 620.

6. (**A**) Potter's syndrome is caused by bilateral renal agenesis. The lack of amniotic fluid leads to anomalies of the face (receded chin, blunted nose, depression between the lower lip and chin, low-set ears, wide-spaced eyes, depressed nasal bridge, prominent epicanthal folds), clubbing or bowing of the feet, and pulmonary hypoplasia. These infants are commonly small for gestational age and have a history of oligohydramnios.

Reference: Bernhardt, J.: Renal and genitourinary disorders. *In* Deacon, J., and O'Neill, P. (Eds.): *Core Curriculum for Neonatal Intensive Care Nursing*, 2nd ed. Philadelphia, W. B. Saunders, 1999, p. 454.

7. (**D**) Potter's syndrome is caused by renal agenesis. A renal ultrasonogram will evaluate for the presence of functioning renal structures, such as the kidneys and bladder.

Reference: Bernhardt, J.: Renal and genitourinary disorders. *In* Deacon, J., and O'Neill, P. (Eds.): *Core Curriculum for Neonatal Intensive Care Nursing*, 2nd ed. Philadelphia, W. B. Saunders, 1999, p. 442.

8. (**C**) Perinatal asphyxia is the most common cause of intrinsic acute renal failure. Cellular damage involves the glomerular, tubular, and collecting systems and leads to dysfunction of these components of the renal system. The hyponatremia is due to the decreased excretion of free water most likely caused by an increase in the secretion of antidiuretic hormone. This also leads to a decrease in plasma osmolality.

Reference: Bernhardt, J.: Renal and genitourinary disorders. *In* Deacon, J., and O'Neill, P. (Eds.): *Core Curriculum for Neonatal Intensive Care Nursing*, 2nd ed. Philadelphia, W. B. Saunders, 1999, p. 442.

9. (**A**) Only 50% of infants void within the first 12 hours of birth, 92% within the first 24 hours, and 99% within the first 48 hours.

Reference: Bonilla-Felix, M., Brannan, P., and Portman, R. J.: Neonatal nephrology. *In* Merenstein, G. B., and Gardner, S. L. (Eds.): *Handbook of Neonatal Intensive Care*, 4th ed. St. Louis, Mosby, 1998, p. 535.

10. (**A**) Circumcision is avoided until the time of surgical repair. The foreskin may be used in the repair process. Performing a circumcision prior to the repair may cause further damage because of the altered anatomy.

Reference: Bernhardt, J.: Renal and genitourinary disorders. *In* Deacon, J., and O'Neill, P. (Eds.): *Core Curricu-*

lum for Neonatal Intensive Care Nursing, 2nd ed. Philadelphia, W. B. Saunders, 1999, p. 442.

CHAPTER 19
GENETICS

1. (**B**) Chromosomes are the structural elements in the cell nucleus that carry the genes and convey genetic information.

Reference: Levine, F.: Genetics. *In* Polin, R., and Fox, W. (Eds.): *Fetal and Neonatal Physiology*, 4th ed. Philadelphia, W. B. Saunders, 1998, p. 1.

2. (**C**) Turner's syndrome is an absence of X chromosomes, caused by non-disjunction, which results in 45 chromosomes. A short webbed neck, low-set ears, broad nasal bridge, and coarctation of the aorta are some of the prominent clinical features of Turner's syndrome seen in the neonatal period.

Reference: Schiefelbein, J.: Genetics and fetal anomalies. *In* Deacon, J., and O'Neill, P. (Eds.): *Core Curriculum for Neonatal Intensive Care Nursing*, 2nd ed. Philadelphia, W. B. Saunders, 1999, p. 540.

3. (**C**) Prominent epicanthal folds, a flat face, protruding tongue, and a herniated umbilicus are some of the prominent clinical features of trisomy 21 seen in the neonatal period.

Reference: Schiefelbein, J.: Genetics and fetal anomalies. *In* Deacon, J., and O'Neill, P. (Eds.): *Core Curriculum for Neonatal Intensive Care Nursing*, 2nd ed. Philadelphia, W. B. Saunders, 1999, p. 540.

4. (**D**) VATER is an acronym for vertebral anomalies, anal atresia, tracheoesophageal fistula, and radial and renal dysplasia. Three or more of the defects are present for diagnosis of VATER association.

Reference: Schiefelbein, J.: Genetics and fetal anomalies. *In* Deacon, J., and O'Neill, P. (Eds.): *Core Curriculum for Neonatal Intensive Care Nursing*, 2nd ed. Philadelphia, W. B. Saunders, 1999, p. 540.

5. (**B**) The genetic term *deletion* is defined as a loss of a chromosomal segment.

Reference: Schiefelbein, J.: Genetics and fetal anomalies. *In* Deacon, J., and O'Neill, P. (Eds.): *Core Curriculum for Neonatal Intensive Care Nursing*, 2nd ed. Philadelphia, W. B. Saunders, 1999, p. 540.

6. (**B**) X-linked recessive disorders are characterized by the male offspring being affected and carrier females transmitting the disorder. The pattern of inheritance of X-linked disorders is distinct because the

mutation occurs on the X chromosome, of which females have two copies, whereas males have only one.

Reference: Schiefelbein, J.: Genetics and fetal anomalies. *In* Deacon, J., and O'Neill, P. (Eds.): *Core Curriculum for Neonatal Intensive Care Nursing,* 2nd ed. Philadelphia, W. B. Saunders, 1999, p. 540.

7. **(A)** Clinical presentation of some of Beckwith-Wiedemann syndrome features include a prominent occiput, omphalocele, macroglossia, polycythemia, and hypoglycemia. Sixty percent are female with this disorder. The cause of the disorder is unknown.

Reference: Schiefelbein, J.: Genetics and fetal anomalies. *In* Deacon, J., and O'Neill, P. (Eds.): *Core Curriculum for Neonatal Intensive Care Nursing,* 2nd ed. Philadelphia, W. B. Saunders, 1999, p. 540.

8. **(B)** An autosomal dominant disorder carries a 50% chance that the offspring of each pregnancy will have the disorder.

Reference: Schiefelbein, J.: Genetics and fetal anomalies. *In* Deacon, J., and O'Neill, P. (Eds.): *Core Curriculum for Neonatal Intensive Care Nursing,* 2nd ed. Philadelphia, W. B. Saunders, 1999, p. 540.

9. **(B)** Cleft lip with or without cleft palate is most commonly seen in males.

Reference: Schiefelbein, J.: Genetics and fetal anomalies. *In* Deacon, J., and O'Neill, P. (Eds.): *Core Curriculum for Neonatal Intensive Care Nursing,* 2nd ed. Philadelphia, W. B. Saunders, 1999, p. 540.

10. **(D)** A disruption is an abnormality of morphogenesis due to disruptive forces acting on the developing structures. Defects that result from amniotic bands are an example of a disruption.

Reference: Schiefelbein, J.: Genetics and fetal anomalies. *In* Deacon, J., and O'Neill, P. (Eds.): *Core Curriculum for Neonatal Intensive Care Nursing,* 2nd ed. Philadelphia, W. B. Saunders, 1999, p. 540.

CHAPTER 20
IMMUNOLOGIC DISORDERS AND INFECTIONS

1. **(A)** IgA is the second most abundant immunoglobulin in serum, but it is the predominant one found in the gastrointestinal and respiratory tracts and in human colostrum and breastmilk.

Reference: Yoder, M. C., and Polin, R. A.: The immune system: Developmental immunology. *In* Fanaroff, A. A., and Martin, R. J. (Eds.): *Neonatal-Perinatal Medicine: Diseases of the Fetus and Infant,* 6th ed. St. Louis, Mosby, 1997, p. 685.

2. **(B)** Diminished or absent increases in the C-reactive protein concentration have been observed during the first 12 to 24 hours of life in infected newborns, particularly in newborns infected with a group B streptococcus. C-reactive protein levels fall rapidly in infants who clinically respond to antimicrobial therapy and return to normal in 5 to 6 days.

Reference: Yoder, M. C., and Polin, R. A.: The immune system: Developmental immunology. *In* Fanaroff, A. A., and Martin, R. J. (Eds.): *Neonatal-Perinatal Medicine: Diseases of the Fetus and Infant,* 6th ed. St. Louis, Mosby, 1997, p. 685.

3. **(D)** The coagulase test is used to differentiate *Staphylococcus aureus* from *Staphylococcus epidermidis.* If *Staphylococcus aureus* is present, a visible clot is produced within 1 to 4 hours (coagulase positive). If no clot is formed (coagulase negative), then the staphylococcus strain is probably epidermidis.

Reference: Lott, J. W., Kenner, C., and Polak, J. D.: General evaluation for suspected infection. *In* Lott, J. W. (Ed.): *Neonatal Infection: Assessment, Diagnosis and Management.* Petaluma, NICU Ink, 1994, p. 23.

4. **(A)** Gentamicin therapeutic serum peak concentration is 5 to 12 µg/mL. Subtherapeutic or elevated peak levels necessitate actual dosing adjustments instead of interval changes.

References: Young, T. E., and Mangum, O. B.: *Neofax: A Manual of Drugs Used in Neonatal Care,* 13th ed. Raleigh, NC, Acorn Publishing, 2000, p. 32.
Wagner, L. T., and Kenreigh, C. A.: Principles of neonatal drug therapy. *In* Kenner, C., Lott, J. W., and Flandermeyer, A. A. (Eds.): *Comprehensive Neonatal Nursing: A Physiologic Perspective.* Philadelphia, W. B. Saunders, 1998, p. 804.

5. **(A)** One of the high-risk circumstances that indicates the need to search for neonatal infection (sepsis, pneumonia, and meningitis) is fetal tachycardia.

Reference: Philip, A. G. S.: *Neonatology: A Practical Guide,* 4th ed. Philadelphia, W. B. Saunders, 1996, p. 182.

6. **(D)** The severity of neonatal disease is determined by the timing of the exposure to varicella. Infections are generally severe if the mother had onset of chickenpox within 4 days before and 2 days after delivery. If the virus is contracted early in pregnancy, the damage is likely to be cutaneous, musculoskeletal, neurologic, and ocular. If maternal varicella oc-

curs 5 to 21 days before delivery, the prognosis is good with no associated mortality.

References: Lott, J. W., and Kenner, C.: Assessment and management of immunologic dysfunction. *In* Kenner, C., Lott, J. W., and Flandermeyer, A. A. (Eds.): *Comprehensive Neonatal Nursing: A Physiologic Perspective,* 2nd ed. Philadelphia, W. B. Saunders, 1998, p. 496.
Freij, B. J., and Sever, J. L.: Chronic infections. *In* Avery, G. B., Fletcher, M. A., and MacDonald, M. G. (Eds.): *Neonatology: Pathophysiology and Management of the Newborn.* Philadelphia, Lippincott Williams & Wilkins, 1999, p. 1123.

7. **(D)** The first clinical signs of respiratory syncytial viral infection transmission include a clear nasal discharge at approximately 10 to 52 days of life, followed by cough and wheezing. Changes compatible with pneumonia may also be found.

Reference: Lott, J. W., and Kenner, C.: Assessment and management of immunologic dysfunction. *In* Kenner, C., Lott, J. W., and Flandermeyer, A. A. (Eds.): *Comprehensive Neonatal Nursing: A Physiologic Perspective,* 2nd ed. Philadelphia, W. B. Saunders, 1998, p. 496.

8. **(A)** Congenital manifestations of cytomegaloviral infection include intrauterine growth retardation, neonatal jaundice secondary to increased direct fraction, and hepatosplenomegaly.

Reference: Merenstein, G. B., Adams, K., and Weisman, L. E.: Infection in the neonate. *In* Merenstein, G. B., and Gardner, S. L. (Eds.): *Handbook of Neonatal Care,* 4th ed. St. Louis, Mosby, 1998, p. 413.

9. **(B)** The care of the infant exposed to human immunodeficiency virus includes implementation of routine neonatal care. Standard (universal) precautions should be followed when required procedures involve actual or potential contact with blood or body fluids. In addition, the skin should be cleansed with antiseptic solutions before any invasive procedures to prevent the potential entry of materials from the skin.

Reference: Kenner, C.: Neonatal acquired immunodeficiency syndrome: Human immunodeficiency virus. *In* Kenner, C., Lott, J. W., and Flandermeyer, A. A. (Eds.): *Comprehensive Neonatal Nursing: A Physiologic Perspective,* 2nd ed. Philadelphia, W. B. Saunders, 1998, p. 815.

10. **(A)** Neonates with infections caused by varicella, MRSA, and outbreaks of resistant organisms should be placed in strict isolation.

Reference: Polak, J. D.: Prevention of infection. *In* Lott,

J. W. (Ed.): *Neonatal Infection: Assessment, Diagnosis and Management.* Petaluma, NICU Ink, 1994, p. 151.

11. **(D)** The recommended route of administration for inactivated poliovirus vaccine is subcutaneous. The other mentioned vaccines are given intramuscularly.

Reference: *2000 Redbook: Report of Committee on Infectious Diseases,* 25th ed. Elk Grove Village, American Academy of Pediatrics, 2000, p. 7.

12. **(A)** The treatment of asymptomatic infected infants in the first 3 months of life is recommended. Uninfected infants with reactive serologic test for syphilis from transplacental transfer of maternal antibody should have decrease in titer by 3 months of age and as nonreactive test by 6 months of age. Cerebrospinal fluid evaluation every 6 months, in addition to serial nontreponemal titers, are recommended for infants with congenital neurosyphilis.

Reference: Hickey, S. M., and McCracken, G.: The immune system: postnatal bacterial infections. *In* Fanaroff, A. A., and Martin, R. J. (Eds.): *Neonatal-Perinatal Medicine: Diseases of the Fetus and Infant,* 6th ed. St. Louis, Mosby, 1997, p. 717.

13. **(B)** A fungal cause for sepsis should be considered strongly in an infant weighing less than 1500 g who has been hospitalized for a prolonged period, is receiving parenteral hyperalimentation through a central vascular catheter, and previously has been treated with multiple antibiotics.

Reference: Freij, B. J., and McCracken, G. H.: Acute infections. *In* Avery, G. B., Fletcher, M. A., and MacDonald, M. G. (Eds.): *Neonatology: Pathophysiology and Management of the Newborn,* 5th ed. Philadelphia, Lippincott Williams & Wilkins, 1999, p. 1189.

14. **(A)** Fungal infection remains a problem because the presence of intravenous fat in the system provides an ideal culture medium for *Candida albicans* and all yeasts, including *Malassezia furfur.* This fungus can cause infection and will also occlude the line.

Reference: Lefrak, L., and Dowling, D. A.: Nutrition: Physiologic basis of metabolism and management of enteral and parenteral nutrition. *In* Kenner, C., Lott, J. W., and Flandermeyer, A. A. (Eds.): *Comprehensive Neonatal Nursing: A Physiologic Perspective,* 2nd ed. Philadelphia, W. B. Saunders, 1998, p. 354.

15. **(C)** The laboratory report shows that the neonate has neutropenia, as evidenced by an absolute neutrophil count (ANC) of

1950 (see calculation below). The normal range of ANC at 12 hours of age is 7800 to 14,400. Neutropenia, especially if it occurs in the early hours of life and is associated with respiratory distress, can be worrisome because of a strong association with early onset GBS sepsis.

$$ANC = \frac{(\% \text{ segs} + \% \text{ immature cells}) \times WBC}{100}$$

$$= \frac{(20 + 10) \times 6500}{100}$$

$$= 1950$$

References: Hall, D. M., Thureen, P. J., and Abzug, M. J.: Infectious diseases. *In* Thureen, P. J., Deacon, J., O'Neill, P., and Hernandez, J. A. (Eds.): *Assessment and Care of the Well Newborn.* Philadelphia, W. B. Saunders, 1999, p. 301.
Hickey, S. M., and McCracken, G.: The immune system: Postnatal bacterial infections. *In* Fanaroff, A. A., and Martin, R. J. (Eds.): *Neonatal-Perinatal Medicine: Diseases of the Fetus and Infant,* 6th ed. St. Louis, Mosby, 1997, p. 717.

16. **(A)** I:T ratio is calculated as follows:

$$I:T = \frac{\% \text{ immature cells (bands, metas, myelos, promyelocytes)}}{\% \text{ mature} + \% \text{ immature cells}}$$

$$= \frac{18}{27 + 18}$$

$$= \frac{18}{45}$$

$$= 0.4$$

Reference: Hall, D. M., Thureen, P. J., and Abzug, M. J.: Infectious diseases. *In* Thureen, P. J., Deacon, J., O'Neill, P., and Hernandez, J. A. (Eds.): *Assessment and Care of the Well Newborn.* Philadelphia, W. B. Saunders, 1999, p. 301.

17. **(B)** An I:T ratio of greater than 0.20 may indicate an infection.

Reference: Hall, D. M., Thureen, P. J., and Abzug, M. J.: Infectious diseases. *In* Thureen, P. J., Deacon, J., O'Neill, P., and Hernandez, J. A. (Eds.): *Assessment and Care of the Well Newborn.* Philadelphia, W. B. Saunders, 1999, p. 301.

CHAPTER 21
ORTHOPEDIC DISORDERS

1. **(B)** Breech positioning in utero increases the risk of developmental dysplasia of the hip (DDH). The others are not identified as risk factors for the development of DDH.

Reference: Butler, J.: Assessment and management of musculoskeletal dysfunction. *In* Kenner, C., Lott, J. W., and Flandermeyer, A. A. (Eds.): *Comprehensive Neonatal Nursing: A Physiologic Perspective,* 2nd ed. Philadelphia, W. B. Saunders, 1998, p. 608.

2. **(C)** The Pavlik harness allows spontaneous movement of the lower extremities and should not be routinely removed by the parents.

Reference: Butler, J.: Assessment and management of musculoskeletal dysfunction. *In* Kenner, C., Lott, J. W., and Flandermeyer, A. A. (Eds.): *Comprehensive Neonatal Nursing: A Physiologic Perspective,* 2nd ed. Philadelphia, W. B. Saunders, 1998, p. 608.

3. **(D)** Fractures cannot be prevented completely, but with careful splinting of the extremities, the occurrence of fractures may be minimized. The cause of osteogenesis imperfecta cannot be treated. Affected infants will not experience normal growth and development.

Reference: Butler, J.: Assessment and management of musculoskeletal dysfunction. *In* Kenner, C., Lott, J. W., and Flandermeyer, A. A. (Eds.): *Comprehensive Neonatal Nursing: A Physiologic Perspective,* 2nd ed. Philadelphia, W. B. Saunders, 1998, p. 608.

CHAPTER 22
DERMATOLOGIC CONCERNS

1. **(C)** Premature infants have increased levels of transepidermal water loss due to an underdeveloped stratum corneum. Raising the ambient humidity decreases water loss caused by evaporation. The other measures are not recommended for the skin care of premature infants.

Reference: Lund, C., Kuller, J., Lane, A., Lott, J. W., and Raines, D. A.: Neonatal skin care: The scientific basis for practice. *Neonatal Network* 18(4):15, 1999.

2. **(A)** Fewer fibrils connect the dermis to the epidermis in the skin of a premature infant. This may cause epidermal stripping and injury following adhesive removal. The other choices are characteristics of premature skin, which predispose the infant to additional problems.

Reference: Lund, C., Kuller, J., Lane, A., Lott, J. W., and Raines, D. A.: Neonatal skin care: The scientific basis for practice. *Neonatal Network* 18(4):15, 1999.

3. **(B)** Epidermolysis bullosa results in blistering of the skin, impairment of skin integrity, and risk of death due to secondary infection.

Reference: Kuller, J. M., and Lund, C. H.: Assessment and management of integumentary dysfunction. *In* Kenner, C., Lott, J. W., and Flandermeyer, A. A. (Eds.): *Comprehensive Neonatal Nursing: A Physiologic Perspective,* 2nd ed. Philadelphia, W. B. Saunders, 1998, p. 648.

4. (**B**) The several subtypes of congenital ich-thyosis are caused by a genetic disorder: X-linked, autosomal recessive, or autosomal dominant inheritance.

Reference: Kuller, J. M., and Lund, C. H.: Assessment and management of integumentary dysfunction. *In* Kenner, C., Lott, J. W., and Flandermeyer, A. A. (Eds.): *Comprehensive Neonatal Nursing: A Physiologic Perspective*, 2nd ed. Philadelphia, W. B. Saunders, 1998, p. 648.

CHAPTER 23
OPHTHALMOLOGIC DISORDERS

1. (**D**) The primary risk factors for retinopathy of prematurity (ROP) are extreme prematurity and extremely low birth weight. ROP may occur in the absence of oxygen therapy.

Reference: Lee, S.: Retinopathy of prematurity in the 1990s. *Neonatal Network* 18(2):31, 1999.

2. (**B**) Retinopathy of prematurity (ROP) comes about when developing retinal blood vessels are exposed to injury, leading to ischemia. This is followed by the process of neovascularization or proliferation of abnormal blood vessels in the retina.

Reference: Lee, S.: Retinopathy of prematurity in the 1990s. *Neonatal Network* 18(2):31, 1999.

3. (**C**) Common complications of surgery for retinopathy of prematurity (ROP) include infection, eyelid edema, and intraocular hemorrhage. Hypotension and arrhythmias are intraoperative complications. Strabismus does not occur as a result of the surgery.

Reference: Lee, S.: Retinopathy of prematurity in the 1990s. *Neonatal Network* 18(2):31, 1999.

CHAPTER 24
MULTISYSTEM

Maternal-Fetal Complications

1. (**D**) A hematocrit of 27% is considered anemia in pregnancy. Chronic anemia limits the amount of oxygen available for fetal consumption and may potentially cause preterm birth and small-for-gestational age infants. Additional interventions would therefore be initiated to attempt to increase the patient's hematocrit.

Reference: Heaman, M.: Other medical complications. *In* Mattson, S., and Smith, J. (Eds.): *Core Curriculum for Maternal-Newborn Nursing*, 2nd ed. Philadelphia, W. B. Saunders, 2000, p. 564.

2. (**D**) Thrombocytopenia is defined as a platelet count of less than 150,000/mm³. Infants born to mothers diagnosed with thrombocytopenia are more likely to be preterm or have low birth weight.

Reference: Heaman, M.: Other medical complications. *In* Mattson, S., and Smith, J. (Eds.): *Core Curriculum for Maternal-Newborn Nursing*, 2nd ed. Philadelphia, W. B. Saunders, 2000, p. 564.

3. (**C**) Infants born to mothers who receive large doses of $MgSO_4$ near delivery are at risk for hypermagnesemia. Signs of hypermagnesemia in the newborn include weakness, lethargy, hypotonia, flaccidity, respiratory depression, poor suck, decrease in gastrointestinal motility, hypotension, and urinary retention.

References: Broussard, A. B.: Antepartum-intrapartum complications. *In* Deacon, J., and O'Neill, P. (Eds.): *Core Curriculum for Neonatal Intensive Care Nursing*, 2nd ed. Philadelphia, W. B. Saunders, 1999, p. 18.
Shannon, D.: Hypertension in pregnancy. *In* Mattson, S., and Smith, J. E. (Eds.): *Core Curriculum for Maternal-Newborn Nursing*, 2nd ed. Philadelphia, W. B. Saunders, 2000, p. 407.

4. (**B**) Administration of magnesium sulfate to the mother crosses the placenta into the fetus. While the fetus is in utero, the maternal kidneys clear the magnesium from the system. Once the infant is born, any magnesium left in its system must be cleared by its own kidneys, which are not as efficient as maternal kidneys, resulting in hypermagnesemia.

References: Broussard, A. B.: Antepartum-intrapartum complications. *In* Deacon, J., and O'Neill, P. (Eds.): *Core Curriculum for Neonatal Intensive Care Nursing*, 2nd ed. Philadelphia, W. B. Saunders, 1999, p. 18.
Olds, S. B., London, M. L., and Lafewig, P. A.: *Maternal Newborn Nursing*, 6th ed. Saddle River, New Jersey: Prentice-Hall Inc., 2000.

5. (**C**) If the onset of maternal infection is within 5 days of delivery of the infant, the infant has not received the varicella-zoster virus antibody because the mother had not yet developed it. Therefore, the VZIG injection is recommended. Airborne and contact precautions are recommended in an active varicella infection. Once the infant has received the VZIG injection, he can room-in with his mother; however, both should be in a negative airflow room used for airborne precautions, and contact precautions are maintained so that infants do not come in di-

rect contact with the mother's weeping lesions.

Reference: Hauth, J. C., and Merenstein, G. B. (Eds.): *Guidelines for Perinatal Care*, 4th ed. Elk Grove Village, Ill, American Academy of Pediatrics, 1997.
American Academy of Pediatrics. Varicella-zoster infections. *In* Pickering, L. K. (Ed.): *2000 Red Book: Report of the Committee on Infectious Diseases*, 25th ed. Elk Grove Village, Ill, American Academy of Pediatrics, 2000, p. 624.

6. (**A**) Signs and symptoms of GBS infection in the infant include: temperature instability, poor feeding, hypoglycemia, and elevated white blood cell (WBC) count persisting after 12 hours of age.

References: Landry, N.: Uncomplicated antepartum, intrapartum, and postpartum care. *In* Deacon, J., and O'Neill, P. (Eds.): *Core Curriculum for Neonatal Intensive Care Nursing*, 2nd ed. Philadelphia, W. B. Saunders, 1999, p. 2.
U.S. Department of Health and Human Services: *Group B Streptococcal Infections*. Atlanta, CDC/NCID, January 1996.

7. (**A**) Renal disease leads to an increased risk of delivering a small for gestational age (SGA) newborn. Gestational diabetes generally results in a macrosomic (large for gestational age [LGA]) infant.

Reference: Broussard, A. B.: Antepartum-intrapartum complications. *In* Deacon, J., and O'Neill, P. (Eds.): *Core Curriculum for Neonatal Intensive Care Nursing*, 2nd ed. Philadelphia, W. B. Saunders, 1999, p. 18.

8. (**D**) Ruptures in the amniotic sac can form floating strands, which are sticky and adhere to the fetus, cutting off circulation and amputating otherwise normal fetal parts. Partial amputation of a foot is not associated with any maternal infection. There is no evidence of genetic defect in an amputation.

Reference: Kellogg, B.: Placental development and functioning. *In* Mattson, S., and Smith, J. E. (Eds.): *Core Curriculum for Maternal-Newborn Nursing*, 2nd ed. Philadelphia, W. B. Saunders, 2000, p. 55.

9. (**C**) Of the choices given, only anomalies of the kidneys are associated with oligohydramnios. Down syndrome, neural tube defects, and tracheoesophageal fistula are associated with polyhydramnios.

References: Blackburn, D. T., and Loper, D. L.: *Maternal, Fetal, and Neonatal Physiology: A Clinical Perspective*. Philadelphia, W. B. Saunders, 1992, p. 91.
Landry, N.: Uncomplicated antepartum, intrapartum, and postpartum care. *In* Deacon, J., and O'Neill, P. (Eds.): *Core Curriculum for Neonatal Intensive Care Nursing*, 2nd ed. Philadelphia, W. B. Saunders, 1999, p. 2.

10. (**D**) Polyhydramnios is associated with congenital anomalies such as central nervous system anomalies (neural tube defects: anencephaly, meningomyelocele), gastrointestinal tract anomalies (gastroschisis, duodenal atresia, tracheoesophageal fistula, diaphragmatic hernia), Down syndrome, and hydrops fetalis. Renal agenesis, hypoplastic lungs, and congenital contractures are all associated with oligohydramnios.

References: Blackburn, S. T., and Loper, D. L.: *Maternal, Fetal, and Neonatal Physiology: A Clinical Perspective*. Philadelphia, W. B. Saunders, 1992, p. 91.
Broussard, A. B.: Antepartum-intrapartum complications. *In* Deacon, J., and O'Neill, P. (Eds.): *Core Curriculum for Neonatal Intensive Care Nursing*, 2nd ed. Philadelphia, W. B. Saunders, 1999, p. 18.

11. (**B**) The mother has had prolonged premature rupture of amniotic membranes, which may predispose the fetus to be exposed to an ascending bacterial infection of the amniotic fluid, which in turn may lead to neonatal sepsis. The complete blood cell count (CBC) with differential is the test that is useful in the diagnosis of infection in the infant.

Reference: Moran, B. A.: Maternal infections. *In* Mattson, S., and Smith, J. E. (Eds.): *Core Curriculum for Maternal-Newborn Nursing*, 2nd ed. Philadelphia, W. B. Saunders, 2000, p. 419.

12. (**D**) The mother has had prolonged rupture of membranes, probably for several days. In pregnancy, a fever in the presence of prolonged rupture of membranes is presumed to be chorioamnionitis until proven otherwise. Prenatal exposure to chorioamnionitis is a major risk factor for the development of neonatal bacterial sepsis.

References: Landry, N.: Uncomplicated antepartum, intrapartum and postpartum care. *In* Deacon, J., and O'Neill, P. (Eds.): *Core Curriculum for Neonatal Intensive Care Nursing*, 2nd ed. Philadelphia, W. B. Saunders, 1999, p. 2.
Moran, B. A.: Maternal infections. *In* Mattson, S., and Smith, J. E. (Eds.): *Core Curriculum for Maternal Newborn Nursing*, 2nd ed. Philadelphia, W. B. Saunders, 2000, p. 419.

13. (**B**) Amniotic fluid aspiration and potential meconium aspiration are complications of vaginal breech delivery. The head or shoulders, not the legs, are at risk of getting stuck during birth. Lacerations of the birth canal and developmental delay are both complications of vaginal breech

delivery but do not require neonatal resuscitation.

Reference: Broussard, A. B.: Antepartum-intrapartum complications. *In* Deacon, J., and O'Neill, P. (Eds.): *Core Curriculum for Neonatal Intensive Care Nursing*, 2nd ed. Philadelphia, W. B. Saunders, 1999, p. 18.

14. **(C)** A second stage of labor longer than 2 hours is one of the clinical presentations of shoulder dystocia. Additionally, the incidence of shoulder dystocia is increased in fetuses weighing 4000 g or more. Shoulder dystocia can result in fracture of one or both of the infant's clavicles during the delivery process.

References: Broussard, A. B.: Antepartum-intrapartum complications. *In* Deacon, J., and O'Neill, P. (Eds.): *Core Curriculum for Neonatal Intensive Care Nursing*, 2nd ed. Philadelphia, W. B. Saunders, 1999, p. 18.

15. **(A)** This patient most likely has a maternal hemorrhage due to placental abruption from the blunt abdominal trauma received in the car accident. The abruption is occult, as no vaginal bleeding was observed. Maternal vital signs indicate that she is responding to an acute blood loss. The fetal heart rate shows nonreassuring signs indicating some degree of fetal compromise. The nurse would expect that the infant will be hypovolemic and expects that fluid resuscitation will be necessary.

Reference: Schmidt, J.: Hemorrhagic disorders. *In* Mattson, S., and Smith, J. E. (Eds.): *Core Curriculum for Maternal-Newborn Nursing*, 2nd ed. Philadelphia, W. B. Saunders, 2000, p. 449.

16. **(C)** The mother has had a maternal hemorrhage due to placental abruption. The infant is at risk for hypovolemia.

Reference: Broussard, A. B.: Antepartum-intrapartum complications. *In* Deacon, J., and O'Neill, P. (Eds.): *Core Curriculum for Neonatal Intensive Care Nursing*, 2nd ed. Philadelphia, W. B. Saunders, 1999, p. 18.

17. **(B)** The patient is in early active labor. She is a multiparous woman whose baby's head has not yet engaged in the pelvis. The baby is small for gestational age. This is a set-up for umbilical cord prolapse, especially at the time of amniotic membrane rupture. Amniotic bands, polylyhydramnios, and gestational diabetes are conditions that develop in the antepartum period.

Reference: Broussard, A. B.: Antepartum-intrapartum complications. *In* Deacon, J., O'Neill, P. (Eds.): *Core*

Curriculum for Neonatal Intensive Care Nursing, 2nd ed. Philadelphia, W. B. Saunders, 1999, p. 18.

18. **(A)** Abruptio placenta is characterized by bright red or dark vaginal bleeding, sharp, continuous abdominal pain, and nonreassuring fetal heart rate patterns. Placenta previa, another cause of vaginal bleeding in the third trimester was ruled out by the ultrasonographic report. Additionally, placenta previa is usually characterized by painless bleeding. Maternal vital signs change as a result of hypovolemic shock and anemia, with an increase in pulse rate and a decrease in blood pressure. This is usually a late sign of hemorrhage.

Reference: Broussard, A. B.: Antepartum-intrapartum complications. *In* Deacon, J., and O'Neill, P. (Eds.): *Core Curriculum for Neonatal Intensive Care Nursing*, 2nd ed. Philadelphia, W. B. Saunders, 1999, p. 18.

19. **(D)** Preparation for emergency treatment maintains a level of safety for mother and fetus. This patient is at high risk. Preparation for the delivery of this infant includes the availability of oxygen and suction for resuscitation. Radiant heat should be provided at a reasonable temperature to provide a thermoneutral environment.

Reference: Broussard, A. B.: Antepartum-intrapartum complications. *In* Deacon, J., and O'Neill, P. (Eds.): *Core Curriculum for Neonatal Intensive Care Nursing*, 2nd ed. Philadelphia, W. B. Saunders, 1999, p. 18.

20. **(B)** Following maternal hemorrhage due to placenta previa, the infant may be hypovolemic. Blood pressure measurement would assist in this diagnosis.

Reference: Olds, S. B., London, M. L., and Lafewig, P. A.: *Maternal Newborn Nursing*, 6th ed. Saddle River, NJ, Prentice-Hall Inc., 2000.

Hydrops

21. **(D)** Pulmonary hypoplasia, caused by severe ascites and hepatosplenomegaly, results in severe respiratory distress requiring intubation and mechanical ventilation.

Reference: White, L. E.: Nonimmune hydrops fetalis. *Neonatal Network* 18(6):25, 1999.

22. **(A)** A fetal cardiac disorder, such as heart block or SVT, is one of the most common causes of nonimmune hydrops fetalis. The others are not recognized as causative

factors of nonimmune hydrops fetalis (NIHF).

Reference: White, L. E.: Nonimmune hydrops fetalis. *Neonatal Network* 18(6):25, 1999.

23. **(C)** Rho-gam is an immunoglobulin given to mothers to prevent the formation of anti-Rh antibodies. Rho-gam does not prevent the development of nonimmune hydrops fetalis.

Reference: Shaw, N.: Assessment and management of hematologic dysfunction. *In* Kenner, C., Lott, J. W., and Flandermeyer, A. A. (Eds.): *Comprehensive Neonatal Nursing: A Physiologic Perspective.* Philadelphia, W. B. Saunders, 1998, p. 520.

Pain

24. **(D)** Since pain is a multidimensional phenomenon, pain tools should incorporate both behavioral and physiologic indices. A composite measure with established reliability and validity provides a more accurate assessment of the neonate in pain than individual physiologic and behavioral indices.

References: Abu-Saad, H., Bours, G., Stevens, B., and Hamers, J.: Assessment of pain in the neonate. *Semin Perinatol* 22(5):1998, p. 402.
U.S. Department of Health and Human Services: *Acute Pain Management in Infants, Children, and Adolescents: Operative and Medical Procedures.* (AHCPR Publication. No. 92–0020). Rockville, Maryland, USDHHS, 1992, p. 1.

25. **(A)** Although analgesia is often withheld because of the fear of opioid-induced cardiorespiratory side effects, very few data are available to support this misconception. Increased intra-abdominal pressure may prolong opioid elimination as a result of reduced hepatic artery and liver blood flow and contribute to an increased risk for cardiorespiratory side effects. Morphine and fentanyl are the most commonly used intravenous opioids in neonates and have the most pharmacokinetic data available for use in neonates. Although neonates can develop physical dependence and tolerance to opioids, it is a misconception that they can become addicted to narcotics.

References: Franck, L.: Identification, management, and prevention of pain in the neonate. *In* Kenner, C., Lott, J. W., and Flandermeyer, A. A. (Eds.): *Comprehensive Neonatal Nursing: A Physiologic Perspective,* 2nd ed. Philadelphia, W. B. Saunders, 1998, p. 788.
Franck, L., and Miaskowski, C.: The use of intravenous opioids to provide analgesia in critically ill, premature neonates: a research critique. *J Pain Sympt Manag* 15(1):41, 1998.

26. **(D)** Although preterm infants were previously thought to be too immature to experience pain, a convincing body of literature substantiates the preterm neonate's anatomic and functional capacity to respond to a noxious stimuli and perceive pain at birth. Furthermore, significantly lower flexor reflex thresholds, the early and abundant expression of putative neurotransmitters, and delayed expression of descending inhibitory neurotransmitters suggest increased sensitivity to pain in preterm neonates. Because of their immature central nervous system and limited ability to withstand stress, preterm infants often demonstrate diminished responsiveness to painful stimuli. The absence of response may only indicate the depletion of response capability and not lack of pain perception. Finally, several studies have found a prolongation in the clearance and elimination half-life in neonates less than 1 month of age as compared with adults or children greater than 1 year of age.

References: Anand, K. J. S.: Clinical importance of pain and stress in preterm neonates. *Biol Neonate* 73(1):1, 1998.
Franck, L.: Identification, management, and prevention of pain in the neonate. *In* Kenner, C., Lott, J. W., and Flandermeyer, A. A. (Eds.): *Comprehensive Neonatal Nursing: A Physiologic Perspective,* 2nd ed. Philadelphia, W. B. Saunders, 1998, p. 788.

27. **(B)** The PIPP is a composite measure developed to assess pain in preterm neonates. The pain tool includes physiologic and behavioral indices as well as contextual factors, which have been shown to modify pain expression in neonates.

References: Bildner, J.: Neonatal pain management. *In* Deacon, J., and O'Neill, P. (Eds.): *Core Curriculum for Neonatal Intensive Care Nursing,* 2nd ed. Philadelphia, W. B. Saunders, 1999, p. 510.
Stevens, B., Johnston, C., Petryshen, P., and Taddio, A.: Premature infant pain profile: Development and initial validation. *Clin J Pain* 12:13, 1996.

28. **(C)** Behavioral state has been shown to act as a moderator of behavioral pain responses in both full-term and preterm infants. Infants in awake or alert states demonstrate a more robust reaction to a painful stimuli than infants in sleep states.

References: Grunau, R., and Craig, K.: Pain expression in neonates: Facial action and cry. *Pain* 28:395, 1987.

Stevens, B., Johnston, C., and Horton, L.: Factors that influence the behavioral pain responses of premature infants. *Pain* 59:101, 1994.

29. **(A)** Opioid analgesics should be used when severe or prolonged pain is assessed or anticipated. Sedatives blunt behavioral responses to noxious stimuli without providing pain relief. Therefore, sedatives should only be used when pain has been ruled out.

References: Bildner, J.: Neonatal pain management. *In* Deacon, J., and O'Neill, P. (Eds.): *Core Curriculum for Neonatal Intensive Care Nursing*, 2nd ed. Philadelphia, W. B. Saunders, 1999, p. 510.
U.S. Department of Health and Human Services: Acute pain management in infants, children, and adolescents: operative and medical procedures (AHCPR Publication. No. 92–0020). Rockville, Maryland, USDHHS, 1992, p. 1.

30. **(C)** Anand and Craig (1996) suggest that pain perception is an inherent quality of life that appears early in ontogeny to serve as a signaling system for tissue damage. In newborns, this signaling includes physiologic and behavioral responses that have been demonstrated to be valid indicators of pain. Although physiologic measures provide greater objectivity in the assessment of pain responses, they reflect the body's nonspecific response to stress and thus are not specific to pain. Emerging evidence suggests that the neonatal intensive care unit (NICU) experience may impact pain responses by contributing to less mature behavioral responses to noxious stimuli as the total number of invasive procedures that a preterm infant encounters increases.

References: Anand, K., and Craig, K.: New perspectives on the definition of pain. *Pain* 67:3, 1996.
Bildner, J.: Neonatal pain management. *In* Deacon, J., O'Neill, P. (Eds.): *Core Curriculum for Neonatal Intensive Care Nursing*, 2nd ed. Philadelphia, W. B. Saunders, 1999, p. 510.
Johnston, C., and Stevens, B.: Experience in a neonatal intensive care unit affects pain response. *Pediatrics* 98(5):925, 1996.

31. **(B)** Clinical signs of opioid withdrawal include neurologic signs such as high-pitched crying and irritability, gastrointestinal signs such as vomiting and diarrhea, and autonomic signs such as increased sweating and fever. Respiratory depression is a potential complication of systemic opioid therapy.

References: Bildner, J.: Neonatal pain management. *In*

Deacon, J., and O'Neill, P. (Eds.): *Core Curriculum for Neonatal Intensive Care Nursing*, 2nd ed. Philadelphia, W. B. Saunders, 1999, p. 510.
Franck, L.: Identification, management, and prevention of pain in the neonate. In Kenner, C., Lott, J. W., and Flandermeyer, A. A. (Eds.): *Comprehensive Neonatal Nursing: A Physiologic Perspective*, 2nd ed. Philadelphia, W. B. Saunders, 1998, p. 788.

32. **(C)** Pain can place increased demands on the cardiorespiratory systems in preterm infants as evidenced by increases in heart rate and decreases in oxygen saturation. Sustained increases in heart rate following the heelstick procedure in preterm infants provide evidence of the procedure's physiologic cost in these infants. Research examining facial as well as bodily activity has demonstrated that the magnitude of infant response has been observed to be less vigorous and robust with decreasing postconceptional age. Decreased pain sensitivity and increased somatization scores have been noted in children who required prolonged neonatal intensive care as a result of extreme prematurity. With appropriate monitoring, analgesics can be safely and effectively administered in neonates.

References: Anand, K. J. S.: Clinical importance of pain and stress in preterm neonates. *Biol Neonate* 73(1):1, 1998.
Bildner, J.: Neonatal pain management. *In* Deacon, J., and O'Neill, P. (Eds.): *Core Curriculum for Neonatal Intensive Care Nursing*, 2nd ed. Philadelphia, W. B. Saunders, 1999, p. 510.
Craig, K., Whitfield, M., Grunau, R., Linton, J., and Hadjistavropoulos, H.: Pain in the preterm neonate: Behavioral and physiological indices. *Pain* 52:287, 1993.

33. **(B)** Emerging evidence suggests that following exposure to a painful stimulus, pain sensitivity of preterm neonates is accentuated by an increased excitability of nociceptive neurons in the dorsal horn of the spinal cord. This finding suggests that for prolonged periods of time after a painful stimulus, other, non-noxious stimuli such as handling, physical examination, and nursing procedures may cause heightened activity in nociceptive pathways, leading to a systemic physiologic stress response. Therefore, the practice of clustered care may be developmentally counterproductive.

Reference: Anand, K. J. S.: Clinical importance of pain and stress in preterm neonates. *Biol Neonate* 73(1):1, 1998.

34. **(A)** Systemic opioid analgesics should be used when severe or prolonged pain is

assessed or anticipated, whereas nonopioid analgesics may provide effective relief for minor procedural pain. Sedatives blunt behavioral responses to noxious stimuli without providing pain relief and should therefore be used only when pain has been ruled out. Sucrose pacifiers have been demonstrated to attenuate pain and distress responses in neonates by activating endogenous opioid pathways. The appropriate dose for oral acetaminophen is 10 to 15 mg/kg.

References: Bildner, J.: Neonatal pain management. *In* Deacon, J., and O'Neill, P. (Eds.): *Core Curriculum for Neonatal Intensive Care Nursing*, 2nd ed. Philadelphia, W. B. Saunders, 1999, p. 510.
Blass, E., and Hoffemeyer, L.: Sucrose as an analgesic for newborn infants. *Pediatrics* 87:215, 1991.

Substance Abuse

35. **(A)** The vasoconstrictive and hypertensive effects of cocaine may lead to placental abruption. The other complications are not associated with cocaine use during pregnancy.

Reference: Flandermeyer, A. A.: The drug-exposed neonate. *In* Kenner, C., Lott, J. W., and Flandermeyer, A. A. (Eds.): *Comprehensive Neonatal Nursing: A Physiologic Perspective*, 2nd ed. W. B. Saunders, Philadelphia, 1998, p. 864.

36. **(B)** The effect of cocaine on the infant's central nervous system in utero causes these signs of cocaine exposure.

Reference: Flandermeyer, A. A.: The drug-exposed neonate. *In* Kenner, C., Lott, J. W., and Flandermeyer, A. A. (Eds.): *Comprehensive Neonatal Nursing: A Physiologic Perspective*, 2nd ed. W. B. Saunders, Philadelphia, 1998, p. 864.

37. **(D)** Central nervous system irritability caused by exposure to cocaine in utero causes infants to be easily overstimulated. Decreasing environmental stimuli (bright lights and noise) and swaddling assist the infant in adapting to its environment. Methadone may be indicated for the infant exposed to opiates as a fetus, but there is no indication for the use of methadone in the cocaine-exposed fetus.

Reference: Flandermeyer, A. A.: The drug-exposed neonate. *In* Kenner, C., Lott, J. W., and Flandermeyer, A. A. (Eds.): *Comprehensive Neonatal Nursing: A Physiologic Perspective*, 2nd ed. W. B. Saunders, Philadelphia, 1998, p. 864.

38. **(A)** Alcohol is a known teratogen with no minimal safe limit of ingestion during pregnancy. The other drugs are not known to be teratogens.

Reference: Flandermeyer, A. A.: The drug-exposed neonate. *In* Kenner, C., Lott, J. W., and Flandermeyer, A. A. (Eds.): *Comprehensive Neonatal Nursing: A Physiologic Perspective*, 2nd ed. W. B. Saunders, Philadelphia, 1998, p. 864.

39. **(C)** The minimal dose of alcohol during pregnancy that produces adverse effects in the fetus is unknown. Neonatal symptoms of alcohol exposure, such as irritability, may be misinterpreted by parents. Mothers of infants exposed to substance abuse need early education and support to facilitate a positive parent-infant relationship.

Reference: Flandermeyer, A. A.: The drug-exposed neonate. *In* Kenner, C., Lott, J. W., and Flandermeyer, A. A. (Eds.): *Comprehensive Neonatal Nursing: A Physiologic Perspective*, 2nd ed. W. B. Saunders, Philadelphia, 1998, p. 864.

40. **(B)** The diagnosis of fetal alcohol syndrome (FAS) is based on the following criteria: dysmorphic facial features, prenatal and postnatal growth retardation, and central nervous system involvement. The other signs and symptoms may be associated with fetal alcohol effects or exposure to other illicit drugs.

Reference: Kenner, C., and D'Apolito, K.: Outcomes for children exposed to drugs in utero. *J Obstet Gynecol Neonatal Nurs* 26(5):595, 1997.

41. **(D)** Smoking cigarettes during pregnancy increases the incidence of sudden infant death syndrome (SIDS) in the infant. Prenatal nicotine exposure causes loss of neonatal hypoxia tolerance.

Reference: Martinez, A., Partridge, C., Bean, X., and Taeusch, H. W.: Perinatal substance abuse. *In* Taeusch, H. W., and Ballard, R. A. (Eds.): *Avery's Diseases of the Newborn*, 7th ed. Philadelphia, W. B. Saunders, 1998, p. 103.

42. **(A)** In addition to crossing the placenta, nicotine also has vasoconstrictive effects on the placenta, resulting in prematurity and low birth weight.

Reference: Flandermeyer, A. A.: The drug-exposed neonate. *In* Kenner, C., Lott, J. W., and Flandermeyer, A. A. (Eds.): *Comprehensive Neonatal Nursing: A Physiologic Perspective*, 2nd ed. W. B. Saunders, Philadelphia, 1998, p. 864.

43. **(A)** An advantage of methadone maintenance over heroin abuse during pregnancy is that the dose of drug is con-

trolled and consistent, resulting in prevention of repeated episodes of fetal withdrawal from heroin.

Reference: Kenner, C., and D'Apolito, K.: Outcomes for children exposed to drugs in utero. *J Obstet Gynecol Neonatal Nurs* 26(5):595, 1997.

44. **(C)** Neonates exposed to heroin in utero may be at decreased risk of respiratory distress syndrome secondary to accelerated lung maturation due to chronic stress or a direct effect of heroin.

Reference: Martinez, A., Partridge, C., Bean, X., and Taeusch, H. W.: Perinatal substance abuse. *In* Taeusch, H. W., and Ballard, R. A. (Eds.): *Avery's Diseases of the Newborn*, 7th ed. Philadelphia, W. B. Saunders, 1998, p. 103.

45. **(D)** The Neonatal Abstinence Scoring System is useful to detect opioid withdrawal symptoms in neonates, determine severity of withdrawal, and evaluate efficacy of treatment.

Reference: Franck, L., and Vilardi, J.: Assessment and management of opioid withdrawal in ill neonates. *Neonatal Network* 14(2):39, 1995.

46. **(B)** The nurse should recognize that all infants are at risk for perinatal exposure to drugs and alcohol. Although more prevalent in some aspects of society, drug and alcohol use may cross all socioeconomic barriers.

Reference: Flandermeyer, A. A.: The drug-exposed neonate. *In* Kenner, C., Lott, J. W., and Flandermeyer, A. A. (Eds.): *Comprehensive Neonatal Nursing: A Physiologic Perspective*, 2nd ed. W. B. Saunders, Philadelphia, 1998, p. 864.

Section III
Professional Issues

CHAPTER 25
RESEARCH

1. **(B)** The problem statement should specify the population and the variables that are being studied. It should contain information about what will be examined by the researcher, or the content of the study.

Reference: Nieswiadomy, R.: *Foundation of Nursing Research*, 3rd ed. Stanford, CT, Appleton & Lange, 1998, p. 26 and p. 61.

2. **(C)** Assumptions are beliefs that are held to be true but have not necessarily been proven. All research is based on assump-

tions that may be either explicitly stated or implied.

Reference: Nieswiadomy, R.: *Foundation of Nursing Research*, 3rd ed. Stanford, CT, Appleton & Lange, 1998, p. 28.

3. **(D)** Hypotheses describe the prediction of relationships between variables.

Reference: Polit, D., and Hungler, B.: *Nursing Research: Principles and Methods*, 5th ed. Chestnut Hill, MA, Boston College School of Nursing, 1995, p. 32.

4. **(C)** The research process is organized. It guides the researcher through the project.

Reference: Polit, D., and Hungler, B.: *Nursing Research: Principles and Methods*, 5th ed. Chestnut Hill, MA, Boston College School of Nursing, 1995, p. 31.

5. **(A)** The purpose statement explains why the study is being undertaken.

Reference: Nieswiadomy, R.: *Foundation of Nursing Research*, 3rd ed. Stanford, CT, Appleton & Lange, 1998, p. 61.

6. **(A)** The presumed cause (tactile and verbal stimulation) of an effect (physiologic arousal) is the independent variable.

Reference: Polit, D., and Hungler, B.: *Nursing Research: Principles and Methods*, 5th ed. Chestnut Hill, MA, Boston College School of Nursing, 1995, p. 23.

7. **(B)** The presumed effect (physiologic arousal) is the dependent variable.

Reference: Polit, D., and Hungler, B.: *Nursing Research: Principles and Methods*, 5th ed. Chestnut Hill, MA, Boston College School of Nursing, 1995, p. 23.

8. **(B)** Qualitative research is concerned with descriptions of people or events. Qualitative research focuses on gaining insight and understanding about individuals' perceptions of events.

Reference: Nieswiadomy, R.: *Foundation of Nursing Research*, 3rd ed. Stanford, CT, Appleton & Lange, 1998, p. 150.

9. **(D)** The results showed no difference, which means each treatment was equally effective in maintaining the patency of the catheter in rabbits. The results of this study support designing a similar study with neonates.

Reference: Kyle, L., and Turner, B.: Efficacy of saline vs. heparin in maintaining 24 gauge intermittent intravenous catheters in a rabbit model. *Neonatal Network* 18(6):49, 1999.

10. **(B)** The results of the study are limited by

their applicability of an animal model to humans.

Reference: Kyle, L., and Turner, B.: Efficacy of saline vs. heparin in maintaining 24 gauge intermittent intravenous catheters in a rabbit model. *Neonatal Network* 18(6):49, 1999.

CHAPTER 26
LEGAL ISSUES IN NEONATAL NURSING

1. **(B)** The foundation of nursing is the nursing process. The five steps of the nursing process—assessment, diagnosis, planning, implementation, and evaluation—should be evident in nurses' documentation, regardless of the charting format utilized. Errors occur when the nursing process is not followed. In legal proceedings involving nursing care, attorneys will look at all pieces of documentation and use the nursing process as one of the guides in determining liability.

References: Meissner-Cutler, S., and Gardner, S. L.: Maternal-child nursing and the law. *In* Gardner, S. L., and Hagedorn, M. I. E. (Eds.): *Legal Aspects of Maternal-Child Nursing Practice: Concepts and Strategies in Risk Management.* Menlo Park, CA, Addison Wesley, 1997, p. 25.
Verklan, M. T.: Legal Issues in the NICU. *In* Deacon, J., and O'Neill, P. (Eds.): *Core Curriculum for Neonatal Intensive Care Nursing,* 2nd ed. Philadelphia, W. B. Saunders, 1999, p. 753.

2. **(C)** The standard of care is established by determining what a reasonable and prudent nurse would have done under similar circumstances. As educational programs and training for neonatal intensive care nurses have become similar across the nation and because technology has made information readily accessible to all people, it is expected that care given to neonates will be similar across the country. Nurses are held to the standards created by the policies, procedures, and protocols of their institutions. These standards should reflect evidence-based practice that has been derived from current nursing research, professional organizations' guidelines, and regulatory agencies' mandates.

References: Meissner-Cutler, S., and Gardner, S. L.: Maternal-child nursing and the law. *In* Gardner, S. L., and Hagedorn, M. I. E. (Eds.): *Legal Aspects of Maternal-Child Nursing Practice: Concepts and Strategies in Risk Management.* Menlo Park, CA, Addison Wesley, 1997, p. 25.
Verklan, M. T.: Legal Issues in the NICU. *In* Deacon, J., and O'Neill, P. (Eds.): *Core Curriculum for Neonatal*

Intensive Care Nursing, 2nd ed. Philadelphia, W. B. Saunders, 1999, p. 754.

3. **(D)** The plaintiff must be able to prove each of four elements in order to win a suit. The elements are
   a. duty—there was a professional relationship between the health care provider and the patient,
   b. breach of duty—there was a break in the professional relationship (also known as negligence),
   c. harm—harm or damages occurred to the patient, and
   d. proximal cause—it was the breach of duty that caused the harm

References: Meissner-Cutler, S., and Gardner, S. L.: Maternal-child nursing and the law. *In* Gardner, S. L., and Hagedorn, M. I. E. (Eds.): *Legal Aspects of Maternal-Child Nursing Practice: Concepts and Strategies in Risk Management.* Menlo Park, CA, Addison Wesley, 1997, p. 25.
Milazzo, V. L.: *How to Screen Medical Malpractice Cases Effectively and Efficiently.* Houston, Medical-Legal Consulting Institute, 1994, p. 3.
Verklan, M. T.: Legal issues in the NICU. *In* Deacon, J., and O'Neill, P. (Eds.): *Core Curriculum for Neonatal Intensive Care Nursing,* 2nd ed. Philadelphia, W. B. Saunders, 1999, p. 758.

4. **(A)** A reasonable and prudent nurse should provide the same level, or standard, of care to similar patients. It is also expected that other reasonable and prudent nurses (who have similar education, backgrounds, and experience) would provide like care if the conditions were similar. Some sources for determining the standards of care include current nursing literature, standards put forth by professional organizations, expert nurse testimony, state and federal regulations, and a particular health care institution's policies and procedures.

References: Carroll, M. M.: Nursing malpractice and corporate negligence: How is the standard of care determined? *J Nurs Law* 3(3):53, 1996.
Meissner-Cutler, S., and Gardner, S. L.: Maternal-child nursing and the law. *In* Gardner, S. L., and Hagedorn, M. I. E. (Eds.): *Legal Aspects of Maternal-Child Nursing Practice: Concepts and Strategies in Risk Management.* Menlo Park, CA, Addison Wesley, 1997, p. 31.
Verklan, M. T.: Legal issues in the NICU. *In* Deacon, J., and O'Neill, P. (Eds.): *Core Curriculum for Neonatal Intensive Care Nursing,* 2nd ed. Philadelphia, W. B. Saunders, 1999, p. 754.

5. **(C)** When a nurse assumes responsibility for a patient's care, a relationship is established. The nurse now has a duty to provide care to this patient. If the nurse fails to provide this care, he/she breaches his/

her duty to the patient, and the nurse is negligent.

Reference: Milazzo, V. L.: *How to Screen Medical Malpractice Cases Effectively and Efficiently*. Houston, Medical-Legal Consulting Institute, 1994, p. 3.

6. (**C**) Charting "physician aware" or "Dr. notified" does not remove the nurse from further responsibility. It is also not complete documentation related to the event. Other components of the nursing process should be evident. What does a sodium level of 121 mean? Which doctor was notified? What was the doctor told? Were orders received? What is the plan of care regarding this occurrence? If an attempt to reach the physician was unsuccessful, each attempt should be documented. If the physician does not respond in a reasonable time frame, there should be documented evidence of using the chain of command to provide for the patient's care. The same documented use of the chain of command should occur if the nurse believes the physician's orders (or lack of orders) is detrimental to the patient.

References: Meissner-Cutler, S., and Gardner, S. L.: Maternal-child nursing and the law. *In* Gardner, S. L., and Hagedorn, M. I. E. (Eds.): *Legal Aspects of Maternal-Child Nursing Practice: Concepts and Strategies in Risk Management*. Menlo Park, CA, Addison Wesley, 1997, p. 35.
Verklan, M. T.: Legal issues in the NICU. *In* Deacon, J., and O'Neill, P. (Eds.): *Core Curriculum for Neonatal Intensive Care Nursing*, 2nd ed. Philadelphia, W. B. Saunders, 1999, p. 764.

7. (**B**) The nurse's role in obtaining consent for procedures or treatments is to ask the parents if the physician has spoken to them about the procedure or treatment and if they are ready to give their permission for the procedure or treatment by signing the Consent Form. If the parents still have questions, the nurse should inform the physician. When a nurse signs a Consent Form as a witness, she is only verifying the parents' signature.

Reference: Verklan, M. T.: Legal issues in the NICU. *In* Deacon, J., and O'Neill, P. (Eds.): *Core Curriculum for Neonatal Intensive Care Nursing*, 2nd ed. Philadelphia, W. B. Saunders, 1999, p. 767.

8. (**D**) The nurse who performed the transcription and the nurse who initialed it are both responsible. Cosigning an item signifies that it has been reviewed and approved as correct or appropriate. It places the cosigner in a position of joint responsibility, as well as liability, if something goes wrong. The nurse giving the medication (if different from the one who transcribed the order) may also be accountable for the error, but not solely responsible.

Reference: Verklan, M. T.: Legal issues in the NICU. *In* Deacon, J., and O'Neill, P. (Eds.): *Core Curriculum for Neonatal Intensive Care Nursing*, 2nd ed. Philadelphia, W. B. Saunders, 1999, p. 765.

9. (**A**) A nurse remains accountable and liable for tasks he/she delegates to unlicenced assistive personnel (UAP). Delegated tasks must be (a) within the scope of the nurse's practice, (b) something that is known to be done properly and safely by the UAP, and (c) unlikely to have risk of harm to the patient. A licensed professional nurse may not delegate a task that requires nursing judgment. Checking for residuals before feeding a baby requires the assessment of data (i.e., type and quantity of residuals) and analysis of that data (i.e., clinical significance of the residuals, safety in proceeding with the feeding). If the nurse evaluated these items personally, and then asked the UAP to feed the infant, that delegation would be appropriate. Provided state law allows tube feeding to be done by an UAP, the nurse knows the UAP is competent to perform the other tasks listed, and the nurse provides appropriate supervision, the items may be delegated.

Reference: Meissner-Cutler, S., and Gardner, S. L.: Maternal-child nursing and the law. *In* Gardner, S. L., and Hagedorn, M. I. E. (Eds.): *Legal Aspects of Maternal-Child Nursing Practice: Concepts and Strategies in Risk Management*. Menlo Park, CA, Addison Wesley, 1997, p. 41.

10. (**A**) A policy statement issued by the American Academy of Pediatrics (AAP) urges that all healthy newborns be placed on their backs or sides when going to sleep to decrease the risk of sudden infant death syndrome (SIDS). The AAP has had an extensive educational campaign, called "Back to Sleep," regarding this issue. Both the nurse and the hospital should have been aware of the AAP's guidelines. The nurse is accountable for continuing her education to keep her practice at the current standard of care. The hospital is accountable for having policies in place that reflect the current standard of care. Being

unaware of a policy does not remove accountability.

References: American Academy of Pediatrics Task Force on Infant Positioning and SIDS: Positioning and SIDS. *Pediatrics* 89:1120, 1992.
Verklan, M. T.: Legal issues in the NICU. *In* Deacon, J., and O'Neill, P. (Eds.): *Core Curriculum for Neonatal Intensive Care Nursing*, 2nd ed. Philadelphia, W. B. Saunders, 1999, p. 755.

CHAPTER 27
ETHICAL ISSUES IN NEONATAL NURSING

1. **(C)** A moral dilemma is a choice between alternatives that can be justified by moral rules or principles.

Reference: Beauchamp, T., and Childress, J.: *Principles of Biomedical Ethics*, 4th ed. New York, Oxford University Press, 1994.

2. **(B)** Ethical theories each have goals, duties, and rights.

Reference: Benjamin, M., and Curtis, J.: *Ethics in Nursing*, 3rd ed. New York, Oxford University Press, 1992, p. 29.

3. **(D)** Practitioners have an obligation of veracity, an obligation to tell the truth and not lie or deceive. Practitioners must disclose factual information so patient and families can exercise their autonomy and judgment.

Reference: Beauchamp, T., and Childress, J.: *Principles of Biomedical Ethics*, 4th ed. New York, Oxford University Press, 1994.

4. **(C)** Parents are legal decision makers and must bear the consequences of their decision.

Reference: Edge, R., and Groves, J.: *The Ethics of Health Care: A Guide for Clinical Practice*. Albany, Delmar Publishers, 1994, p. 107.

5. **(A)** Ethical conflicts are often more about communication than a true conflict in competing moral views. Regular and frequent communication with parents is essential for maintaining clear communication.

References: Rushton, C., and Glover, J.: Involving parents in decisions to forego life-sustaining treatment for critically ill infants and children. *AACN Clin Issues Crit Care Nurs* 1(1):206, 1990.
Pierce, S.: Neonatal intensive care. Decision making in the face of prognostic uncertainty. *Nurs Clin North Am* 33(2):287, 1998.

6. **(A)** Informed consent requires disclosure of benefits, risks, and alternatives.

Reference: Beauchamp, T., and Childress, J.: *Principles of Biomedical Ethics*, 4th ed. New York, Oxford University Press, 1994.

7. **(B)** When members of the health care team believe they know what is best and restrict choices, or make decisions with no input from patients or families, they are acting paternalistically.

Reference: Edge, R., and Groves, J.: *The Ethics of Health Care: A Guide for Clinical Practice*. Albany, Delmar Publishers, 1994, p. 48.

8. **(D)** Telling the truth is veracity. Doing no harm is nonmaleficence.

Reference: Edge, R., and Groves, J.: *The Ethics of Health Care: A Guide for Clinical Practice*. Albany, Delmar Publishers, 1994, p. 28.

9. **(D)** The scenario clearly demonstrates a need for initial information exchange between physicians and parents about treatment options. The nurse has an obligation to facilitate exchange of information. In the initial sharing of options, it is the primary responsibility of the physician to discuss treatment options. There is not enough information to suggest an ethical conflict.

Reference: Benjamin, M., and Curtis, J.: *Ethics in Nursing*, 3rd ed. New York, Oxford University Press, 1992, p. 52.

10. **(B)** Nurses have a duty to their patients and families and their colleagues to explore all reasonable options and seek assistance when necessary. This situation describes a conflict between parents' wishes and physicians' wishes.

Reference: Benjamin, M., and Curtis, J.: *Ethics in Nursing*, 3rd ed. New York, Oxford University Press, 1992, p. 159.

Section IV
Family Care

CHAPTER 28
FAMILIES IN CRISIS

1. **(B)** The birth of a premature or sick infant and the death of an infant are unexpected stressful life events for which a person or family is often physiologically unprepared. Such events are referred to as situational or accidental stressors.

Reference: Kenner, C., and Amlung, S.: Families in crisis. *In* Deacon, J., and O'Neill, P. (Eds.): *Core Curriculum* *for Neonatal Intensive Care Nursing*, 2nd ed. Philadelphia, W. B. Saunders, 1999, p. 635.

2. (**C**) Predictors of poor maternal parenting outcomes include an inappropriately low anxiety level, infrequent visits not related to a lack of transportation, and personalization of the infant's behavior as a failure of parenting abilities or that the baby is "bad." Worries about maternal competency are a predictor of good maternal parenting outcomes.

Reference: Kenner, C., and Amlung, S.: Families in crisis. *In* Deacon, J., and O'Neill, P. (Eds.): *Core Curriculum for Neonatal Intensive Care Nursing*, 2nd ed. Philadelphia, W. B. Saunders, 1999, p. 635.

3. (**A**) Bonding is a gradual, reciprocal process that begins with acquaintance. Although mothers experience a sharp increase in bonding around the fifth month of pregnancy, the father's feelings usually tend to develop more slowly and become congruent after birth, when infant caretaking begins. Attachment is the quality of the bond. Touching is an example of attachment behavior.

Reference: Kenner, C., and Amlung, S.: Families in crisis. *In* Deacon, J., and O'Neill, P. (Eds.): *Core Curriculum for Neonatal Intensive Care Nursing*, 2nd ed. Philadelphia, W. B. Saunders, 1999, p. 635.

4. (**D**) Anticipatory grief is grieving that occurs before an actual loss. Chronic grief, also called unresolved or blocked grief, is frequently seen in parents of a disabled child, who is a constant reminder of loss.

Reference: Kenner, C., and Amlung, S.: Families in crisis. *In* Deacon, J., and O'Neill, P. (Eds.): *Core Curriculum for Neonatal Intensive Care Nursing*, 2nd ed. Philadelphia, W. B. Saunders, 1999, p. 635.

5. (**D**) Interventions for parents experiencing a perinatal loss include encouraging the family to see, hold, and spend time with the infant before and after death, being sensitive to individual and cultural differences, physically bringing the family together and offering privacy, keeping mementos in a file for future retrieval should parents not take them immediately, and helping parents understand the importance of informing siblings about the death of the infant.

Reference: Kenner, C., and Amlung, S.: Families in crisis. *In* Deacon, J., and O'Neill, P. (Eds.): *Core Curriculum for Neonatal Intensive Care Nursing*, 2nd ed. Philadelphia, W. B. Saunders, 1999, p. 635.

6. (**C**) If at all possible, allow the parents to see and touch their infant in the delivery room, if only for a few moments. This helps to establish the reality of the infant for the parents.

Reference: Kenner, C., and Amlung, S.: Families in crisis. *In* Deacon, J., and O'Neill, P. (Eds.): *Core Curriculum for Neonatal Intensive Care Nursing*, 2nd ed. Philadelphia, W. B. Saunders, 1999, p. 635.

7. (**B**) When teenagers become pregnant, they often experience a disruption of family ties. Adolescent parents may be trying to take on adult responsibilities while feeling they are being treated as children. Independence from adults is a developmental task at this age. Teenaged parents often have unrealistic expectations of their role as parents and may lack parenting skills. Teenagers have difficulty anticipating long-term implications of their actions.

Reference: Kenner, C., and Amlung, S.: Families in crisis. *In* Deacon, J., and O'Neill, P. (Eds.): *Core Curriculum for Neonatal Intensive Care Nursing*, 2nd ed. Philadelphia, W. B. Saunders, 1999, p. 635.

8. (**C**) Assisting adolescent parents in defining their roles with their own parents by helping them learn how to talk with their parents is an intervention that supports their efforts to assume a parental role and may foster the positive social support the adolescent parents need from their parents during this critical time.

Reference: Kenner, C., and Amlung, S.: Families in crisis. *In* Deacon, J., and O'Neill, P. (Eds.): *Core Curriculum for Neonatal Intensive Care Nursing*, 2nd ed. Philadelphia, W. B. Saunders, 1999, p. 635.

9. (**A**) Mothers and fathers usually have incongruent grieving. They do not grieve at the same place. This frequently leads to marital discord because of misconceptions about feelings and an inability to communicate.

Reference: Kenner, C., and Amlung, S.: Families in crisis. *In* Deacon, J., and O'Neill, P. (Eds.): *Core Curriculum for Neonatal Intensive Care Nursing*, 2nd ed. Philadelphia, W. B. Saunders, 1999, p. 635.

10. (**B**) Acknowledging the pain of their loss gives parents permission to talk about their loss and provides support for acknowledging and working through their grief. Grieving parents need to be given the opportunity to express their feelings. Conveying an attitude of availability to

the family gives parents permission to experience their feelings regardless of how uncomfortable or unpleasant. A sense of loss may persist even after grief responses are resolved.

Reference: Kenner, C., and Amlung, S.: Families in crisis. *In* Deacon, J., and O'Neill, P. (Eds.): *Core Curriculum for Neonatal Intensive Care Nursing*, 2nd ed. Philadelphia, W. B. Saunders, 1999, p. 635.

CHAPTER 29
TRANSITION OF THE HIGH RISK NEONATE TO HOME

1. **(C)** Transition process begins at admission and actively involves parents in a meaningful caregiving and decision-making role throughout the hospital stay.

Reference: Forsythe, P. L.: Transition of the high-risk neonate to home care. *In* Deacon, J., and O'Neill, P. (Eds.): *Core Curriculum for Neonatal Intensive Care Nursing*, 2nd ed. Philadelphia, W. B. Saunders, 1999, p. 772.

2. **(B)** Nurses play a critical role in the education and modeling of interventions for parents. Modeled interventions assist parents in their ability to assimilate what is taught in the hospital and to apply these skills in the home environment. Sequencing required education helps parents build on previously acquired skills and confidences. Involving home care service providers in transition planning helps families become familiar with the use of equipment before discharge. All patients and families require individualized transition to home planning.

Reference: Forsythe, P. L.: Transition of the high-risk neonate to home care. *In* Deacon, J., and O'Neill, P. (Eds.): *Core Curriculum for Neonatal Intensive Care Nursing*, 2nd ed. Philadelphia, W. B. Saunders, 1999, p. 772.

3. **(D)** Although outcome-oriented and cost-conscious, the primary focus of managed care is the integration, coordination, and advocacy provided for neonates and their families requiring extensive health care services. Case managers may use clinical pathways to monitor the anticipated progress of neonates and their families and to identify variables that affect the transition to home. Case managers collaborate with other health care providers and with families to ensure that individual needs are met in a timely fashion. The process of case-managed care extends beyond the neonatal intensive care unit (NICU) into long-term follow-up care settings.

References: Forsythe, P. L.: Transition of the high-risk neonate to home care. *In* Deacon, J., and O'Neill, P. (Eds.): *Core Curriculum for Neonatal Intensive Care Nursing*, 2nd ed. Philadelphia, W. B. Saunders, 1999, p. 772.

4. **(D)** If an infant is still in the hospital at 2 months of age, the immunizations routinely scheduled at that age should be given, including DTaP (or DTP), *Haemophilus influenzae* conjugate (HiB), and poliovirus vaccines (IPV). To avoid nosocomial transmission of poliovirus vaccine strains in the nursery, IPV should be given.

References: American Academy of Pediatrics. Immunization in special clinical circumstances. *In* Pickering, L. K. (Ed.) *2000 Red Book. Report of the Committee on Infectious Diseases*, 25th ed. Elk Grove Village, IL, American Academy of Pediatrics, 2000, p. 54.
American Academy of Pediatrics, Committee on Infectious Diseases: Recommended childhood immunization schedule: United States, January–December 2000. *Pediatrics* 105:148, 2000.

5. **(C)** The parent is recognized as the most constant person in the neonate's life and therefore as the best person to care for the infant. However, parents also need complex support and education during the hospital stay and after discharge. Advances in home care technology programs and resources support the complex clinical problems that parents must deal with in the home environment. Numerous legislative initiatives and active involvement of third-party payers are affecting health care delivery both in the hospital and at home.

Reference: Forsythe, P. L.: Transition of the high-risk neonate to home care. *In* Deacon, J., and O'Neill, P. (Eds.): *Core Curriculum for Neonatal Intensive Care Nursing*, 2nd ed. Philadelphia, W. B. Saunders, 1999, p. 772.

6. **(A)** Prematurity and illness represent a major event in life and motivate families to learn. Parents require anticipatory guidance to alleviate unnecessary concerns and to prepare for the reality of the neonate's effect on home life.

Reference: Forsythe, P. L.: Transition of the high-risk neonate to home care. *In* Deacon, J., and O'Neill, P. (Eds.): *Core Curriculum for Neonatal Intensive Care Nursing*, 2nd ed. Philadelphia, W. B. Saunders, 1999, p. 772.

7. **(B)** Parents learn about parenting by ob-

serving caregivers and actively participating in and demonstrating care on a daily basis. Ongoing instruction, encouragement, and participation in care during hospitalization enable parents to practice and successfully demonstrate their caregiving skills and to gain confidence in their ability to make decisions independently and to care competently for their infant at home.

Reference: Forsythe, P. L.: Transition of the high-risk neonate to home care. *In* Deacon, J., and O'Neill, P. (Eds.): *Core Curriculum for Neonatal Intensive Care Nursing,* 2nd ed. Philadelphia, W. B. Saunders, 1999, p. 772.

8. **(C)** The eye examination, hearing screen, and car seat test are recommended because of the infant's gestational age at birth. Based on this case study, there is no indication that a bilirubin level is needed at 68 days of life.

References: American Academy of Pediatrics, Committee on Injury and Poison Prevention and Committee on Fetus and Newborn: Safe transportation of premature and low birthweight infants. *Pediatrics* 97:758, 1996.
Forsythe, P. L.: Transition of the high-risk neonate to home care. *In* Deacon, J., and O'Neill, P. (Eds.): *Core Curriculum for Neonatal Intensive Care Nursing,* 2nd ed. Philadelphia, W. B. Saunders, 1999, p. 772.

9. **(D)** Premature and low birth weight infants may be at risk for oxygen desaturation when placed in semi-upright car seats. The American Academy of Pediatrics recommends that premature infants have a period of observation in a car safety seat before discharge. An infant's ability to sit in a car seat for a period of observation without evidence of respiratory distress indicates a successful car seat safety observation.

Reference: American Academy of Pediatrics, Committee on Injury and Poison Prevention and Committee on Fetus and Newborn: Safe transportation of premature and low birth weight infants. *Pediatrics* 97:758, 1996.

10. **(A)** Effectiveness of the transitional plan is best evaluated by correlating how well the processes of care match the patient outcomes. No care complications or liabilities were incurred. The infant was not readmitted to the hospital within the first month of discharge. The institution's outcome data compare favorably with those of equivalent neonatal centers.

Reference: Forsythe, P. L.: Transition of the high-risk neonate to home care. *In* Deacon, J., and O'Neill, P.

(Eds.): *Core Curriculum for Neonatal Intensive Care Nursing,* 2nd ed. Philadelphia, W. B. Saunders, 1999, p. 772.

CHAPTER 30
FOLLOW-UP AND OUTCOME IN PREMATURE INFANTS

1. **(D)** A saturation of 97% or greater will allow for maximal reversal of pulmonary vasoconstriction and optimal pulmonary vasodilation.

Reference: Louch, G.: Follow-up of the preterm infant and outcome of prematurity. *In* Deacon, J., and O'Neill, P. (Eds.): *Core Curriculum for Neonatal Intensive Care Nursing,* 2nd ed. Philadelphia, W. B. Saunders, 1999, p. 781.

2. **(C)** An intelligence quotient of greater than 85 has been found in 66% of infants with a birth weight less than 750 g.

Reference: Hack, M., Friedman, H., and Fanaroff, A. A.: Outcomes of extremely low birth weight infant. *Pediatrics* 98:931, 1996.

3. **(B)** The preterm infant's immune response is most closely related to postdelivery age, not corrected age.

Reference: Louch, G.: Follow-up of the preterm infant and outcome of prematurity. *In* Deacon, J., and O'Neill, P. (Eds.): *Core Curriculum for Neonatal Intensive Care Nursing,* 2nd ed. Philadelphia, W. B. Saunders, 1999, p. 781.

4. **(C)** Eye appearance and social interactions may be unaffected, which accounts for why parents are sometimes unable to detect visual impairment with cortical blindness.

Reference: Louch, G.: Follow-up of the preterm infant and outcome of prematurity. *In* Deacon, J., and O'Neill, P. (Eds.): *Core Curriculum for Neonatal Intensive Care Nursing,* 2nd ed. Philadelphia, W. B. Saunders, 1999, p. 781.

5. **(D)** Symptoms of gastroesophageal reflux include feeding problems, arching back during feeding, irritability, vomiting, and poor weight gain.

Reference: Louch, G.: Follow-up of the preterm infant and outcome of prematurity. *In* Deacon, J., and O'Neill, P. (Eds.): *Core Curriculum for Neonatal Intensive Care Nursing,* 2nd ed. Philadelphia, W. B. Saunders, 1999, p. 781.

6. **(A)** The adjusted age is calculated by subtracting the birth date from "today's" date and then subtracting the number of weeks premature. The infant is 7 months

chronologic age and 4 months adjusted age.

	Year	Month	Day
		9	33
"Today's" Date	2001	~~10~~	~~3~~
Birth Date	2001	−2	−4
Chronologic Age		7 mo	9 days
Subtract Weeks Premature		−3	−7
Adjusted Age		4 mo	2 days

(Today's date [in stem] is 10/3/01, but to subtract 4 from 3, you have to "borrow" 30 days [1 mo] from October)

Reference: Louch, G.: Follow-up of the preterm infant and outcome of prematurity. *In* Deacon, J., and O'Neill, P. (Eds.): *Core Curriculum for Neonatal Intensive Care Nursing*, 2nd ed. Philadelphia, W. B. Saunders, 1999, p. 781.

7. **(D)** Premature infants may be at less than the 5th percentile on premature growth curves at discharge. Growth may follow the infant's own growth curve, and show "catch up", but may still fall below the 5th percentile.

Reference: Louch, G.: Follow-up of the preterm infant and outcome of prematurity. *In* Deacon, J., and O'Neill, P. (Eds.): *Core Curriculum for Neonatal Intensive Care Nursing*, 2nd ed. Philadelphia, W. B. Saunders, 1999, p. 781.

8. **(C)** Gestational age should be considered when evaluating the growth of preterm infants. After approximately 2 1/2 years of age, differences in growth between adjusted and chronologic age become insignificant. Adjusted age should be used when plotting a preterm infant's growth up until 2 1/2 years of age.

Reference: Bernbaum, J. C.: Medical care after discharge. *In* Avery, G. B., Fletcher, M. A., and MacDonald, M. G. (Eds.): *Neonatology: Pathophysiology and Management of the Newborn*, 5th ed. Philadelphia, Lippincott, Williams & Wilkins, 1999, p. 1463.

9. **(A)** Hearing deficits can affect speech, behavior, and parent/child interaction.

Reference: Louch, G.: Follow-up of the preterm infant and outcome of prematurity. *In* Deacon, J., and O'Neill, P. (Eds.): *Core Curriculum for Neonatal Intensive Care Nursing*, 2nd ed. Philadelphia, W. B. Saunders, 1999, p. 781.

10. **(A)** Diplegia cerebral palsy affects the lower extremities and is found in infants who were born prematurely.

Reference: Louch, G.: Follow-up of the preterm infant and outcome of prematurity. *In* Deacon, J., and O'Neill, P.: *Core Curriculum for Neonatal Intensive Care Nursing*, 2nd ed. Philadelphia, W. B. Saunders, 1999, p. 781.